SPORTS NUTRITION

Judy A. Driskell

CRC Press
Boca Raton London New York Washington, D.C.

NUTRITION in EXERCISE and SPORT

Edited by Ira Wolinsky and James F. Hickson, Jr.

Published Titles

Exercise and Disease,
Ronald R. Watson and Marianne Eisinger

Nutrients as Ergogenic Aids for Sports and Exercise,
Luke Bucci

Nutrition in Exercise and Sport, Second Edition,
Ira Wolinsky and James F. Hickson, Jr.

Nutrition Applied to Injury Rehabilitation and Sports Medicine,
Luke Bucci

Nutrition for the Recreational Athlete,
Catherine G.R. Jackson

NUTRITION in EXERCISE and SPORT

Edited by Ira Wolinsky

Published Titles

Sports Nutrition: Minerals and Electrolytes,
Constance V. Kies and Judy A. Driskell

Nutrition, Physical Activity, and Health in Early Life:
Studies in Preschool Children,
Jana Parizkova

Exercise and Immune Function,
Laurie Hoffman-Goetz

Body Fluid Balance: Exercise and Sport,
E.R. Buskirk and S. Puhl

Nutrition and the Female Athlete,
Jaime S. Ruud

Sports Nutrition: Vitamins and Trace Elements,
Ira Wolinsky and Judy A. Driskell

Amino Acids and Proteins for the Athlete—The Anabolic Edge,
Mauro G. DiPasquale

Nutrition in Exercise and Sport, Third Edition,
Ira Wolinsky

Published Titles Continued

Gender Differences in Metabolism: Practical and Nutritional Implications,
Mark Tarnopolsky

Macroelements, Water, and Electrolytes in Sports Nutrition,
Judy A. Driskell

Sports Nutrition,
Judy A. Driskell

NUTRITION in EXERCISE and SPORT

Edited by Ira Wolinsky

Forthcoming Titles

Energy-Yielding Macronutrients and Energy Metabolism in Sports Nutrition,
Judy A. Driskell and Ira Wolinsky

High Performance Nutrition: Diets and Supplements for the Competitive Athlete,
Mauro DiPasquale

Physique and Fitness,
Thomas Battinelli

Nutrition and the Strength Athlete,
Catherine R. Jackson

Sports Drinks: Basic Science and Practical Aspects,
Ron Maughan

Nutrition and Exercise Immunology,
David C. Nieman

Nutritional Applications in Exercise and Sport,
Ira Wolinsky

Nutrients as Ergogenic Aids for Sports and Exercise, Second Edition,
Luke R. Bucci

Contact Editor:	Lourdes Franco
Project Editor:	Ibrey Woodall
Cover design:	Dawn Boyd

Library of Congress Cataloging-in-Publication Data

Driskell, Judy A. (Judy Anne)
   Sports nutrition / Judy A. Driskell.
        p. cm. — (Nutrition in exercise and sport)
    Includes bibliographical references and index.
    ISBN 0-8493-8197-5 (alk. paper)
    1. Athletes — Nutrition. 2. Physical fitness — Nutritional aspects.
I. Title. II. Series.
TX361. A8D75 1999
613.2′024′796—dc21
                                                      99-26360
                                                        CIP

© 2000 by CRC Press LLC

No claim to original U.S. Government works
International Standard Book Number 0-8493-8197-5
Library of Congress Card Number 99-26360
Printed in the United States of America 1 2 3 4 5 6 7 8 9 0
Printed on acid-free paper

Series Preface

The CRC series, Nutrition in Exercise and Sport, provides a setting for in-depth exploration of the many and varied aspects of nutrition and exercise, including sports. The topic of exercise and sports nutrition has been a focus of research among scientists since the 1960s, and the healthful benefits of good nutrition and exercise have been appreciated. As our knowledge expands, it will be necessary to remember that there must be a range of diets and exercise regimes that will support excellent physical condition and performance. There is not a single diet-exercise treatment that can be the common denominator, or the single formula for health, or panacea for performance.

This series is dedicated to providing a stage upon which to explore these issues. Each volume provides a detailed and scholarly examination of some aspect of the topic.

Contributors from any bona fide area of nutrition and physical activity, including sports and the controversial, are welcome.

This book is the contribution of my creative, energetic, and talented colleague, Judy Driskell, on the subject of sports nutrition. This book will certainly find approval as an excellent text as well as a valuable reference work.

Ira Wolinsky, Ph.D.
Series Editor
University of Houston

Dedication

This textbook is dedicated to my former students, particularly my graduate students, who were curious about nutrition as it relates to physical performance. Appreciation is also expressed to the students, primarily in exercise science, at the University of Nebraska who utilized the book manuscript as a text in a Nutrition and Exercise course, undergraduate-graduate level, Fall semester of 1998. The comments and suggestions made by several of these students were utilized in preparing the final draft of the book.

Preface

The media extols the health benefits of good nutrition and exercise. This book is designed to be utilized as a textbook for college/university students wanting to learn more about nutrition as it relates to exercise and sport. The book also addresses how nutrition and physical activity are related to health. The book has been student-tested in an undergraduate–graduate level Nutrition and Exercise course. The book may also be of interest to sport and fitness educators, nutritionists and dietitians, coaches, trainers, and other health professionals. Lay individuals interested in improving or maintaining their own health or that of others may also find the book to be of value.

The book begins by briefly reviewing the nutrients and their digestion and absorption. The next few chapters describe each of the nutrients in detail with emphasis being placed on function (particularly as it relates to energy metabolism), food sources, deficiency, pharmacology, toxicity, and health interrelationships. Energy requirements and the importance of controlling body weight to health follow. The role of body composition in physical performance and health is discussed with emphasis being placed on obesity, eating disorders, and conditioning. Information is provided as to what is known regarding the nutritional status of athletes. The guidelines/recommendations of various nutrition, exercise, and health organizations are included with emphasis being placed on the health benefits of good nutrition and exercise habits throughout one's life. Exercise programs are vital in helping individuals obtain and maintain good health and are also being utilized as therapy for several of the degenerative diseases. The book concludes with summarizing discussions of nutrition and exercise as they relate to the health of individuals and public health objectives.

Hippocrates wrote about the interrelationships between nutrition, exercise, and health over 2,000 years ago. During the last decade or so, an explosion of information is available in all forms of the media on nutrition, exercise, and health interrelationships. Though more scientific research is needed before these interrelationships are conclusively understood, the existing research and resulting guidelines/recommendations of how nutrition, exercise, and health interrelate are presented in course format in this book.

Judy A. Driskell
January, 1999

The Author

Judy A. Driskell, PhD, RD, received her Bachelor of Science degree in biology in 1965 from the University of Southern Mississippi and her Master of Science and Doctor of Philosophy degrees in nutrition from Purdue University in Indiana in 1967 and 1970, respectively. She has served in research/teaching and research/teaching/extension positions at Auburn University, Florida State University, Virginia Polytechnic Institute and State University, and is presently at the University of Nebraska. She has also served as the Nutrition Scientist for the U.S. Department of Agriculture/Cooperative State Research Service in Washington, D.C.

Dr. Driskell is a member of numerous professional organizations including the American Society for Nutritional Sciences, the Institute of Food Technologists, the American College of Sports Medicine and the American Dietetic Association. She was the 1987 recipient of the Borden Award for Research in Applied Fundamental Knowledge of Human Nutrition. In 1993, she received the Professional Scientist Award of the Food Science and Human Nutrition Section of the Southern Association of Agricultural Scientists.

Dr. Driskell recently coedited the following books: *Sports Nutrition: Minerals and Electrolytes*; *Sports Nutrition: Vitamins and Trace Elements*; *Macroelements, Water, and Electrolytes in Sports Nutrition*; and *Energy-Yielding Macronutrients and Energy Metabolism in Sports Nutrition*. She also was a coauthor for the advanced nutrition textbook *Nutrition: Chemistry and Biology*. She has published over 100 refereed research articles and 15 book chapters as well as several publications intended for lay audiences and has given numerous professional and lay presentations.

Dr. Driskell is presently Professor of Nutritional Science and Dietetics. Her research interests center around vitamin metabolism and requirements, including the interrelationships between exercise and vitamin requirements.

Contents

Introduction

1. The Nutrients 5

    Nutritional Habits 5
    Nutrients 6
    Classes of Nutrients 6
    Disease Relationships 7

2. Digestion, Absorption, and Circulation of Nutrients 9

    GI Tract Function 9
    Absorption 12
    Absorptive Mechanisms 12
    Absorption of the Nutrients 13
    Intestinal Microflora 14
    Lymphatic System 14
    Circulatory System 14

The Most Important Nutrient

3. Water 19

    Body Distribution 19
    Functions 19
    Water Balance 21
    Dietary Recommendations 22

The Energy-Yielding Nutrients

4. Carbohydrates 29

    Classification 29
    Digestion 30
    Functions 30
    Blood Glucose Homeostasis 31
    Recommended Intakes 31
    Carbohydrate and Fiber Consumption Habits 32
    Glycogen Loading 32
    Endurance Capacity 32

5. Lipids 35

    Classification 35
    Digestion 35
    Lipid Transport 36

Functions 36
Recommended Intakes 37
Lipid Consumption Habits..37
Health Effects of Fats 38
Fat Substitutes 38

6. Proteins 39
Amino Acids: The Building Blocks of Protein 39
Protein Structure 39
Classification of Amino Acids By Function................................40
Protein Quality 41
Digestion 41
Protein Status 41
Functions of Proteins in the Body..42
Protein Catabolism..42
Protein-Energy Malnutrition 43
Recommended Intakes 43
Protein Consumption Habits...44
Excessive Protein Intakes 44
Processed Proteins 44

Micronutrients: The Catalysts

7. Vitamins.. 49
Fat-Soluble and Water-Soluble Vitamins 49
Vitamin A 50
Vitamin D 53
Vitamin E...56
Vitamin K 59
Vitamin C...61
Thiamin..63
Riboflavin 65
Niacin..67
Vitamin B_6...69
Folic Acid..72
Vitamin B_{12} 75
Biotin...77
Pantothenic Acid 79
Choline..81

8. Minerals 85
Calcium...87
Phosphorus 91
Magnesium 93
Sulfur..95
Potassium 95
Sodium..97
Chloride..99
Iron 100
Copper 104
Zinc..106

Iodine 108
Selenium 109
Fluoride 111
Manganese 113
Chromium 114
Molybdenum 116

9. Other Substances in Foods and Exercise **119**
Nutrients Essential for Some Higher Animals That May Be Related to
    Athletic Performance in Humans 119
Taurine 119
Carnitine 120
Myo-inositol 120
Arsenic 121
Nickel 121
Silicon 122
Boron 122
Other Trace Elements 123
Coenzymes, Growth Factors, Amino Acids, and Buffers That May Be
    Related to Athletic Performance in Humans 123
Coenzyme Q10 123
Creatine 124
Arginine, Ornithine, and Citrulline 124
Aspartate and Asparagine 124
Branched-Chain Amino Acids 125
Inosine 125
Bicarbonate, Phosphate, and Citrate Salts (Buffers) 125
Substances Not Determined Essential for Animals or Humans That May
    Be Related to Athletic Performance in Humans 125
Dimethylglycine 126
Lecithin 126
Oryzanoles and Ferulic Acid 126
Octacosanol 126
Gamma Hydroxybutyrate and Hydroxymethylbutyrate 126
Glandulars 126
Smilax Compounds 126
Yohimbine 127
Ginsengs 127
Bioflavonoid Derivatives 127
Glutathione 127
Carotenoids 127
Bee Pollen 128
Caffeine 128
Ethanol 128

Energy Requirements

10. Assessment of Energy Intake **133**
Hunger, Appetite, and Satiety 133
Calories 133

Dietary Intakes 135
Caloric Density of Foods...136

11. Assessment of Energy Expenditure...137
Body Calorimetry..137
Components of Energy Expenditure...137
Basal and Resting Metabolism 138
Thermic Effect of Food 138
Thermic Effect of Exercise..138
Estimating Energy Expenditure..139

12. Energy Production in the Body...145
Energy Currency 145
Energy Reservoir 145
Aerobic and Anaerobic Energy Release 146
Anaerobic and Aerobic Energy from Foods 146
Brief Description of Energy Pathways 147
Feasting...149
Fasting...149
Detailed Description of Energy Pathways 150
Catabolic Pathways of Carbohydrates 150
Catabolic Pathways of Lipids...161
Catabolic Pathways of Proteins...164
Elimination of Ammonia: The Urea Cycle 165
Energy, ATP, and the Catabolic Pathways 168

13. Weight Control 171
Healthy Body Weight 171
Energy Balance 175
Caloric Intake and Body Weight Changes...176
Weight Loss..177
Weight Gain 178
Behavior Modification...178

Body Composition

14. Assessment of Body Composition..183
Direct Assessment of Body Composition 183
Indirect Assessment of Body Composition 183
Hydrostatic Weighing..183
Other Methods for Evaluating Body Density 184
Skinfold Thickness Measurements 185
Girth Measurements 193
Breadth Measurements..194

15. Overweight and Obesity 197
Body Fat Distribution 200
Health Concerns of Overweight Individuals...200
Obesity as a Familial Trait..200

Determinants of Obesity 201
Obesity as a Lifestyle 203
Treatment of Obesity 203

16. Underweight and Eating Disorders 205
Health Concerns 205
Anorexia Nervosa 205
Bulimia 206
Exercise Dependency 206
Nutritional and Exercise Therapy 206

17. Conditioning 209
Fitness and Health 209
Muscle Contraction 210
Principles of Conditioning 210
Conditioning for Muscular Strength 211
Resistance Training Programs 211
Conditioning for Muscle Endurance 211
Cardiovascular Endurance Training 212
Training Programs 213

Diet and Exercise Recommendations

18. Nutritional Status of Athletes 219
Median Daily Nutrient Intakes of Adults 219
Use of Vitamin/Mineral Supplements by Athletes 219
Nutritional Status of Athletes 221

19. Nutrition and Exercise Recommendations 223
Dietary Recommendations 223
Recommended Dietary Allowances 223
Dietary Reference Intakes 225
Dietary Guidelines for Americans 230
Food Guide Pyramid 231
Nutritional Labeling 234
Dietary Supplements 237
Exercise Recommendations 240
Evolution of Physical Activity Guidelines 240
Physical Activity Guidelines 241

20. Recommendations for Individuals in the Various Stages of Their
Life Cycles 243
Pregnancy 243
Lactation 243
Infancy 244
Childhood 245
Adolescence 245
Young and Middle Adulthood 245
Older Adulthood 247

21. Health Benefits of Exercise...**249**
    Beneficial Effects of Exercise on Health and Disease.................................249
    Adverse Effects of Exercise on Health 251
    Improved Fitness...251

22. Exercise as Therapy for Degenerative Diseases..................................**253**
    Coronary Artery Disease...253
    Hypertension 254
    Diabetes Mellitus..254
    Osteoporosis 254
    Neuromuscular Disease 255
    Physical Effects 255

Summary

23. Interrelationships Between Nutrition and Exercise **259**
    Body Weight..259
    Disease 259
    Healthy People 2000 260
    Nutrition and Exercise Guidelines 261

References...**263**
Index...**267**

Introduction

Introduction

Good nutritional practices can enhance physical performance. Exercise and sport are becoming concerns for health professionals and a large segment of the general public. The pursuit of excellence in exercise and sports necessitates that all the body's systems perform in such a manner that the bioenergetic functions of the muscles can be sustained as well as function at peak levels.

The energy-yielding nutrients, carbohydrates, lipids (frequently referred to as fats), and proteins, provide the fuel for bioenergetic reactions. Vitamins and minerals catalyze these reactions. Water is the body solvent in which these reactions take place. Water also functions in cooling the body from the heat produced by these reactions. All of the essential nutrients are needed in appropriate quantities in order for the body to function efficiently, particularly in exercise and sport.

The body gets its nutrients primarily from the food one consumes, though some nutrients may come from nutrient supplements. The digestive tract breaks down foods into smaller components, and varying amounts of the nutrients are absorbed. The cells of the body then utilize the absorbed nutrients for all their metabolic reactions including energy production. Some of the food you eat today becomes part of you in the future.

Exercise is important in obtaining and maintaining good health. Exercise also enhances one's nutritional state. For the first time in 1995, one of the Dietary Guidelines for Americans was to "balance the food you eat with physical activity — maintain or improve your weight." In the United States, the President's Council on Physical Fitness and Sports and the Center for Disease Control and Prevention collaboratively developed a report of the Surgeon General in 1996 entitled *Physical Activity and Health*. This report indicated "that people of all ages can improve the quality of their lives through a lifelong practice of moderate physical activity." So physical activity joined proper nutrition as being essential health objectives. Physical activity and proper nutrition actually function synergistically in helping individuals obtain and maintain good health and reduce the risk of chronic diseases. Actually, this was recognized as early as 480 B.C. by Hippocrates, who wrote that "eating alone is not enough for health. There must be exercise of which the effects must likewise be known. The combination of these two things makes regimen, when proper attention is given to the season of the year, the changes of the winds, the age of the individual, and the situation of his home. If there is any deficiency in food or exercise the body will fall sick."

1

The Nutrients

Nutrition affected your life before you were born and will affect it until you die. You must obtain nutrients in order to survive. *Nutrition* may be defined as the science of nourishing the body properly. Nutrition is both a physical and a behavioral science. Nutritionists are concerned with the changes that occur in food and the way the body uses food from the time it is selected and ingested until it is eventually incorporated into body tissues, participates in metabolic reactions, or is excreted from the body. The Council on Food and Nutrition of the American Medical Association has a more detailed definition of nutrition, which follows: nutrition is "the science of food, the nutrients and the substances therein, their action, interaction, and balance in relation to health and disease, and the process by which the organism ingests, digests, absorbs, transports, utilizes, and excretes food substances." The American Dietetic Association adds the word "selects" in that appropriate food selection is an important component to obtaining and maintaining a good state of nutrition or nutritional status.

Every day you make food choices that may affect your health for better or worse. If beneficial choices are made, these may decrease the chances of getting various diseases including chronic diseases like cancer and heart disease. Good nutrition is one of the most important factors in obtaining and maintaining good health. Good nutrition can help you meet your genetic potential.

Nutritional Habits

Nutritional habits are affected by many factors, including those which are inborn, cultural (family, caregivers), religious, ethical, economic, convenience, social, emotional, and psychological. We choose what we eat for many varied reasons. Economic and convenience factors are usually major influences for college students. Sometimes, we experience social pressure to eat certain foods. We also have positive as well as negative associations related to the eating of certain foods. We may choose to eat or not eat some foods with other foods. For example, individuals in a certain religion may not eat meat and dairy foods in the same meal. What we eat may be related to our personal values and the image we want to portray to friends, family, and even strangers. When deciding whether to eat a certain food, one should consider the nutritional value of that food.

Social and cultural traditions may also be associated with the preparation, serving, and eating of food. The sharing of food can be symbolic. Eating is a *social behavior*.

The taste, flavor, aroma, texture, color, and appearance of a food may affect whether or not we choose to eat that food. These characteristics are called *sensory attributes*. Our likes and dislikes for various foods are formed early in our childhood.

Nutrients

Foods are carriers of nutrients. Nutrient supplements also provide nutrients. *Nutrients* are chemicals that have specific functions in the body. Nutrients provide the body with energy, structural components to build and maintain the body, and regulators for various functions. *Essential nutrients* are those that the body can not synthesize for itself in adequate quantities. Essential nutrients must be obtained from the diet. The body will develop deficiencies if not provided with adequate quantities of essential nutrients. Nutrients essential to some animal species may not be needed by other species. For example, the laboratory rat can synthesize adequate quantities of ascorbic acid, but humans can not.

Classes of Nutrients

The six classes of nutrients are water, carbohydrates, lipids (fats and oils), proteins, vitamins, and minerals. Water, carbohydrates, lipids, and proteins are known as *macronutrients* in that these nutrients are found in large amounts in our bodies and our bodies require large quantities (over a few grams) of these nutrients daily. Conversely, vitamins and minerals are known as *micronutrients* in that small amounts of these nutrients are found in our bodies and our bodies require small quantities (mg or μg) of these nutrients on a daily basis. Carbohydrates, lipids, proteins, and vitamins are *organic*; that is, these nutrients are from living things that have captured solar energy and converted this energy into carbon-containing compounds. Minerals and water are *inorganic*.

Water is the most vital essential nutrient. A person would die sooner if water was not consumed than if any other nutrient was not consumed. On a weight basis, more water than any other nutrient is present in the body. Water is continuously being lost from the body and must be replaced, particularly during exercise.

Carbohydrates, lipids, and *proteins* are energy-yielding nutrients. *Energy-yielding nutrients* are broken down by the cells of the body to produce energy. Similar forms of energy are produced from carbohydrates, lipids, and proteins. When energy is produced, heat, water, and carbon dioxide are released. The energy from food supports all of the body's activities including exercise.

The unit in which energy is measured in known as a *calorie*. Food energy is measured in kilocalories (kcal) or 1,000 calories. As used in nutrition, calorie is a misnomer and actually refers to a kilocalorie. So the term calorie, in popular use, is really 1,000 calories or a kilocalorie.

The energy content of a food depends on how much carbohydrate, lipid, and protein are present in that food. Carbohydrates provide the body with 4 calories (actually kilocalories, but commonly called calories) per gram. Proteins also provide the body with 4 calories per gram; however, the major function of dietary protein is the synthesis of body proteins, including those in muscles. Lipids provide the body with 9 calories per gram and are referred to as being energy-dense or calorie-dense (also energy-rich or calorie-rich). The *449 rule* is often utilized in remembering the energy contributions of carbohydrates, proteins, and lipids, respectively. Though not classified as a nutrient, alcohol also contains food energy. The body is provided with 7 calories per gram of alcohol. Sometimes, energy is measured using kilojoules (kJ). One can multiply calories (which actually are kilocalories) by 4.2 to get kilojoules.

Carbohydrates consist primarily of sugars and starches. Sugars impart sweetness to many of the foods we eat. Carbohydrates, once broken down by the body and absorbed, provide *glucose*. The body must have a certain amount of glucose daily. *Fibers* are primarily indigestible carbohydrates. Fibers provide bulk to the diet and help keep the gastrointestinal tract healthy.

There are two fatty acids which are essential to the body. These *essential fatty acids* are linoleic acid (an omega-6 or N-6 fatty acid) and linolenic acid (an omega-3 or N-3 fatty acid). Arachidonic acid (another omega-6 or N-6 fatty acid) is sometimes considered a semiessential fatty acid in that it can be synthesized only from the essential fatty acid linoleic acid after linoleic acid needs are met.

Nine amino acids are essential or indispensable to the body. These *essential amino acids* are histidine, isoleucine, leucine, lysine, methionine, phenylalanine, threonine, tryptophan, and valine. Some evidence exists, though considered inconclusive, that arginine may also be an essential amino acid. The amino acids cystine (and cysteine) and tyrosine are sometimes considered semiessential amino acids in that they can only be synthesized from methionine and phenylalanine, respectively, once needs for methionine and phenylalanine are met.

Vitamins are organic catalysts and micronutrients. Vitamins function as body regulators. We require four fat-soluble vitamins (vitamins A, D, E, and K) as well as the water-soluble vitamins ascorbic acid and B-complex vitamins (thiamin, riboflavin, niacin, vitamin B_6, folate, vitamin B_{12}, biotin, and pantothenic acid). Some evidence exists, though inconclusive, that some other organic nutrients may be needed by humans in small amounts.

Minerals are inorganic catalysts and micronutrients. Minerals function as body regulators. *Essential minerals* are those which, when added to a purified diet, cause a demonstrable improvement in growth. Minerals are frequently subcategorized as macrominerals (or macroelements or major minerals or major elements), electrolytes, and trace minerals (or trace elements). The essential macrominerals are calcium, phosphorus, and magnesium. The essential electrolytes are sodium, potassium, and chloride; these electrolytes may also be classified as macrominerals. The essential trace minerals are iron, copper, zinc, iodine, selenium, manganese, fluoride, chromium, and molybdenum. There is some evidence, though inconclusive, that other minerals may be essential for humans.

Foods also contain *nonnutrients*, or substances other than the six classes of nutrients. *Phytochemicals*, meaning chemicals found in plants, are nonnutrients of interest in today's world. Phytochemicals may be responsible for some of the sensory attributes of foods. Some of the phytochemicals also may have drug or medicinal effects.

Elemental diets, those having precise chemical composition, have been fed to individuals, particularly hospitalized persons who can not eat ordinary foods. These diets seem to be beneficial in continuing life and helping in recovery. However, these diets do not enable individuals to thrive. There may be some substances present in foods, not identified as being essential, that the body needs. There appear to be physical and psychological effects that food has that are not met by elemental diets to date. Food may give us more than just nutrients known to be essential. Nutrient supplements alone, though they may contain sufficient vitamins and minerals, are not able to replace food in its role in nourishing the body.

Disease Relationships

An inadequate intake of any or a combination of the essential nutrients is associated with disturbed body metabolism and certain diseases. Current research indicates that the same can be said with regard to excessive intakes of many of these essential nutrients. The consumption of too little or too many calories also has been associated with certain diseases,

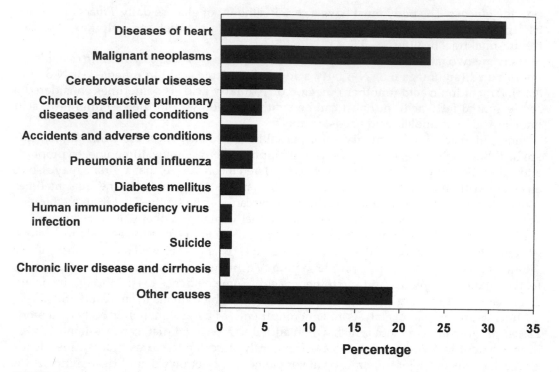

FIGURE 1.1
Top 10 causes of death (U.S.) (1996).

particularly *chronic diseases*. Before the 1980s nutritional research and nutritional surveys were concerned primarily with nutrient deficiencies. Currently, the emphasis is on the relationships between diet and diseases and on the possible effects of nutrient toxicities.

The 10 *leading causes of death* in the United States in 1996 are given in Figure 1.1 Among these, diseases of the heart, malignant neoplasms, cerebrovascular diseases, and diabetes mellitus are definitely nutrition-related. The remaining causes of death may also have some association with nutrition. Poor nutrition can accelerate the development of degenerative diseases. Healthful nutrition can aid in the prevention of diseases, or perhaps forestall diseases. Nutritional therapy can frequently ease the impact of many diseases. Good nutrition throughout life is important to having good health.

2

Digestion, Absorption, and Circulation of Nutrients

The complex food particles that you consume are broken down into smaller, readily absorbable nutrient products by *digestion*. Most nutrients are soluble in body fluids (which are composed predominantly of water), but some insoluble nutrients must be converted into soluble forms. The smaller nutrient products are then absorbed into the body proper, where they are transported via the circulatory system (lymphatic system may also be involved) to the individual cells of the body where they perform their functions or are stored. The nutrient products may be excreted by the body. Malfunctions in digestion, absorption, transport, cellular metabolism, and excretion can result in malnutrition.

Nutrient digestion and absorption takes place in the *gastrointestinal (GI) tract* or alimentary system. The GI tract (see Figure 2.1) is comprised of tubular organs that extend from the mouth to the anus. Mucus protects the linings of the GI tract and serves as a lubricant for the food materials passing through the tract. The liver, gallbladder, and pancreas also function in digestion. Digestion gets the food residues ready for absorption. Absorption also takes place in the GI tract.

GI Tract Function

The GI tract performs many functions. The GI tract receives, macerates, and transports consumed substances; secretes mucus, several digestive enzymes, acid, and bile; digests the consumed foods; absorbs and transports the products formed by digestion; promotes the synthesis of some nutrients by microorganisms; reabsorbs some nutrients from the body proper; and transports, stores, and excretes waste products. These processes are primarily under the control of the autonomic (involuntary) nervous and the endocrine systems. Hormones that function in the GI tract are known as *enterogastrones*. There are more than one hundred million neurons in the nervous system of humans. There are several *neurotransmitters* that function in the regulation of GI activity. These include bombesin, enkaphalin, neurotensin, somatostatin, substance P (for pain), the vasoactive inhibitory polypeptide, catecholamines, acetycholine, serotonin, purines, pancreatic polypeptide, and encephalins. These neurotransmitters are released from the GI tract and nervous system and function in stimulating and inhibiting the release of gastric hormones, acid, and enzymes. Scientists are just beginning to understand the relationships between these neurotransmitters and GI function.

Digestion begins in the mouth, where maceration reduces the size of the ingested food. The tongue aids in chewing and contains taste receptors for bitter, salt, sour, and sweet. The ingested food is mixed with *saliva*. Saliva contains *ptyalin* (salivary amylase), which hydrolyzes starch to smaller carbohydrate units (oligosaccharides and disaccharides). The food material is then swallowed into the esophagus. The epiglottis prevents the food that

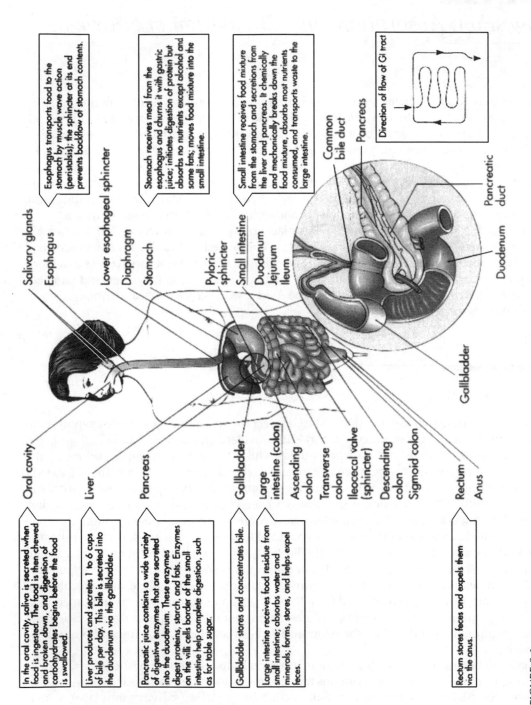

In the oral cavity, saliva is secreted when food is ingested. The food is then chewed and broken down, and digestion of carbohydrates begins before the food is swallowed.

Liver produces and secretes 1 to 6 cups of bile per day. This bile is secreted into the duodenum via the gallbladder.

Pancreatic juice contains a wide variety of digestive enzymes that are secreted into the duodenum. These enzymes digest proteins, starch, and fats. Enzymes on the villi cells border of the small intestine help complete digestion, such as for table sugar.

Gallbladder stores and concentrates bile.

Large intestine receives food residue from small intestine; absorbs water and minerals; forms, stores, and helps expel feces.

Rectum stores feces and expels them via the anus.

Esophagus transports food to the stomach by muscle wave action (peristalsis); the sphincter at its end prevents backflow of stomach contents.

Stomach receives meal from the esophagus and churns it with gastric juice; initiates digestion of protein but absorbs no nutrients except alcohol and some fats; moves food mixture into the small intestine.

Small intestine receives food mixture from the stomach and secretions from the liver and pancreas. It chemically and mechanically breaks down the food mixture, absorbs most nutrients consumed, and transports waste to the large intestine.

Oral cavity

Salivary glands

Esophagus

Lower esophageal sphincter

Diaphragm

Stomach

Pyloric sphincter

Small intestine

Duodenum
Jejunum
Ileum

Liver

Pancreas

Gallbladder

Large intestine (colon)

Ascending colon

Transverse colon

Ileocecal valve (sphincter)

Descending colon

Sigmoid colon

Rectum

Anus

Common bile duct

Pancreas

Pancreatic duct

Duodenum

Gallbladder

Direction of flow of GI tract

FIGURE 2.1

The gastrointestinal (GI) tract. Reprinted with permission from McGraw-Hill Companies. Wardlaw, G., *Contemporary Nutrition: Issues and Insights*, Brown & Benchmark, Dubuque, IA, © 1997.

is being swallowed from going into the trachea (windpipe). The swallowed food material is called a **bolus. Peristalsis**, wave-like muscular contractions, carry the bolus through the esophagus and the cardiac sphincter to the stomach.

The distension of the stomach by the bolus promotes the secretion of the hormone **gastrin**. The presence of gastrin and of "secretatogues" (proteins, alcohol, caffeine), stimulates the secretion of gastric enzymes and hydrochloric acid. The parietal cells of the stomach secrete **hydrochloric acid**, making the pH become about 1.5. Rennin, pepsin, and gastric lipase are enzymes secreted by the stomach. **Rennin** acts on casein (milk protein), curdling it so that pepsin can hydrolyze it. **Pepsin** hydrolyzes protein in the presence of hydrochloric acid to smaller protein components (polypeptides). **Gastric lipase** hydrolyzes tributyrin (a lipid) to free fatty acids. **Intrinsic factor,** which functions in the absorption of vitamin B_{12}, is synthesized by the chief cells of the stomach. The stomach converts the bolus to **chyme**. The stomach also temporarily stores food materials. The stomach empties in one to four hours after the food was consumed. Carbohydrates leave the stomach first, followed by proteins, and then by lipids. Also, liquid food stuffs leave the stomach before those that are solid. When the pH of the stomach is too low, gastrin release is reduced. Chyme leaves the stomach via the pyloric sphincter, which is controlled by antral peristaltic waves and the pyloric pump.

The chyme then moves into the small intestine. The upper small intestine is known as the duodenum; the middle portion, the jejenum; and the lower portion, the ileum. **Secretin**, a hormone released from the duodenal mucosa in response to acidity in the duodenum, opposes the action of gastrin. Secretin stimulates the **pancreas** to secrete **bicarbon**ate and water, which flow into the duodenum via the pancreatic duct. Neutralization of the acidity to about pH 8 provides the proper pH for the activity of intestinal and pancreatic enzymes and also protects the intestinal mucosa. The **gastric inhibitory polypeptide**, a hormone released from the duodenal mucosa in response to lipid residues and glucose, inhibits hydrochloric acid secretion in the stomach and stimulates the release of insulin. **Motilin** is another hormone released by the duodenal mucosa in response to alkalinity. Motilin slows the emptying of the stomach and stimulates intestinal motility. **Somatostatin**, a hormone released by the stomach and duodenum, inhibits the release of insulin and glucagon by the pancreas. Pancreatic **glucagon**, released by the pancreas, stimulates hepatic glucose output and inhibits pancreatic enzyme secretion.

The hormone **cholecystokinin** is released by the intestinal mucosa in response to the presence of lipid and protein components in the chyme. Cholecystokinin causes the gallbladder to release bile which goes into the duodenum via the bile duct. Cholecystokinin also stimulates the pancreas to secrete digestive enzymes into the duodenum and to a limited extent, bicarbonate and water. Cholecystokinin also slows the emptying of the stomach.

Bile is synthesized by the liver, stored in the gallbladder, and performs its function in the duodenum. Bile emulsifies lipids, and thus facilitates lipid digestion and absorption.

Pancreatic enzymes that function in the duodenum are trypsin (secreted in the inactive form as trypsinogen), chymotrypsin (secreted in the inactive form as chymotrypsinogen), carboxypolypeptidase, elastase, ribonuclease, deoxyribonuclease, pancreatic lipase, pancreatic amylase, and cholesterol esterase. **Trypsin, chymotrypsin**, and **carboxypolypeptidase** function in the breakdown of proteins. Elastase acts on fibrous proteins. Ribonuclease and **deoxyribonuclease** act upon RNA and DNA. **Pancreatic lipase** acts on lipids, while **pancreatic amylase** acts on starch and dextrins. **Cholesterol esterase** converts cholesterol to cholesterol esters and fatty acids.

The duodenum also secretes some of its own enzymes. The intestinal enzymes are enterokinase, four peptidases, intestinal amylase, dextrinase, three disaccharidases, alkaline phosphatase, and intestinal lipase. **Enterokinase** activates the pancreatic enzymes trypsinogen and chymotrypsinogen to trypsin and chymotrypsin, respectively, thus enabling these two pancreatic enzymes to hydrolyze proteins. The peptidases *polypeptidase, aminopeptidase, carboxypeptidase,* and *dipeptidase* act upon smaller proteins. *Intestinal amylase* and *dextrinase* break down starches and dextrins. The disaccharidases *sucrase, maltase,* and *lactase* break these carbohydrates into smaller units. *Alkaline phosphatase* removes phosphate from organic compounds such as proteins. *Intestinal lipase* breaks down lipids.

Chyme moves through the small intestine via peristalsis, taking between 3 to 10 hours. Most of the digestive process is completed in the small intestine. Much of the vitamin K, vitamin B_{12}, and biotin that are synthesized by the *intestinal microflora* is absorbed, primarily in the ileum, and can be utilized by humans. The quantity of each of these vitamins that is absorbed varies greatly from individual to individual. Nutrient absorption takes place primarily in the small intestine, mostly in the duodenum. Normally 92 to 98 percent of the mixed Western diet is digested and absorbed.

The unabsorbed food residues then passes through the ileocecal valve to the large intestine or colon. There is some reabsorption of water and electrolytes in the large intestine. There is also some absorption in the large intestine of short-chain fatty acids formed by colonic bacteria. Unabsorbed nutrients, desquamated cells, mucus, digestive secretions, bacteria, yeast, and fungi pass through the large intestine (ascending, transverse, and descending colon) for excretion as *feces. Defecation* is the term used for the expulsion of feces from the body.

Absorption

Following digestion, nutrients are in smaller units and may be absorbed. Most *nutrient absorption*, the transfer of nutrients from the intestinal lumen (interior) across the intestinal mucosa into the circulatory or lymphatic systems, takes place in the small intestine. A small amount of nutrient absorption does occur in the stomach and large intestine. The mucosal cells are selective as to what nutrients and how much of each nutrient is absorbed.

The convulsions (folds) of the intestinal mucosa (see Figure 2.2) contain many *villi,* which are finger-like projections. Every cell on each villus contains a brushlike covering which is covered by tiny hairs called the brush border or *microvilli. Capillaries* and *lacteals* extend into the villi. Water-soluble substances are absorbed into the capillaries and enter the circulatory system. Fat-soluble substances are absorbed into the lacteals and enter the lymphatic system. The lymphatic system eventually delivers the fat-soluble nutrients into the circulatory system via the thoracic duct.

Absorptive Mechanisms

Nutrients may be absorbed by diffusion, osmosis, and active transport. When the concentration of a substance is higher in the intestinal lumen than in the absorptive cells, the substance will naturally move from the higher to the lower concentration; this process is called *simple diffusion* or passive absorption. Simple diffusion involving just water is known as *osmosis. Facilitated diffusion* occurs when a carrier protein is involved in the substance moving from the higher to the lower concentration. Sometimes, energy must be expended in getting substances to cross membranes. *Active transport* or active absorption is when energy (usually as adenosine triphosphate, ATP) is required to move substances in combination with a carrier protein across a membrane. In active transport, the substance is generally

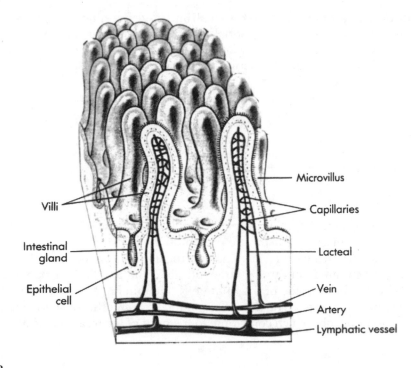

FIGURE 2.2
Structure of villi. Reprinted with permission from McGraw-Hill Companies. Gottfried, S.S., *Biology Today*, Mosby-Year Book, Inc., St. Louis, MO, © 1993.

going from a higher concentration to a lower one. In phagocytosis, a substance is engulfed by first forming an indentation in the cell membrane and then surrounding the substance and incorporating the substance into the inside of the cell. If the substance undergoing phagocytosis is liquid, the process is called pinocytosis.

Absorption of the Nutrients

Monosaccharides and, occasionally, disaccharides from carbohydrate digestion are absorbed by the small intestine. The monosaccharides glucose and galactose are absorbed by active transport utilizing a sodium-dependent carrier. The monosaccharide fructose is absorbed by sodium-dependent facilitated diffusion. The indigestible carbohydrates cellulose, hemicellulose, pectin, and other forms of fiber are not absorbed, but are excreted in the feces.

The free fatty acids and monoglycerides from fat digestion complex with bile salts as micelles. The micelles then facilitate the passage of these lipids through the intestinal lumen to the microvilli where the bile salts are released. In the microvilli, the fatty acids and monoglycerides are reassembled into new triglycerides. These triglycerides, as well as cholesterol and phospholipids, are surrounded by a β-lipoprotein coat, thus forming *chylomicrons*. These globules then pass into the lacteals of the intestinal villi by *exocytosis*. The fat-soluble vitamins are absorbed in the same manner as lipids.

Individual amino acids and sometimes dipeptides from protein digestion are absorbed in the small intestine by sodium-dependent active transport. There are four carriers for the amino acids; one each for acidic, basic, and neutral amino acids, and one for the amino acids proline and hydroxyproline. Immunoglobulins from breast milk are probably absorbed by pinocytosis.

Water is absorbed by osmosis in both the small and large intestine. Most of the water-soluble vitamins are absorbed by the intestinal villi by passive diffusion, though the water-soluble vitamins can also be absorbed by active transport. Most of the cationic minerals are absorbed by facilitated diffusion involving carriers or by active transport. The anionic minerals are generally absorbed by simple diffusion, though the mechanism can be active transport. Many of the minerals have common carriers. Electrolytes and sometimes vitamins are absorbed in the large intestine.

Intestinal Microflora

Around a hundred different species of microorganisms have been identified in the intestines of humans. Few microorganisms are present in the intestines in the newborn. There is little bacterial activity in the stomach in that hydrochloric acid is a germicidal agent. Most of the microorganisms are found in the large intestine, and to a limited extent, the ileum. Humans are able to absorb some of the vitamin K, vitamin B_{12}, and biotin that is synthesized by these microorganisms. The microflora of the large intestine also synthesize gases, acids, indoles, and phenols, which contribute to the odor of the fecal materials.

Lymphatic System

The lymphatic system consists of circulatory vessels that carry lymph. *Lymph* is a fluid similar to blood, but it does not contain erythrocytes. Fat-soluble substances in the intestines are absorbed into the lacteals and go on into the lymphatic system. The lymphatic system may also be of importance with regard to the transportation of immunity factors. The lymphatic system drains into the thoracic duct of the circulatory system.

Circulatory System

All blood that leaves the digestive system goes first to the *liver*. The liver may alter the absorbed nutrients and other substances before sending it on to the heart via the circulatory system.

The circulatory system provides the tissues of the body with nutrients including water, and oxygen. It also takes carbon dioxide and waste products including nutrient end-products away from the tissues (see Figure 2.3). The *heart* is the muscle that pumps blood throughout the circulatory system. Blood basically travels in two routes. Blood is pumped from the right side of the heart to the lungs where it exchanges carbon dioxide for oxygen; this is known as *pulmonary circulation*. The oxygenated blood goes back to the heart. The oxygenated blood is pumped from the left side of the heart to all the other tissues of the body where nutrients from the blood are exchanged in the capillaries for waste products; this is known as *systemic circulation*. There are capillaries in every part of the body.

The fluid surrounding each cell is known as *extracellular fluid* or interstitial fluid. This extracellular fluid is derived from the blood that squeezes out of the capillaries and flows

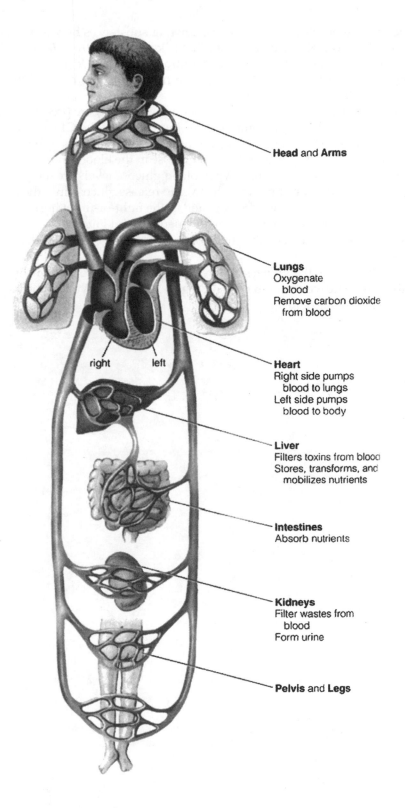

Head and **Arms**

Lungs
Oxygenate
    blood
Remove carbon dioxide
    from blood

Heart
Right side pumps
    blood to lungs
Left side pumps
    blood to body

Liver
Filters toxins from blood
Stores, transforms, and
    mobilizes nutrients

Intestines
Absorb nutrients

Kidneys
Filter wastes from
    blood
Form urine

Pelvis and **Legs**

right   left

FIGURE 2.3
The circulatory system. Reprinted with permission from Wadsworth Publishing Companies. Sizer, F., and Whitney, E., *Nutrition Concepts and Controversies*, 7th ed., West/Wadsworth, Belmont, CA, © 1997.

around the outside of cells. There is an exchange of substances between the extracellular fluid and the fluid located inside each cell that is known as *intracellular fluid*. The metabolic reactions inside the cell take place in the intracellular fluid (cytoplasmin) or in subcellular components suspended in the cytoplasmin. Some of the extracellular fluid again enters the capillaries.

The blood also carries *hormones* from the glands, where they are produced, to their target organs. Earlier in this chapter, enterogastrones (hormones of the GI tract) were discussed. Other hormones also affect the utilization of nutrients by the body. The pancreas secretes *insulin* in response to high concentrations of glucose in the blood (hyperglycemia). Insulin aids in the cellular uptake of glucose. When blood glucose levels are too low, the pancreas secretes *glucagon*. Glucagon stimulates the liver to release glucose into the circulatory system. *Epinephrine* (also known as adrenalin and as the fight-or-flight hormone) and *norepinephrine* (also known as noradrenalin) also influence blood glucose levels as well as stress responses. The body produces other hormones that directly or indirectly affect nutrient metabolism.

The blood also goes to the *kidneys*, where it is filtered. Many of the waste products, particularly those that are water-soluble, including water, are removed by the kidneys and are excreted as components of *urine*.

The Most Important Nutrient

3

Water

No other compound is more essential to life than water, for without it there would be no life of any kind. Bacteria, plants, animals, and humans all require exogenous water. Without water we would die in a few days. *Water*, H_2O, contains hydrogen and oxygen and is an inorganic *solvent*. Different life forms contain different anatomical proportions of water. Wheat and corn, properly dried, contain only a small amount of water. Fresh fruits and vegetables may be 80 to 90 percent water. The water content of a food affects its *caloric density.* Generally, foods that are high in water are low in calories.

Body Distribution

The human body contains more water than any other component. The water content in the body varies according to age, sex, bone density, lean body mass, and gross body weight. It usually varies between 45 and 75 percent of total body weight with the water content being generally higher in the young, in men, and in lean people. Gender differences in body water content are mainly due to differences in body fat. Most of the water in the body is localized in cells (about 60 percent), particularly those in the muscles and viscera, and is called *intracellular water.* Most of the remaining body water is *extracellular water* (about 38 percent) consisting of interstitial fluids and blood. About 2 percent of the body water is in the transcellular fluid compartment, which consists of cerebrospinal fluid, synovial fluid, vitreous fluid, and that in peritoneal and pericardial spaces. Smaller amounts of water are to be found in bone, adipose tissue, the gallbladder (as bile), and secretory glands. The water content of skeletal muscles is about 65 to 75 percent by weight. Adipose tissue contains about 10 percent water by weight. Bone has about the same amount of fat as adipose tissue. Typical fluid volumes for the average female and male are given in Figure 3.1.

Functions

Water is biologically important because of its many unusual physical and chemical properties. It has been called the universal solvent, for it is capable of dissolving not only polar molecules and inorganic salts, but also large organic molecules which may be either polar or contain hydrophobic components. Water has a high specific heat (1 cal/g) and a high heat of vaporization (80 cal/g). These physical properties of water help to prevent rapid fluctuations in body temperature, either hot or cold, and permit small amounts of water (perspiration and transpiration) to remove large amounts of body heat during exercise.

55 kg female
25% body fat — 41.3 kg lean body mass
Total body water 30.7 L

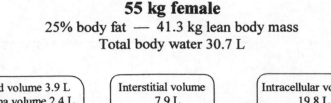
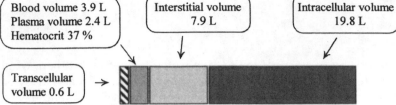

70 kg male
15% body fat — 59.5 kg lean body mass
Total body water 43.6 L

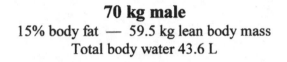
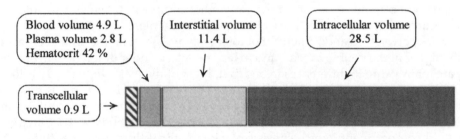

FIGURE 3.1
Fluid volumes for the average woman and man. Adapted form Minson and Halliwill, 1999.

Water's large dielectric constant and extensive intermolecular hydrogen bonding relative to other organic liquids (e.g., alcohols) are factors contributing to its special properties.

Other characteristics that make water physiologically important include its low viscosity and moderate surface tension, permitting blood flow and lubrication for eyelids, articulating joints, movement of muscle filaments, and peristalsis. Water also permits transmission of light (eye) and sound (ear).

While the primary function of water remains as a solvent for the myriads of biochemical reactions in cells and blood, water also enters directly into some biochemical reactions. Molecular water is consumed during the hydrolysis of proteins, lipids, and carbohydrates undergoing digestion and metabolism. It is also consumed during hydroxylation reactions and is produced as the terminal product of oxidative phosphorylation. Water is consumed in photosynthesis in plants. Water produced in this manner is often referred to as *metabolic water*. About 10 percent of our daily water need is fulfilled by the formation of metabolic water. The remaining 90 percent of our daily water requirement is ingested in foods (about 30 percent) and as various liquids (about 60 percent). Some foods are high in water content while others are low (Table 3.1).

TABLE 3.1

Approximate Water Content of Selected Foods

	% Water
Skim milk	91
Broccoli, cooked, drained	90
Orange juice	88
Spaghetti with tomato sauce and cheese	80
Potatoes, mashed	78
Hard-cooked egg	75
Tuna, canned, drained	61
Beef patty, lean, broiled	56
Bread, white, enriched	37
Italian salad dressing	34
Bagel, plain	29
Cheddar cheese	28
Butter	16
Raisin bran	9
Crackers, saltines	4
Corn oil	0

Water helps the body rid itself of *waste products*. Water is eliminated from the body primarily as urine or as *insensible perspiration* via epidermal and pulmonary evaporation. Urine is about 95 percent water by weight. About 5 percent of the total elimination of body water is contained in feces, providing lubrication and a soft stool. Urinary water provides the solvent for the elimination of the metabolic end-products of most nutrients and other substances. Insensible perspiration of skin provides for elimination of some body salts, and insensible perspiration of both skin and lungs carries away body heat by way of *evaporation*. Diffusion of gases in the body takes place across membranes moistened by water. The evaporation of water as sweat helps the body cool itself. Sedentary adults typically excrete 1,000 to 1,500 ml of urine, 500 to 700 ml of sweat, 250 to 350 ml of small water droplets in exhaled air, and 100 to 200 ml of water in the feces. Exercise greatly increases the amount of water lost via *perspiration* and *expiration*. In fact, body metabolism during endurance exercise can exceed resting metabolism by 15-fold. About 80 percent of this increase in metabolism is converted to heat and needs to be dissipated or the body's core temperature will be elevated. The amount of water lost in perspiration and expiration is affected by environmental temperature and humidity.

Water Balance

The water intake should approximate the water output on a daily basis. Figure 3.2 illustrates the routes and approximate quantities of water intake and outgo in a 70 kg male without sweating. Euhydration exists when water intake and output are equal. The body has essentially no water reserves. The kidneys along with the gastrointestinal tract and brain homeostatically regulate the amount of water in the body, at least the fat-free components.

When total body water decreases by about 1 to 2 percent, the normal individual has a sensation of thirst with the message coming from the hypothalamus. The thirst sensation may be blunted in the elderly and in individuals performing vigorous exercise. If individuals become dehydrated, their *heat tolerance* is affected. The *antidiuretic hormone* is released and the kidneys conserve water and electrolytes during dehydration. The individual may experience a *heat stroke*. The symptoms of a heat stroke are headache, nausea, dizziness,

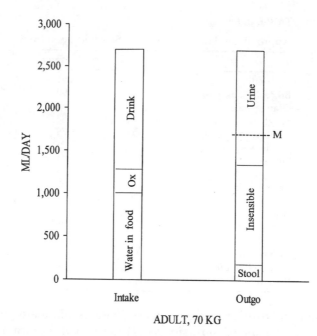

ADULT, 70 KG

FIGURE 3.2

Routes and quantities of water intake and output without sweating. M is minimal urine volume at maximal solute concentration. Ox is water of oxidation. Reprinted with permission from National Research Council, *Recommended Dietary Allowances.* © 1989 by the National Academy of Sciences. Courtesy of the National Academy Press, Washington, DC.

clumsiness, stumbling, excessive or insufficient sweating, mental confusion, and loss of consciousness. An individual experiencing extreme dehydration may go into a coma and even die. *Hypohydration* is the term used when the body has a water deficit. Physical performance begins to decline soon after the body's water loss exceeds the intake. In fact, for every 1 percent of body weight in water lost, plasma volume decreases about 2.5 percent and the fluid in the muscles decrease 1 percent. Long-term hypohydration also affects oxygen transport. Hypohydration is frequently observed in the elderly and in individuals participating in vigorous exercise, particularly in hot humid environments.

On the other hand, *water intoxication* occurs if one is given excessive water or has excessive water or electrolyte loss, resulting in hyposmolarity. Once again, the antidiuretic hormone and the kidneys try to respond, but if fluid homeostasis can not be obtained, there is headache, nausea, blurring of vision, muscle twitching, gradual mental dulling, convulsion, and even death. Water intoxication is rarely observed in normal adults. *Hyperhydration* (too much water in the body) has been reported in athletes who become overhydrated by consuming excessive fluids.

Both hypohydration and hyperhydration compromise the cardiovascular system. The cardiovascular system is then less able to accommodate stresses including heat stress. Hypohydration is much more prevalent in the athletic population than hyperhydration.

Dietary Recommendations

The recommended water intake is 1 to 1.5 ml/kcal expended or about ½ cup/100 kcal. This is equivalent to about 2 to 3 quarts for the person expending 2,000 kcal daily. As indicated

TABLE 3.2

Guidelines for Fluid Replacement

1. Consume a balanced diet and drink adequate fluids during the 24 hours preceding exercise.
2. Drink 500 mL of fluid two hours before exercise.
3. During exercise, drink fluids early and at regular intervals. The goal is to replace fluid at a rate equal to what is lost in sweating (up to what can be tolerated).
4. Fluid should be cooler than ambient temperature (15 to 22°C or 59 to 72°F), flavored for palatability, and readily available.
5. Additionally, if exercise will be longer than one hour, proper amounts of carbohydrates and/or electrolytes should be included in fluids.
   A. The addition of carbohydrates should allow for 30 to 60 g/h. This can be achieved by consuming 600 to 1200 mL/h of a 4 to 8 percent carbohydrate solution.
   B. The addition of sodium at 0.5 to 0.7 g/L increases palatability, promotes fluid retention, and avoids hyponatremia.

Reprinted with permission from CRC Press. Minson, C.T. and Halliwill, J.R., Fluid and Electrolyte Replacement, In: Driskell, J.A., and Wolinsky, I., Eds., *Macroelements, Water and Electrolytes in Sports Nutrition*, © 1999 by CRC Press, Boca Raton, FL, as adapted from the American College of Sports Medicine position stand on exercise and fluid replacement, 1996.

earlier, food consumption does contribute to the water intake. Some water, referred to as *metabolic water*, can also come from metabolism. For a sedentary adult, about 300 to 400 ml of water is provided each day through metabolic reactions. Additional water is needed for extended physical activity. The suggestion has been made that physically active individuals should consume 1.5 mL water per kcal expended. Water is important to athletic performance as well as life itself.

When engaging in strenuous exercise of over 0.5 to 1 hour's duration, one should drink water before, during (every 15 minutes or so), and after the event. A typical water intake recommendation for the adult endurance athlete is to drink 2 to 3 cups about 2 hours before an event, 1 to 2 cups 10 to 15 minutes before the event, ½ to 1 cup every 10 to 15 minutes during the event, and 1 to 2 cups after the event at about 15 minute intervals. Furthermore, the water should be cooler than ambient temperature. The American College of Sports Medicine in 1996 released a position stand on exercise and fluid replacement. These guidelines are summarized in Table 3.2. Well before exercise begins, athletes should hydrate their bodies. The American College of Sports Medicine indicates that water itself is sufficient for rehydration in exercise lasting less than one hour. However, some research indicates that sugar and electrolyte replacement may also be beneficial in strenuous exercise lasting less than one hour. Water and electrolyte replacement should occur throughout exercises lasting more than one hour. The drinking schedule should be selected so as to maximize fluid absorption in the gastrointestinal tract. Research also indicates that voluntary fluid consumption can be increased by having beverages readily available, having beverages at 15 to 22°C (59 to 72°F), and adding sweeteners and flavoring (increases palatability) to the beverages. Fluid replacement should continue after the exercise bout until the body is completely rehydrated and core body temperature returns to normal. One could consume a beverage containing water, sugar, and electrolytes together as these are all needed in additional quantities during vigorous exercise. The presence of sugar in the beverage slows gastric emptying. The use of glucose polymers, such as maltodextrins, rather than simple sugars reduces the negative effect on gastric emptying. Adult athletes can lose ½ to 1 gallon of fluid every hour during heavy exercise. The relative humidity affects the cooling efficiency of sweating. Blood volume becomes reduced when sweating and causes a fluid loss of 2 to 3 percent of body mass, which puts a strain on the circulatory system and can impair one's capacity for exercise and for thermoregulation. Fluid replacement is important to individuals performing prolonged exercise in the heat. Fluid replacement is also of importance to individuals exercising in cold temperatures where the fluids consumed should be warmer than when one exercises in hotter environments (between 25 and 30°C or 77 and 86°F). Individuals who exercise at high altitudes for long periods of time also need additional fluids. Research indicates that voluntary fluid consumption can be increased by having beverages readily available, having beverages at appropriate temperatures, and adding sweeteners and flavorings (increases palatability) to the beverages.

The consumption of large quantities of protein facilitates water loss through urea production and excretion. This increased excretion of urine can hasten body dehydration. Diarrhea and vomiting can also cause body dehydration.

The Energy-Yielding Nutrients

The Energy-Yielding Nutrients

The body can obtain its energy or fuel from carbohydrates, lipids, and proteins. The body functions best if the energy comes from carbohydrates and lipids. Dietary protein is best utilized for the synthesis of body proteins.

At the cellular level, carbohydrates, lipids, and proteins can be catabolized to energy, water, and carbon dioxide. These nutrients share some of the same metabolic pathways. From a caloric viewpoint, it makes little difference whether dietary energy is obtained from high- or low-carbohydrate diets, from plant oils or animal fats, or from high- or low-quality proteins. All living beings need energy. Energy needs vary from person to person, depending primarily upon age and level of physical activity.

Adults should consume as many calories (food energy) as they expend. Children need to consume slightly more calories than they expend. When caloric intake and expenditure are not balanced and intake exceeds expenditure, an individual gains weight. Obesity is a major health problem in the United States. The vast majority of the time, obesity is caused by the caloric intake exceeding the expenditure over a period of time.

4

Carbohydrates

Carbohydrates contain carbon, hydrogen, and oxygen. The ratio of hydrogen to oxygen in carbohydrates is 2:1, the same as water; hence, the name *carbohydrates.*

Classification

Carbohydrates are either sugars (simple carbohydrates) or complex carbohydrates (starches, fibers). Monosaccharides are the simplest units of carbohydrates. This is the unit from which all more complex carbohydrates are built.

The most common *monosaccharides* are glucose (blood sugar), fructose (sweetest sugar), and galactose (a component of milk sugar). Glucose is also called dextrose. Glucose, fructose, and galactose are known as hexoses, or 6-carbon sugars. Pentoses, 5-carbon sugars, are components of nucleic acids and other nucleotides.

The most common *disaccharides* (made up of two monosaccharide units linked together) are sucrose, maltose, and lactose. Sucrose (table or granulated sugar) is made up of glucose plus fructose. The consumption of sucrose in the American diet is high and is a contributing factor to *tooth decay.* Lactose (milk sugar) is composed of glucose plus galactose. Maltose (malt sugar) is composed of two molecules of glucose and is found in germinating cereals.

Sugars are monosaccharides and disaccharides. Artificial sweeteners, such as saccharin, aspartame, and acesulfame are not true sugars, but they do have the sweetness qualities of sugars without having as many calories.

Polysaccharides contain three or more monosaccharides. This is the form of most carbohydrates. Common polysaccharides include starch, fiber, and glycogen. Starch is generally referred to as *complex carbohydrate.* Starch is found in corn, beans, peas, potatoes, and pasta, as well as breads, cereals, and pastries. *Dextrins* are intermediates in the breakdown of starches. Dextrins are found in some processed foods and sports beverages. *Glycogen* (animal starch) is stored in liver and muscle and consumed as a component of meat. Glycogen is not a significant food source of carbohydrate and is not counted as a complex carbohydrate in diet planning, but technically it is a complex carbohydrate. *Dietary fiber* (including cellulose) is the structural framework of plant tissues. Humans lack the enzyme necessary to break down cellulose. Cellulose, also known as indigestible carbohydrate, contributes to bulk in the diet and helps maintain gastric motility. Dietary fibers (such as cellulose, hemicelluloses, lignins, pectins, lignins, and gums) are needed by the body primarily for bulk. The vast majority of the dietary fibers are carbohydrates.

Digestion

Carbohydrate digestion is initiated with salivary amylase. Limited digestion of carbohydrates occur in the acidic environment of the stomach. In the small intestine, pancreatic amylase, intestinal amylase, maltase, sucrase, and lactase break down the carbohydrates to monosaccharides. Monosaccharides are absorbed through the intestinal mucosa into the circulatory system. The circulatory system supplies the cells of the body with monosaccharides. *Available carbohydrates* are those digested and absorbed by the body. Undigested carbohydrates (mainly dietary fiber) are excreted in the feces.

Some individuals are *lactose intolerant*, meaning that they can not adequately digest lactose or milk sugar. Infants may be born with inadequate quantities of lactase to digest lactose though intolerance can also occur with aging. Lactose intolerance is more common in persons of color including Native Americans, Blacks, Hispanics, and Orientals, though Whites may also be lactose intolerant. Lactose intolerance may be treated with lactose-free diets and formulas as well as Lact-aid®-type products. Lactose-intolerant individuals can avoid eating foods that contain lactose, primarily dairy products, and get the nutrients contained in dairy products (particularly calcium) from other food sources.

Functions

The major function of carbohydrates is to provide *energy*. One gram of carbohydrate provides on the average ~4 calories. Most American adults get 40 to 50 percent of their energy from carbohydrates, and much of that is from sugars. Adults should get at least 55 percent or more of their calories from carbohydrates and these should be primarily complex carbohydrates. Energy is formed when energy-yielding nutrients, including carbohydrates, are broken down to CO_2 and H_2O. Dietary fat and protein can also be used for energy formation. The *central nervous system* uses glucose (and perhaps also short-chain fatty acids) almost exclusively for energy formation.

Dietary carbohydrate may be converted to *glycogen* and stored in the body. The body stores only enough glycogen to provide energy for a few hours to a day.

Dietary carbohydrate can also be converted to fat; the liver breaks glucose into smaller molecules and then synthesizes fat. Dietary carbohydrate which is not needed for other purposes is converted to *adipose tissue*.

Dietary carbohydrates spare protein in that protein will not be used for energy formation if adequate carbohydrate is available for this function. Dietary carbohydrate also spares fat or serves as a "primer" for fat metabolism. If carbohydrate breakdown products are not available, the body will mobilize fat to a greater extent than it can use. This results in the accumulation of ketone bodies, which leads to ketosis, which affects the acid-base balance of the body. To avoid ketosis, an adult should eat a minimum of 50 to 100 g carbohydrates daily.

The following health effects have been reported for dietary fiber: relieves constipation, increases intestinal transit time, increases fecal weight, helps control body weight, relieves diverticulitis in most people, decreases hemorrhoids in most people, may decrease blood cholesterol concentration, may increase blood glucose concentration, may decrease the incidence of colon cancer, and may decrease the incidence of cardiovascular disease. Intestinal discomfort can occur when large quantities of fiber are consumed. The microflora of the large intestines have enzymes that break down the dietary fiber to fatty acids, gases, H_2O, and CO_2. The consumption of large quantities of dietary fiber has been reported to interfere with the absorption of the minerals iron, copper, and zinc; however, this has been questioned, particularly when dietary fiber is consumed in reasonable amounts.

Blood Glucose Homeostasis

The normal physiologic response of carbohydrate ingestion, digestion, and absorption is the postprandial increase in blood glucose followed by increased glucose uptake by tissues. The timing and magnitude of this glycemic response is variable with different foods. Glucose ingestion induces a rapid and large increase in blood glucose; whereas, consumption of fructose results in a much slower and lower glycemic response. The *Glycemic Index* is a ranking of the postprandial blood glucose response to a specific food as compared to a reference food, containing 50 g of available carbohydrate (frequently glucose itself). In determining the Glycemic Index the amount of carbohydrate in the two foods being compared are the same. The Glycemic Index of glucose is 100, while that of fructose is 23. Contradictory evidence exists as to whether dietary fiber consumption influences the Glycemic Index.

Blood glucose must be maintained at optimal levels, not too high or too low. If blood glucose levels are too low (*hypoglycemia*), the person becomes dizzy and weak, and if too high (*hyperglycemia*), the person becomes confused and has difficulties breathing. Both extremes can be fatal. Insulin, a hormone produced by the pancreas, decreases blood glucose levels. In *diabetes mellitus*, blood glucose levels are too high. The diabetic does not produce enough insulin (Type I or insulin-dependent), the insulin receptors may become inactive, or for some reason, the insulin that is produced does not perform its function (Type II or non-insulin-dependent). Hypoglycemia impairs exercise performance. A diet rich in complex carbohydrates and dietary fibers and low in concentrated sugars helps in the regulation of blood glucose levels.

Recommended Intakes

The recommended carbohydrate intake for adults, according to the American Heart Association, is 55 to 60 percent of calories, with an emphasis on complex carbohydrates. The American and Canadian Dietetic Associations recommend that the carbohydrate content of the diet should be 60 to 65 percent of calories and be elevated to 65 to 70 percent if the individual is involved in exhaustive training. Research indicates that the diet may need to contain up to 7 to 10 g carbohydrates per kg body weight for athletes involved in different levels of physical activity. Generally, the *recommended carbohydrate intake* is 55 to 65 percent calories, with power and endurance athletes consuming 65 to 75 percent calories as carbohydrates. Carbohydrates should be consumed mainly as complex carbohydrates. *Sugars* should be consumed sparingly. The bacteria that are present in the mouth can produce acids from sugars (particularly those in sticky candies). These acids can break down the enamel of teeth and lead to increased *dental caries*. Sugars are also "empty calories" in that little to no vitamins and minerals are found in most foods that have high sugar content. The *recommended fiber intake* is 20 to 35 g daily according to an expert panel of the Federation of American Societies of Experimental Biology. The *Dietary Guidelines for Americans* includes the guideline choice of a diet with plenty of grain products, vegetables, and fruits. Research indicates that there is no health hazard in consuming chiefly complex carbohydrates provided that the essential amino and fatty acids, vitamins, and minerals are also present in the diet.

Carbohydrate and Fiber Consumption Habits

The median daily carbohydrate intakes of men and women, 20 to 50 years old, in the United States are 46.8 and 49.5 percent of calories, respectively, according to NHANES III (*Third National Health and Nutrition Examination Survey*) data for 1988-91. The median daily dietary fiber intakes of these same individuals are 16.5 and 11.9 g, respectively. American adults are not consuming as much carbohydrate (as percent of calories) or dietary fiber as is recommended.

Glycogen Loading

"Staleness" is a physiologic state caused by gradual depletion of the glycogen reserves in the body by strenuous endurance workouts even though the person may be consuming a typical carbohydrate intake. An athlete can optimize his/her glycogen reserves by gradually decreasing the intensity of exercise workouts several days prior to a competition while maintaining a high complex carbohydrate intake. Glycogen replenishment is of importance to the athlete. After much of the glycogen has been utilized for energy formation, muscle glycogen is restored by consumption of a diet high in complex carbohydrates and having relative physical rest.

In *glycogen loading* (also called "carboloading"), the athlete trains at a high aerobic intensity and about one week before the event gradually reduces or tapers the duration of exercise on successive days. Carbohydrates represent ~50 to 55 percent of calories during the first three days and then are increased to ~70 to 75 percent of calories for the last three days before the competition. The *precompetition meal* is light, but high in complex carbohydrates and is consumed about three hours before the competition. Sometimes liquid or formula meals are utilized. The pre-event meal should be largely digested and absorbed before the event so as to minimize gastric upset and energy being expended to digest and absorb the food during the event. It is important to consume a *post-event high-complex carbohydrate meal* after the body has returned to a resting state. This post-event meal is of importance to athletes who participate in frequent activities (daily, weekly) where fast recovery is critical to performance.

Endurance Capacity

The endurance athlete should glycogen load. Drinking a sugar drink prior to the endurance event hinders endurance capacity. However, during intense exercise lasting longer than one hour, carbohydrates should be consumed at a rate of 30 to 60 g/hour in order to maintain oxidation of carbohydrates and delay fatigue. This may be accomplished by drinking 600 to 1200 ml/hour of fluid solutions containing 4 to 8 percent carbohydrates as sugars (sucrose or glucose) or starch (maltodextrin). Sugar drinks need not be consumed during moderate exercise. Sports drinks generally contain 2 to 8 percent sugar.

Carbohydrate manipulation seems to be most effective for endurance activities lasting over two hours, though some studies, but not all studies, indicate beneficial effects for shorter-duration, high-intensity activity. Generally, simple carbohydrates in beverages have been utilized for carbohydrate manipulation. Numerous studies indicate that the consumption of carbohydrates during long-term endurance exercise improves endurance capacity and performance. Glucose, sucrose, and maltodextrins (containing multiple glucose units) seem to be equally effective in improving athletic performance according to most studies. Inconclusive evidence exists that maltodextrins may empty rapidly from the stomach, and thus, more readily supply glucose. Also, maltodextrins are not very sweet tasting, and many individuals find maltodextrins more palatable than monosaccharides.

5

Lipids

Lipids are fatty substances that are organic and do not dissolve in water because of their chemical structure. *Fats* is frequently used as another name for lipids. However, lipids can be either fats or oils. *Fats* are lipids that are solid at room temperature; fats usually are derived from animals. *Oils* are lipids that are liquid at room temperature; oils usually are derived from plants.

Classification

Lipids, like carbohydrates, contain carbon, hydrogen, and oxygen. Most lipids are referred to as *simple lipids* and contain the 3-carbon alcohol *glycerol* linked to one to three *fatty acids* or their derivatives. Glycerol when linked to a fatty acid is known as a *glyceride*. Glycerides containing one fatty acid are known as monoglycerides, those with two fatty acids are diglycerides, and those with three fatty acids are triglycerides. The most common lipids are triglycerides. The fatty acids can be short- (contain 2 to 6 carbons), medium- (contain 6 to 10 or 12 carbons), and long- (contain 10 or 12 or more carbons) chain. Generally, the shorter chain fatty acids are more liquid at room temperature and are also more water-soluble. The fatty acids can be saturated or unsaturated. *Saturated fatty acids* have only single bonds linking the carbons together while *unsaturated fatty acids* contain at least one double bond in the carbon chain. *Monounsaturated fatty acids* have one double bond in the carbon chain while *polyunsaturated fatty acids* have many double bonds. Olive, canola, and peanut oils contain monounsaturated fatty acids. Soybean, corn, sunflower, and safflower oils contain polyunsaturated fatty acids.

Compound lipids are composed of simple lipids linked with other substances. Common compound lipids are phospholipids, glucolipids, and lipoproteins. *Derived lipids* are composed of derivatives of simple and compound lipids. Derived lipids include cholesterol as well as many of the hormones which are steroids. Fat-soluble vitamins are sometimes considered to be lipids.

Digestion

Fats are hydrophobic and hydrophilic. There is some, but little, digestion of fat by lingual lipase in the mouth and gastric lipase. *Bile* is needed for the digestion of fat. Bile is synthesized from cholesterol. Fats are digested primarily by pancreatic and intestinal lipases. Usually 95 percent of all fats are absorbed as glycerol, fatty acids, and monoglycerides. Cholesterol in foods often has a fatty acid attached which is removed, then 25 to 75 percent (average is 55 percent) of dietary cholesterol is absorbed. Glycerol and the short- and medium-chain fatty acids are actually water-soluble and go directly into the circulatory system following absorption via the portal vein and on to the liver. Following absorption, the long-chain fatty acids and monoglycerides are made into triglycerides in the intestinal cells. Triglycerides, cholesterol, and phospholipids are assembled into *chylomicrons* and are transported via the lymphatic system to the circulatory system. Chylomicrons transport the diet-derived lipids (mainly triglycerides) from the intestine to the rest of the body. The liver cells remove remnants of the chylomicrons after about 14 hours.

The cholesterol that is found in the body may come from foods of animal origin that are consumed (*exogenous cholesterol*) or cholesterol can be synthesized by the body. In general, the more cholesterol one eats, the less cholesterol one synthesizes. However, some people have trouble with the feedback mechanism that regulates the synthesis of cholesterol.

Lipid Transport

Once the chylomicrons enter the circulatory system, their lipoproteins are degraded by *lipoprotein lipase* into free fatty acids and glycerol. These "freed" fatty acids can be used for energy formation or resynthesis to triglycerides and stored as adipose tissue. Meanwhile, liver cells are synthesizing other fats to be transported out to other body tissues. The liver is the most active site of lipid synthesis. The lipids that are synthesized in the liver are transported by very low density lipoproteins (*VLDL*). As VLDL travels through the body, cells remove triglycerides and VLDL shrinks and it gathers cholesterol from other lipoproteins circulating in the blood stream and becomes low density lipoprotein (*LDL*).

LDL circulates through the body making its contents (lipids including cholesterol) available to all cells (muscle, adipose stores, mammary glands, etc.). Special LDL receptors in the liver cells remove LDL from circulation; this is important in controlling blood lipid levels. High density lipoprotein (*HDL*) carries cholesterol and phospholipids from tissues to the liver for recycling or disposal. LDL and HDL work in opposition to each other. HDL is frequently referred to as being the "good" cholesterol and LDL, the "bad" cholesterol.

Functions

Fats are the most *energy-dense* class of nutrients. The body converts 1 g of fat to an average of 9 calories. During rest and moderate exercise, well-nourished adults obtain about half of their energy from fats and half from carbohydrates. More fat than carbohydrate is used for energy formation in exercise of one hour or longer; in fact, lipids can supply as much as 90 percent of the energy. In intense but short-term exercise, the vast majority of the energy comes from glycogen. *Adipose tissue* is the major body reserve or storehouse for excess nutrient energy. One pound of body fat provides approximately 3,500 calories; glucose is needed for this conversion.

Fat, as subcutaneous adipose tissue, *insulates* the body against the environmental stress of hot and cold temperatures, sometimes referred to as temperature shock. Adipose tissue also protects the vital organs of the body serving as a *shock absorber*.

The body needs *essential fatty acids*; these must be provided by the diet as the body can not synthesize them in adequate amounts. *Linoleic* (an omega-6 fatty acid) and *linolenic* (an omega-3 fatty acid) *acids* are essential fatty acids. If the body is deficient in linoleic acid, then arachidonic acid becomes an essential fatty acid. Normally, vegetable oils and meats supply enough of these essential fatty acids to meet body needs. Symptoms of essential fatty acid deficiency include skin lesions, neurological and visual problems, growth retardation, reproductive failure, skin abnormalities, kidney and liver disorders, and death. Essential fatty acid deficiency is rare and historically is seen only in infants and hospitalized patients fed formulas.

Fats function in carrying and storing the fat-soluble vitamins A, D, E, and K. Foods that contain fat often contain these fat-soluble vitamins.

Fats, as phospholipids and as cholesterol, are components of all *biologic membranes* as well as neural tissues. Phospholipids enable the cell membranes to allow both water- and fat-soluble substances to pass through the membrane into the interior of the cells. Fats are components of the retina of the eye, some hormones, and some digestive secretions. A derivative of cholesterol can be used by the body in the synthesis of vitamin D. *Eicosanoids* (including prostaglandins and thromboxanes) are fatty acid derivatives which help regulate blood pressure, blood clotting, and may perhaps have other functions. Eicosanoids may play protective roles against the development of heart disease and cancers.

Fats also have *satiety value*. Fats take longer for the body to digest than carbohydrates and proteins. Hence, some fat in the diet helps to delay "hunger pains" and promotes a feeling of fullness. Fats also add *palatability* to the diet. Many of the flavors in food are fat-soluble and their smell can be sensed by the nose and mouth. Weight-reduction diets containing moderate levels of fat generally lead to more weight loss than diets that are very low in fat.

Recommended Intakes

The Diet and Health Report of the National Research Council (1989) recommends that "total fat intake be less than 30 percent of calories," that "saturated fat intake be less than 10 percent of calories," and that "cholesterol intake be less than 300 mg daily." Other health groups and organizations have made similar recommendations, though some indicate that these recommendations are equal or less than these values, such as equal to or less than 30 percent of calories for total fat. One of the *Dietary Guidelines for Americans* is to choose a diet low in fat, saturated fat, and cholesterol. The American Heart Association recommends that one consume less than 30 percent of calories as total fat with equal proportions being saturated, monounsaturated, and polyunsaturated. The recommended intakes for power and endurance athletes are the same as for the nonathlete.

Lipid Consumption Habits

In Western countries, people generally consume more lipid than is recommended. The median daily total, saturated, monounsaturated, and polyunsaturated lipid and cholesterol intakes of men and women, 20 to 59 years old, in the United States are 35.2 and 34.5 percent of calories, 11.8 and 11.9 percent of calories, 13.0 and 12.4 percent of calories, 6.4 and 6.7 percent of calories, and 283 and 187 mg, respectively, according to NHANES III data for 1988-91. Though lipid intakes of American adults have decreased over the last decade, median intakes are still higher than recommended.

Health Effects of Fats

Research indicates that the cholesterol content of foods is not as influential in increasing blood cholesterol (specifically LDL) as total fat, especially saturated fat. The priority is in the following order: avoid excess fat, saturated fat, and cholesterol. This tends to reduce *coronary heart disease* (CHD). The consumption of fish oils has a questionable effect on blood cholesterol levels.

An expert panel of the National Cholesterol Education Program has indicated that adults should have their blood cholesterol levels checked at least every five years. Desirable blood lipid levels for adults 20+ years of age are as follows: <200 mg/dL total cholesterol, <130 mg/dL LDL-cholesterol, >60 mg/dL HDL-cholesterol, and <200 mg/dL triglycerides. Blood total cholesterol levels of 200 to 239 mg/dL and LDL-cholesterol levels of 130 to 159 mg/dL are "borderline-high." Blood total cholesterol levels of 240+ mg/dL are "high" as are LDL-cholesterol levels of 160+ mg/dL. According to surveys about 20 percent of American adults have high blood cholesterol levels. Many studies indicate that lowering blood cholesterol levels reduces the risk of heart disease.

The higher one's blood cholesterol level, the more likely that cholesterol will be deposited in the arteries. Ways to control blood cholesterol levels include quit smoking, exercise (increases HDL levels and helps control body weight), diet, and medications. The following recommendations have been made with respect to controlling blood cholesterol levels with diet: increase complex carbohydrates; increase soluble fiber; if obese, lose weight; decrease total fat intake to less than 30 percent of calories; decrease saturated fat intake to less than 10 percent of calories; increase polyunsaturated fat intake (decreases coronary heart disease, but may increase cancer); consume equal quantities of saturated, monounsaturated, and polyunsaturated fatty acids; decrease dietary cholesterol to less than 300 mg daily, do not eat trans-fatty acids (as in margarine); and replace some animal proteins with vegetable proteins or eat leaner meats. Factors that increase HDL-cholesterol levels include: gender (female higher than male, estrogen therapy should be considered); increased exercise; moderate alcohol consumption may increase; some dietary fibers may increase; and chromium may increase, but it can also be carcinogenic.

The consumption of high-fat diets has also been associated with increased incidence of cancer of the colon, breast, prostate, and endometrium. The consumption of excessive calories has also been associated with increased incidence of these cancers. Several studies involving blood cholesterol levels and incidence of all types of cancer together suggest that if blood cholesterol is low, the statistical risk of cancers is increased. Other studies have not shown this relationship. Additional research is needed on this association.

Fat Substitutes

Fat substitutes on the market include Simplesse, Olestra, and Maltodextrin. Simplesse is physically modified milk and/or egg white protein with added water. Olestra is the chemical union of sucrose and fatty acid components. Maltodextrin is hydrolyzed cornstarch with added water. Other fat substitutes are also available commercially.

6

Proteins

The nitrogen-containing class of foods is called **proteins**. Like carbohydrates and lipids, proteins contain carbon, hydrogen, and oxygen. Proteins contain about 16 percent nitrogen. Proteins, a term derived from the mythological Greek god Proteus, means "first." Proteins were the first substance to be recognized as a vital part of living tissue. Proteins are essential nutritionally.

Amino Acids: The Building Blocks of Protein

Proteins are assembled from their basic units, the **amino acids**. The body uses amino acids to synthesize its own variety of proteins. Amino acids or organic compounds of similar nature were probably first formed in that primordial soup at the beginning of biological time. About 20 to 22 amino acids are commonly found in proteins. All the amino acids except proline and hydroxyproline (which are really imino acids) are α-amino carboxylic acids. They contain a basic amino group and an acidic carboxyl group both attached to the α-carbon (see Figure 6.1). They differ from each other by the remainder of the molecule (R). The basic and acidic portions of the molecule enable amino acids and proteins to function as **buffers**.

Protein Structure

All amino acids needed for synthesis of a protein in the body must be in the same cell at the same time. Proteins are assembled from their constituent amino acids, one by one and one at a time. Two amino acids are initially combined, forming a dipeptide by the exclusion of a molecule of water from the carboxylic acid and the amino group of the second amino acid. The result is the formation of a dipeptide with its amide, "**peptide bond.**" Addition of

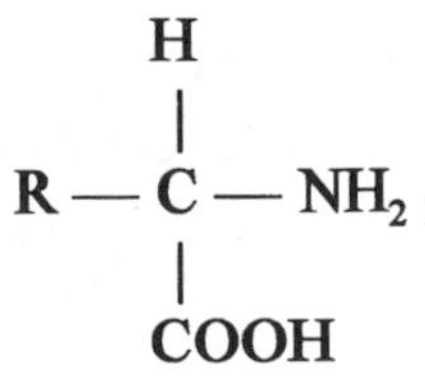

$$R - \overset{\displaystyle \overset{H}{|}}{\underset{\displaystyle \underset{COOH}{|}}{C}} - NH_2$$

FIGURE 6.1
Structure of an amino acid.

a third amino acid to the dipeptide results in the formation of a second peptide bond and a tripeptide. To the tripeptide is added, in similar fashion, another amino acid, forming a tetrapeptide, and so, one by one, polypeptides are assembled from amino acids. When polypeptides begin approaching 50 amino acids in length they are called proteins. Proteins do not always exist singularly, but are often associated with other compounds. Such complex proteins in association with nucleic acids, lipids, carbohydrates, and minerals are often classified according to the molecule with which the protein associates. These protein complexes, often called *conjugated proteins*, perform specific functions which neither constituent could properly perform alone. Derived proteins come from protein metabolism and include peptides, peptones, and proteoses.

Classification of Amino Acids By Function

Rose, during the 1930s, demonstrated that some of the amino acids found in proteins were *essential* or indispensable while others were *nonessential* or dispensable. The essential amino acids can not be synthesized *in vivo* from nonprotein sources in sufficient quantity to meet the body's needs, and so must be supplied to humans from either plant or animal proteins. There are nine essential amino acids required in the diet of the human infant. A decade or so ago, there were eight amino acids considered to be essential for the human adult; now there are considered to be nine. These essential amino acids are given in Table 6.1. The human infant requires histidine; it is controversial whether adults also require histidine. Kopple and Swendseid have suggested that histidine may also be essential for adults. Arginine is not synthesized in amounts sufficient to meet the needs of the young of most mammalian species. It appears that arginine is not required by the human infant, but the need by the premature infant is unknown. The amino acids tyrosine and cysteine (cystine too) are sometimes classified as *semiessential amino acids* or conditionally-essential amino acids. Tyrosine can be synthesized *in vivo* only from the essential amino acid phenylalanine, while cysteine (cystine) can be synthesized *in vivo* only from the essential amino acid methionine. Frequently, humans consume phenylalanine and methionine in low amounts and these two amino acids may not be available for conversion to tyrosine and cysteine (cystine). There is some evidence that arginine, proline, and glycine are conditionally essential for low-birth-weight infants.

The body is able to synthesize the nonessential amino acids by *transamination* utilizing amino groups from other nonessential amino acids and unneeded essential amino acids. A certain quantity of nonessential amino acids is considered to be a dietary essential. The body's protein needs are both qualitative and quantitative. The body needs each of the essential amino acids in certain proportions and also needs a sufficient quantity of protein.

TABLE 6.1

Essential Amino Acids*

Histidine	Phenylalanine
Isoleucine	Threonine
Leucine	Tryptophan
Lysine	Valine
Methionine	

* Some evidence exists that arginine may be an essential amino acid.

Protein Quality

The essential amino acid content of protein foods determines the quality of the protein (know as *protein quality*). Most protein foods contain many different proteins, so the quality of a protein food reflects a composite of the amino acid content of several different proteins. For example, milk contains the proteins lactoalbumin and casein.

Complete proteins contain all the essential amino acids needed by the body in amounts that are adequate. Complete proteins are high-quality proteins. Generally, proteins from animal-derived foods are complete; these include meat, poultry, fish, cheese, eggs, and milk. Gelatin is an animal protein that is incomplete.

Incomplete proteins do not contain all the essential amino acids needed by the body in amounts that are adequate. Incomplete proteins contain one or more essential amino acid(s) in insufficient quantities to meet the body's needs. Most plant proteins are incomplete. The essential amino acid that is present in the shortest supply relative to the amount needed for protein synthesis is called the *limiting amino acid*. The lack of even one essential amino acid can stop protein from being synthesized.

Complementary proteins are two or more incomplete proteins whose essential amino acid assortments complement each other in such a way that the essential amino acid(s) missing from one protein (the limiting amino acid) is supplied by the other. The following are general statements about limiting amino acids as some exceptions exist: vegetables are low in methionine, legumes are low in methionine and tryptophan, grains are low in lysine, seeds are low in lysine, and nuts are low in threonine and sometimes lysine. Combinations which are complementary include the following: legumes + grains, legumes + seeds, vegetables + grains, vegetables + seeds, vegetables + nuts, and grains + nuts. Individuals can obtain adequate protein quality and quantity by eating complementary proteins.

Cooking with moist heat softens connective tissue. This increases the digestibility of protein. Overheating, particularly in a dry environment, tends to make the protein harder to digest and may destroy or alter some of the amino acids such as lysine.

Digestion

Protein digestion begins in the stomach by the enzyme pepsin. Pepsinogen is converted to pepsin by the hormone gastrin. Pepsin is particularly effective in the acid environment of the stomach; the acidity is due to the presence of hydrochloric acid. The peptide fragments leaving the stomach are broken down by trypsin, which is produced in the pancreas and performs its function in the duodenum. These peptide fragments are degraded to single amino acids, di- and tri-peptides, which are absorbed in the small intestine and delivered into the circulatory system.

Protein Status

In a research setting, the protein status of humans is most commonly determined via nitrogen balance studies. Most of the body's nitrogen is found in protein. *Nitrogen balance* is equal to the nitrogen intake minus the nitrogen output (in urine and feces; sometimes sweat is also included). Adults should maintain nitrogen balance, while children should have a positive nitrogen balance (eat more nitrogen than is excreted). The aged and individuals with some diseases have negative nitrogen balance (eat less nitrogen than is excreted).

Unfortunately, no satisfactory measurement is available for assessment of protein status. Parameters other than nitrogen balance that are utilized for evaluation of protein status of humans include serum total protein, albumin, prealbumin, or transferrin concentrations; serum amino acid ratios; urinary hydroxyproline indices or 3-methylhistidine levels, and fasting urinary urea:creatinine ratios. Several muscle function tests and immunological measurements may also be used in evaluating protein status. Generally, the most often used biochemical method for assessing protein status in a hospital or clinic setting is the determination of serum albumin concentration.

Somatotrophin (or growth hormone), insulin, testosterone, and estrogen stimulate protein synthesis. Thyroxine increases the metabolic rate, and thus influences both the anabolism and catabolism of proteins. Both gluconeogenesis and ketogenesis of proteins are increased by glucocorticoids. Several reports exist that acute or chronic alcohol intake decreases protein synthesis and affects muscle fibers.

Functions of Proteins in the Body

Amino acids and their specific order in the primary protein structure provides the chemical specificity that dictates their function. Dietary protein provides the amino acids needed for synthesis of body proteins; this is an anabolic process which builds and maintains body tissues. These body proteins include those needed for cellular structure, enzymes, transport proteins (usually lipoproteins), nucleic acids and nucleoproteins, antibodies, blood-clotting factors, visual pigments, glutathione, taurine, some hormones, and some neurotransmitters. *Body protein* is constantly being synthesized and degraded; this is known as protein turnover. Body proteins also function in the maintenance of acid-base balance (as *buffers*) and in fluid and electrolyte regulation. Proteins can also be used to provide the body with *energy* and *heat*; proteins contain approximately 4 kcal/g. Proteins may also be converted to *adipose tissue*.

Protein Catabolism

Only a small reserve of amino acids exists in the body. Amino acids which are not needed for protein synthesis are deaminated primarily in the liver with the resulting carbon skeleton being used for either energy production or adipose tissue formation. The deaminated amino group is converted to *urea* in the liver and excreted in the urine. The quantity of urea excreted by an individual varies with the protein intake. The metabolism of protein consumed in excess of the body's requirement is referred to as *exogenous protein metabolism*.

Uric acid is the end-product of purine catabolism. Purines are components of nucleic acids. A disorder of the catabolism of purines to uric acid is gout.

Creatinine is the end-product of creatine catabolism. Creatine is found in all muscle tissues. Creatine phosphate is a high-energy phosphate reserve. The quantity of creatinine which is excreted is reflective of the lean body mass of an individual. Each individual excretes a relatively constant quantity of creatinine daily; hence, it is frequently utilized in ascertaining the completeness of 24-hour urine collections. The metabolism of protein which was once part of the body is referred to as *endogenous protein metabolism.*

Protein-Energy Malnutrition

Protein-Energy Malnutrition (PEM), formerly known as Protein-Calorie Malnutrition (PCM), is the most widespread form of *malnutrition* in the world. Around a quarter of the world's population experiences pain from hunger due to lack of food. PEM is prevalent in underdeveloped countries including those in Africa, Asia, and Central and South America. Some cases have been reported in the United States.

Kwashiorkor, or protein deficiency, is caused by insufficient good quality protein. Kwashiorkor occurs primarily among 2- to 5-year-old children who are weaned to diets of starch cereal pastes. Individuals with kwashiorkor have edema, scaly skin, red flag (reddish pigmentation of the formerly dark hair), fatty liver, decreased immunity, decreased growth, decreased intelligence, and eventually, death. Individuals with kwashiorkor frequently have secondary infections which generally are related to their deaths.

Marasmus is a condition in which there is insufficiency of both protein and food energy. Marasmus is starvation. In marasmus, there is a deficiency of many essential nutrients. The clinical symptoms of marasmus are different from those of kwashiorkor. Symptoms of marasmus include severe muscle wasting, absence of subcutaneous fat, dermatosis, reduced growth, hepatomegaly, anxiety, and decreased intelligence.

The clinical symptoms of PEM can be reversed in four to six weeks with a diet adequate in food energy, nutrients, and high-quality protein. Unfortunately, the effects of PEM on mental development in children are nonreversible. Frequently, individuals with PEM also have intestinal parasites and other infectious disorders which also require treatment as well as psychologic problems.

Recommended Intakes

The 1989 Recommended Dietary Allowance (RDA) for protein is 0.75 g/kg body weight for adults. Younger individuals require more protein per kg body weight than adults. The *Daily Value* (DV) for protein for individuals four years of age and older (not including pregnant and lactating women), based on 0.8 g protein/kg body weight, is 50 grams.

Power and endurance athletes appear to need 1.2 to 1.5 g/kg body weight. For strength athletes, an allowance for making gains in skeletal muscle with training is justified and appropriate. Endurance athletes may need additional protein for repair of damaged muscle fibers. The International Center for Sports Nutrition endorses the range of 1.0 to 1.5 g/kg body weight/day. Endurance athletes need a little more protein than power athletes as they retain some of this protein in their muscles. Some evidence refutes this and indicates that the protein needs of both endurance and power athletes are the same as for less active persons.

Power-lifters and body builders frequently consume proteins that have been chemically "predigested" in the form of liquids, powders, or pills. Some evidence exists that creatine, formed from glycine plus arginine and methionine, may be beneficial to the athlete.

Protein Consumption Habits

The median protein intakes of men and women, 20 to 59 years old, in the United States are 94 and 64 g, respectively, according to NHANES III data for 1988-91. These median intakes are equivalent to 14.7 and 14.6 percent of kcal. Median intakes of other age-sex groups over a year of age ranged from 12.9 to 16.3 percent of kcal. Median protein intakes of all age-sex groups were well above the 1989 RDAs, but less than twice the 1989 RDAs.

Excessive Protein Intakes

In Western countries, people generally consume more protein than they require; the protein is frequently of high quality. Individuals can add adipose tissue by consumption of diets high in protein. Many foods which are high in protein are also high in fat. Individuals can get *dehydrated* if they consume too much protein. Some studies indicate that there may be an increased excretion of calcium in those consuming high levels of protein. The consumption of high levels of protein can create a problem for individuals having liver or kidney disorders. The National Research Council Committee on Diet and Health recommends that "protein intakes not exceed twice the RDA."

Processed Proteins

Soy protein isolates are frequently used as meat analogues or substitutes. Soy protein concentrates are sometimes added to foods to provide texture and emulsification. Tofu is soybean curd. Miso is soybean paste. Surimi, a slurry made from minced fresh fish (cheap ones), is used in making imitation seafoods. Casein is used in the manufacturing of some dessert toppings and coffee whiteners. Hydrolyzed vegetable proteins are frequently used for flavorings.

Monosodium glutamate (MSG) is made from glutamic acid. MSG is a flavor enhancer. MSG is safe for the vast majority of people, but some people may be sensitive to MSG. If MSG is added to a product, it must be listed on the food label.

Aspartame is a sugar substitute made from phenylalanine plus aspartic acid. Aspartame is used in making diet beverages and foods. People with phenylketonuria (PKU) should avoid consuming foods containing aspartame. Aspartame is marketed as a sugar substitute as Nutrasweet® and Equal®.

Micronutrients: The Catalysts

Micronutrients: The Catalysts

Vitamins and minerals, both micronutrients, function as catalysts in numerous metabolic reactions in the body. Frequently they function along with proteins as components of enzymes. The body is unable to function without the presence of vitamins and essential minerals. Energy production, the synthesis and maintenance of tissues, and even the synthesis and breakdown of adipose tissues, are among these functions. The body requires small amounts of each of the vitamins and essential minerals. Evidence exists that the recreational and competitive athlete may need more of some of these vitamins and essential minerals than nonathletes.

The most recent national survey of food intakes in the United States is the *Third National Health and Nutrition Examination Survey* (NHANES III) of 1988-91. Median intakes of men, 20 to 59 years of age, for vitamin A, vitamin E, vitamin B_6, magnesium, and zinc were lower than the 1989 Recommended Dietary Allowances for these nutrients. Median intakes of women, 20 to 59 years of age, for vitamin A, vitamin E, vitamin B_6, calcium, magnesium, iron, and zinc were lower than the 1989 Recommended Dietary Allowances for these nutrients. Median copper intakes were lower than the 1989 Estimated Safe and Adequate Daily Dietary Intake for copper. On the other hand, median sodium intakes of these individuals were higher than recommended. Not all vitamins and essential minerals were included in this survey. The nutrient contributions of vitamin/mineral supplements were included in these intake estimations. The few studies that have been done with athletic populations (all had small sample sizes), indicate that the intakes of athletes are rather similar to those of the total population with regard to vitamins and minerals. An individual or a group of people are not deficient or marginally deficient in a nutrient just because of consumption of less than recommended quantities of that nutrient. However, individuals who habitually consume **less than two-thirds of the Recommended Dietary Allowance** for a nutrient are likely to be deficient or marginally deficient in that vitamin.

Surveys indicate that about one-fourth to one-half of the U.S. population take *vitamin/mineral* supplements at least occasionally. Most reports indicate higher supplement usage among athletes. Some individuals take individual vitamins and minerals as opposed to multivitamins/multiminerals. The amount consumed of some vitamins and minerals in relation to that of other vitamins and minerals is known to be of importance from a nutritional viewpoint. For example, the consumption of large amounts of phosphorus can affect the absorption and utilization of calcium.

Many of the vitamins and essential minerals function as *pharmacologic agents*. Sometimes the vitamin or mineral is successful in treating or alleviating the symptoms of certain diseases or conditions in some individuals, but not in others. Many of the vitamins and essential minerals are known to be toxic when consumed in large quantities.

Several of the *Other Substances in Foods* are ergogenic aids. *Ergogenic aids* are thought, usually falsely, to enhance physical performance. There are a variety of ergogenic aids available over the counter. In most cases, these substances are not beneficial to physical performance. However, evidence does exist that a few of these substances, particularly creatine, may positively influence physical performance.

7

Vitamins

Throughout history, people have suffered not always from a lack of food, but also from a lack of certain nutrients in their diets. Ancient world populations were frequently susceptible to the dietary absences, and thus, deficiencies of the organic factors the body needed. These organic dietary factors are called vitamins in today's world. The lack of these dietary organic factors, or vitamin-deficiency diseases, were known to the ancient Greeks and Chinese; the Crusaders of the Middle Ages; the early seafaring explorers; and even to Americans living in the South and those in Central America in the twentieth century. The lack of vitamins in the diets of populations have at times no doubt altered the course of history. Many cultures developed dietary practices to prevent vitamin-deficiency diseases. Such practices have been passed from one generation to the next and are referred to today as traditional medicine, folklore, and "old wives' tales." In the twentieth century, Western populations have replaced most of these practices with fortified foods available year round and vitamin supplements.

No specific chemical knowledge of any vitamin was known before 1900, with one interesting exception. Nicotinic acid was prepared from nicotine in 1867 by C. Huber, though it remained on the chemist's shelf for many years. Dietary growth factors later known as vitamins were initially discovered and separated based on their solubility in oils (fat) or water. In 1912, C. Funk coined the term "vitamine" to describe the newly discovered growth factors because they were thought to be vital to life and quite mistakenly amines. The term "vitamine," with the omission of the "e," is used today. A *vitamin* is an organic substance needed in very small amounts for normal functioning that can not be synthesized by the body in adequate amounts.

Fat-Soluble and Water-Soluble Vitamins

The *fat-soluble vitamins* are vitamins A, D, E, and K. These vitamins possess characteristics which, in addition to their solubility, are much different from those of the water-soluble vitamins. The *water-soluble vitamins* are vitamin C, the B-complex vitamins or B-vitamins, and perhaps choline. The B-vitamins are thiamin, riboflavin, niacin, vitamin B_6, folacin, vitamin B_{12}, pantothenic acid, and biotin. The water-soluble B vitamins generally function as coenzymes in enzyme systems, are required in the diet, do not exhibit appreciable tissue storage, and are relatively nontoxic except at quite high levels. Deficiencies of water-soluble vitamins develop rapidly. The water-soluble vitamins are also more labile than those which are fat-soluble, meaning that there is generally greater loss of water-soluble vitamins during food preparation. In contrast, fat-soluble vitamins are not known to function as coenzymes. Most of the fat-soluble vitamins are absorbed with lipids in the small intestine; bile and pancreatic secretions are required for efficient absorption. Provitamin D, 7-dehydrocholesterol, is synthesized in the skin and is converted to

TABLE 7.1

The Vitamins

Fat-Soluble	Water-Soluble	
Vitamin A	Vitamin C	Folic Acid
Vitamin D	Thiamin	Vitamin B$_{12}$
Vitamin E	Riboflavin	Biotin
Vitamin K	Niacin	Pantothenic Acid
	Vitamin B$_6$	Choline[a]

[a] Conclusive data are not available as to the dietary essentiality of choline.

vitamin D in the presence of adequate sunshine. Vitamin E functions as an antioxidant; other antioxidants can replace vitamin E with regard to much of its functioning. Vitamin K can be synthesized by the intestinal flora of mammals and absorbed from the human intestinal tract. Biotin, likewise, is synthesized by the intestinal microflora and absorbed by the human intestinal tract. Fat-soluble vitamins are stored in the lipid components of adipose tissue, liver, and cell membranes. When ingested in large amounts, fat-soluble vitamins A and D can be quite toxic, as they will continuously accumulate in lipid tissues. Deficiencies of fat-soluble vitamins are slow in their development.

Some of the vitamins have known *pharmacologic functions*. Niacin may lower total serum cholesterol and triglyceride and raise HDL cholesterol levels when taken in excess of 1,200 mg daily. Pharmacologic doses of vitamin B$_6$ may be of benefit in the treatment of mental diseases. Some people have overdosed on vitamins, and toxicities were thus noted. For many of the vitamins, optimal, pharmacologic, and toxic intake levels are known to exist.

The concentration of serum homocysteine has been associated with the incidence of coronary heart disease. Folate, vitamin B$_6$, and vitamin B$_{12}$ function with relation to homocysteine metabolism. Hence, a deficiency of any of these three vitamins could possibly increase the incidence of coronary heart disease.

Some vitamins function without biochemical modification. Other vitamins, however, have to be converted by the body into their metabolically active form(s), while other vitamins serve as components of even larger coenzymes. The vitamins are presented in Table 7.1. Each of the vitamins will be discussed beginning with the fat-soluble vitamins followed by those which are water-soluble. Food sources will be given in tabular form for each of the vitamins. *Good sources* of nutrients contain 10 to 19 percent of the Daily Value of that nutrient per serving, while *rich sources* contain 20+ percent.

Vitamin A

Name: Retinoids
Active Form: Retinol, retinal, retinoic acid
Function: Antioxidant, visual cofactor, growth, immunity
Activity: 1 RE = 1 µg all-trans retinol
    6 µg all-trans β-carotene
    12 µg other provitamin A carotenoids
    3.33 IU vitamin activity from retinol
    10 IU vitamin activity from β-carotene
Precursor: Several carotenoids including β-carotene

Vitamin A, as one may guess, was the "first" fat-soluble vitamin to be recognized; it was first separated by E. V. McCollum in 1920. McCollum was later to discover that his vitamin A also contained another lipid-soluble factor, vitamin D.

Forms

Both retinoids and carotenoids have vitamin A activity. The **retinoids** are also known as previtamin A. About 50 of the 600 characterized *carotenoids*, including β-carotene, are known as provitamin A compounds or *vitamin A precursors*, as they can be converted to vitamin A, if needed, by the body. Not all carotenoids are vitamin A precursors. Retinoids are consumed in foods as retinyl esters of fatty acids, usually palmitate (retinyl palmitate), in which the ester stabilizes the molecule from peroxidation. Retinoids are digested and absorbed, as with lipids, with bile and pancreatic secretions and the presence of antioxidants increasing absorption efficiency. Retinol is the major circulating retinoid, and is carried by the retinol-binding protein (RBP) and as transthyretin. Retinal (formerly known as retinene) functions in vision. Retinoic acid, the excretory form of retinoids, can function with regard to tissue growth. Retinoids are stored, primarily in the liver, as retinyl esters along with lipids. If required, carotenoids are converted to retinol in the small intestine and liver via a dioxygenase. One molecule of β-carotene is converted *in vivo* to one molecule of retinol. β-carotene is the most potent form of provitamin A.

Functions

The best known function for vitamin A is its role as a coenzyme with the protein opsin, found in rods and cones, the *photoreceptor* cells of the eye. The visual protein pigments, rhodopsin (rods), responsible for low light vision, and iodopsin (cones), responsible for color and bright light vision, both contain retinol (as 11-cis-retinal). Rhodopsin and iodopsin are the visual pigments of the eye, which in the presence of light are "bleached." Bleaching results in the conversion of vitamin A to the all-trans retinal by light energy, release of opsin, and the interruption of optic nerve electric impulses by calcium (dark current), which are amplified and interpreted by the visual cortex as light. Niacin and riboflavin function in the vitamin A visual cycle.

Vitamin A is required for normal growth of *epithelial* (eyes, skin, respiratory tract, digestive tract, urogenital tract) and *skeletal tissues*, affecting protein synthesis, bone cell differentiation, and enamel formation. Vitamin A also functions in *mucopolysaccharide synthesis*, including that of mucus. Mucus lubricates the linings of all body openings. Vitamin A plays a role in *reproduction* and *immune functioning*.

Vitamin A is a weak *fat-soluble antioxidant*. Vitamin A status most often is evaluated by quantitating plasma levels of retinoids and nutritionally active (capable of being converted to retinoids) carotenoids. High plasma levels of retinoids are associated with a decreased incidence of chronic diseases, particularly coronary heart disease and epithelial cancers. Even stronger evidence exists between high blood levels of both nutritionally active and inactive carotenoids and decreased incidence of chronic disease. Most of these associations have been observed in epidemiological studies. It may be that the carotenoids and retinoids have protective effects in reducing oxidative effects, and thus decreasing the risk of chronic disease.

Food Sources

Table 7.2 gives selected good and rich sources of vitamin A and β-carotene. Preformed vitamin A is found only in animal foods, particularly organ meats, egg yolks, and fortified food products. Nonfat and low-fat dairy products are frequently fortified with retinoids.

TABLE 7.2

Selected Good and Rich Sources of Vitamin A
(including β-Carotene)

Apricots	Broccoli	Butternut squash
Carrots	Cantaloupe	Egg yolks
Fortified cereals	Fortified dairy products	"Greens"
Kale	Liver	Pumpkin
Spinach	Sweet potatoes	Winter squash

Carotenoids are found in dark green, leafy vegetables and yellowish-orange fruits and vegetables. Individuals living in the United States generally get about a quarter of their vitamin A from carotenoids; however, individuals in developing countries get most of their vitamin A from carotenoids. Retinoids and carotenoids are relatively stable in common food preparation procedures, but somewhat sensitive to oxidation.

Dietary Recommendations

The recommendations of the National Research Council for vitamin A intakes are given in *retinol equivalents* (RE) as µg. The 1989 RDA for men and women is 1,000 and 800 RE, respectively. The different forms of the retinoids and carotenoids have different vitamin A activities, with retinoids having higher potencies than carotenoids. Commercial vitamin A supplements are used fairly extensively by the American public. According to NHANES III data, the median vitamin A intakes of men and women, 20 to 59 years, in the United States were 739 and 581 RE, respectively. These intakes were below 1989 RDA levels, but the incidence of this population having low serum vitamin A levels was low. The *1995 Third Report on Nutrition Monitoring in the United States* classified vitamin A as being a "potential public health issue." This is because of the relative prevalence of high and low intakes of the vitamin and their effects on health.

Deficiency

Symptoms characteristic of early vitamin A deficiency include reduced appetite, weight loss, skin disorders, decreased mucus production, and follicular hyperkeratosis. *Night blindness,* a vitamin A deficiency disease, was recognized and treated by the ancient Chinese, the early Egyptians, and even Hippocrates himself. A more severe vitamin A deficiency can lead to xerophthalmia (dry eye) and if untreated, permanent blindness. Xerophthalmia among children of Southeast Asia remains an almost permanent contemporary problem. Vitamin A deficient individuals characteristically have Bitot's spots. Depressed growth and decreased immune function are observed in vitamin A deficient individuals. Vitamin A is transported in the blood by proteins; thus, vitamin A status is influenced by *protein deficiency.* Vitamin A deficiency is usually associated with PEM, low fat intakes and malabsorption, gastrointestinal distress, and respiratory disease. Although rare in the United States, vitamin A deficiency is the most prevalent nutrient deficiency worldwide, and resulting blindness and death are relatively common. Vitamin A status is usually evaluated by measuring plasma levels of the vitamin, and sometimes includes also measuring plasma β-carotene levels.

Pharmacologic Doses

Large oral doses (~60 mg one to three times yearly) of retinoids have been used prophylactically in infants and children in developing countries where vitamin A deficiency is prevalent.

Many retinoids have been used with some efficacy in treating severe acne and other skin disorders and some types of cancer. In that high doses of retinoids are generally required for maximal effectiveness, toxic effects are frequent.

Toxicity

Vitamin A toxicity symptoms are variable, but may include headache, insomnia, dry skin, loss of hair, dryness and fissuring of lips, menstrual irregularities, weight loss, bone abnormalities, spontaneous abortions, birth defects, and hepatomegaly. *Hypervitaminosis A* may also adversely affect the rods and cones in the eyes. Toxicity occurs with sustained daily intakes, from foods and supplements, exceeding about 6,000 RE daily in infants and young children and 15,000 RE daily in adults. Hypervitaminosis A is reversible in its early stages.

Carotenoids are relatively nontoxic when consumed in large quantities, partially because of their reduced absorption efficiency. However, carotenoids are absorbed well enough to produce orangish-yellow adipose tissues including subcutaneous tissues. *Hypercarotenosis* results in yellowish skin, palms of hands, and soles of feet. The yellowish color disappears when high intake is discontinued.

Needs in Exercise

Vitamin A is needed for tissue repair and an increased metabolism of the vitamin would be expected during strenuous exercise. Adult athletes reportedly are well-nourished with regard to total vitamin A. Some athletes take too much vitamin A, which can be harmful and potentially toxic. A few studies indicate that vitamin A may be mobilized from the liver during exercise if the athlete remains on a diet deficient in the vitamin; however, deficiency as assessed by plasma retinal concentrations, will not occur until the liver reserves are severely depleted and exercise may even increase these concentrations.

Strenuous exercise increases oxygen consumption. This increased oxygen consumption causes an increase in free radical production, leading to lipid peroxidation and possible tissue damage. β-carotene, as an antioxidant, may affect exercise-induced lipid peroxidation and skeletal muscle damage. Equivocal results have been reported in supplementation studies of usually several antioxidants combined, not just β-carotene, on exercise performance. Increased plasma antioxidant capacity, measured *in vitro*, has been observed in elderly women given 90 mg β-carotene daily for three weeks. β-carotene has some promise of being beneficial with relation to protection from oxidative damage. Carotenoids, from a variety of vegetables and fruits, should be consumed for antioxidant protection and not just as a source of vitamin A.

Vitamin D

Name: Calciferol
Active form: 1,25-$(OH)_2$D and 24,25-$(OH)_2$D
Function: Facilitates utilization of calcium and phosphorus, insulin secretion, cell differentiation, immunity, and skin cell development
Activity: 1 μg D_2 or D_3 = 40 IU
Precursor: 7-dehydrocholesterol

Vitamin D is known as the *antirachitic vitamin*. Vitamin D deficiency is the cause of *rickets*, a crippling disease of children. In adults, vitamin D deficiency is expressed as *osteomalacia*.

These diseases have been a scourge on humankind throughout history. Especially plagued with the disease have been those people living in the northernmost latitudes of Europe, Asia, and North America. Vitamin D is not a vitamin at all in the classic sense of dietary need and coenzyme function. Vitamin D is a *vitamin-hormone* produced in the skin of people in amounts adequate to prevent rickets and osteomalacia when exposed directly to the ultraviolet light of the sun. Long winters, indoor confinement, overcast skies, heavy clothing, and polluted cities all contribute to reduced ultraviolet light exposure and the reduced vitamin D synthesis. Such environmental circumstances are compounded by the lack of significant vitamin D in the diet. Vitamin D is a vitamin in the classic sense as a result of environmental lifestyle.

In the early part of this century, E. Mellanby produced and then cured rickets with cod-liver oil in dogs. E. V. McCollum, in 1922, found the anti-rachitic factor in cod-liver oil not to be vitamin A, and named the fat-soluble substance vitamin D. In 1919, K. Huldskinsky reported curing rachitic children with ultraviolet light. The ultraviolet light conversion of fat-soluble factors into vitamin D was demonstrated by H. Steenbock and A. Black in 1924. A U.S. patent (1,680,818) covering the irradiation of ergosterol for the synthesis of vitamin D was issued in 1928.

Forms

The precursors of vitamin D are ergosterol in plants and 7-dehydrocholesterol in the skin of animals and humans; these compounds have chemical structures nearly identical to cholesterol. In the presence of ultraviolet light, ergosterol is converted into *vitamin D_2* in plants and 7-dehydrocholesterol, into *vitamin D_3* in animals. Ultraviolet light results in the fission of the β-sterol ring. Vitamins D_2 and D_3 have equivalent vitamin D potency, and both forms are used in supplements. The absorption of dietary vitamin D is enhanced by the presence of dietary lipids and the secretion of bile. Vitamin D from the skin or intestine is carried in the blood by a vitamin D-binding protein. Vitamin D is stored in the liver, skin, muscles, and adipose tissues.

Vitamins D_2 and D_3 are *prohormones* to the active vitamin derivative which is a hormone. In a series of brilliant experiments by J. Lund and H. F. DeLuca, beginning in 1966, the metabolism of vitamin D began to unfold. Following dietary absorption of vitamin D_2 or D_3 or synthesis of vitamin D_3 in the skin, vitamins D_2 and D_3 in mammals are hydroxylated in the liver by enzymes requiring molecular oxygen, magnesium, and niacin (as $NADPH_2$), producing 25-(OH)-vitamin D, often referred to as 25(OH)D. The 25(OH)D transported by the α-globulin from the liver to the kidney undergoes a second renal hydroxylation by a mixed-function oxygenase to yield $1,25(OH)_2$ D, calcitriol, and $24,25(OH)_2D$. $1,25(OH)_2D$ is the most active form of vitamin D, but $24,25(OH)_2D$ does have some vitamin D activity.

Functions

Vitamin D as $1,25(OH)_2D$ along with the *parathyroid hormone* (PTH) functions in the regulation of mineral homeostasis, particularly that of *calcium* and *phosphorus*, by its influence on the intestines, kidneys, bones, and parathyroid glands. $24,25(OH)_2D$ is known to increase absorption of calcium, phosphorus, and perhaps other bone minerals. Serum levels of calcium and phosphorus effectively regulate $1,25(OH)_2D$ and $24,25(OH)_2D$ synthesis. $1,25(OH)_2D$ is also essential for normal insulin secretion, cell differentiation, immunity, skin cell development, and perhaps muscle contraction and relaxation. Vitamin D status may be evaluated by quantitating the various forms of the vitamin in plasma, or indirectly and more frequently evaluated by measuring serum calcium concentrations in that vitamin D is needed to maintain normal serum calcium levels. Status may also be evaluated by quantitating plasma alkaline phosphatase activity.

TABLE 7.3

Selected Good and Rich Sources of Vitamin D

Cod	Egg yolks	Cod-liver oil
Fortified cereals	Fortified dairy products	Fortified margarines
Herring	Liver	Mackerel
Salmon	Sardines	Shrimp

Note: Sunlight promotes the synthesis of vitamin D in the skin. However, overexposure to sunlight should be avoided.

Food Sources

Table 7.3 gives selected good and rich sources of vitamin D. The amount of vitamin D present in unfortified foods is small and variable, with the exception of fatty fish and fish liver oils. Most dairy products and margarines are *fortified with vitamin D* as are many of the cereals and chocolate mixes. Vitamin D is quite stable to various food preparation procedures.

Dietary Recommendations

Individuals whose skins are exposed to sufficient sunlight are able to synthesize sufficient vitamin D to meet their needs. In that many individuals in the United States are not exposed to much light, especially during certain seasons of the year, dietary need for vitamin D exists. The 1997 Adequate Intake for vitamin D given by the National Research Council is 5 µg (200 IU) daily for individuals below the age of 51, 10 µg daily for those 51 to 70 years, and 15 µg for those over 70 years. The 1997 Tolerable Upper Intake Level for vitamin D is 50 µg daily for individuals over one year of age.

Deficiency

Rickets is the vitamin D deficiency disease in children and *osteomalacia* is the deficiency disease in adults. Without vitamin D, calcium, phosphorus, and perhaps other bone minerals are not deposited in the collagen matrix of bones. Rachitic bones are unable to support the body and withstand weight. Bowlegs, knock-knees, enlarged joints, curvature of the spine, pigeon breast, and frontal bossing of the skull result. There is also inadequate mineralization of tooth dentin and enamel. Deformities of the chest, pelvis, spine, and limbs and even bone fractures are seen in osteomalacia, where there is an inability of reabsorbed bone to recalcify. Vitamin D deficiency is rare in the United States today, primarily due to the fortification of foods with the vitamin. However, rickets and osteomalacia are still observed world-wide.

Pharmacologic Doses

In that toxicities of vitamin D have been observed at relative low doses (~40 µg daily), vitamins D_2 and D_3 are not utilized therapeutically. Individuals with bone diseases due to bone, kidney, or parathyroid malfunctioning have been successfully treated with 25(OH)D and 1,25(OH)$_2$D. These individuals are unable to synthesize 25(OH)D or 1,25(OH)$_2$D.

Toxicity

Vitamin D toxicity is a serious consequence of excessive vitamin intake. Early symptoms include nausea, vomiting, excessive thirst and urination, muscular weakness, and joint pain. Consequences of severe *hypervitaminosis D* included hypercalcemia and hypercalciuria, with death possible from irreversible calcification of the heart, lungs, major arteries, and kidneys. It is not possible to get hypervitaminosis D by overexposure to sunlight.

Needs in Exercise

A few studies have been conducted with regard to vitamin D and exercise performance. There is little evidence that vitamin D is extensively involved in physical performance. The ingestion of large doses of vitamin D can result in toxicity.

Vitamin E

Name: Tocopherols and Tocotrienols
Active form: α-, β-, γ-, and δ-tocopherols and tocotrienols
Function: Antioxidant
Activity: 1 RE = 1 mg d-α-tocopherol
           2 mg β-tocopherol
           10 mg γ-tocopherol
           3.34 mg α-tocotrienol
           1.49 IU

Vitamin E was recognized and named by H. Evans in 1925 as the fertility factor that prevented reproductive failure in female rats fed a rancid diet and whole wheat. Present in the oil of the wheat germ was vitamin E. Isolated as a pale yellow oil and identified structurally in 1938 by Fernholz, vitamin E was found to be a derivative of tocol and was named α-tocopherol, meaning childbirth (tokos, Greek) and to carry or bear (pherin), in that it was required for pregnant rats to bear young. It is also required for reproduction in male rats.

Forms

Eight compounds have been isolated that have vitamin E activity; these are α-, β-, γ- and δ-tocopherols and tocotrienols. The most active form of vitamin E is d-α-tocopherol. In plants and seeds (oils), α-tocopherol may constitute only 10 to 15 percent of the total tocopherols, but in animals and fish, α-tocopherol normally accounts for >90 percent of all tocopherols. The various forms of the vitamin have different amounts of vitamin E activity. Commercial tocopherols are stabilized and supplied as either the acetate or succinate esters. Absorption of dietary tocopherols is about 20 to 40 percent, and is facilitated by lipids, bile, and pancreatic secretions. Absorbed into the lymph and subsequently, the blood, vitamin E circulates with all the lipoproteins and membranes of erythrocytes. In general, vitamin E penetrates and is found associated with the lipid fraction of cells and membranes. Its concentration is particularly high in association with adipose tissue, adrenals, liver, and muscles.

Functions

The only function attributed to vitamin E is its role as an ***antioxidant***. Vitamin E protects unsaturated lipid components of cells from free-radical attack by itself becoming oxidized. Vitamin E is found in cellular membranes and subcellular membranes associated with polyunsaturated fatty acids. Vitamin E is the body's major defense against potentially harmful oxidations. Vitamin C, β-carotene, and selenium frequently function with vitamin E as antioxidants. Vitamin E also protects the skeletal muscles, nervous system, and ocular retina from oxidation via its functioning as an antioxidant. Vitamin E, a potent fat-soluble antioxidant, protects lipoprotein membranes in the various kinds of tissues from oxidation.

TABLE 7.4

Selected Good and Rich Sources of Vitamin E

Almonds	Canola oil	Safflower oil
Peanuts	Sunflower seeds	Wheat germ
Shrimp	Corn oil	

Male and female rats need vitamin E for reproduction. There is no good evidence to relate malfunction of the reproductive process in humans with an increased need for vitamin E.

Vitamin E is essential for normal *immune function*. High plasma levels of vitamin E, particularly α-tocopherol, have been associated with decreased incidence of coronary heart disease and certain cancers. Most of these associations were observed in epidemiological studies, though some were from clinical studies. Vitamin E protects LDL from oxidation.

Vitamin E may reduce the toxicity of metals, particular iron and lead, likely owing to its antioxidant properties. Vitamin E may also protect against environmental pollutants such as ozone, and the effects of tobacco usage. Vitamin E is also protective against the hepato-toxicity of alcohol and certain drugs.

Vitamin E affects arachidonic and prostaglandin metabolism. Several, but not all, studies indicate that vitamin E inhibits platelet aggregation. The suggestion has been made that vitamin E may serve as a repressor for the synthesis of some enzymes. The suggestion has also been made that vitamin E may serve as an electron acceptor in the electron transport chain. It may be that vitamin E is performing these functions as an antioxidant or perhaps the vitamin has other functions.

Food Sources

The richest food sources of vitamin E are vegetable oils and products made from them. Nuts, wheat germ, and seeds also are rich sources of vitamin E (Table 7.4). Frequently as much as half of the vitamin E in a food is lost during food processing and cooking. Vitamin E is particularly susceptible to destruction by oxygen, light, and repeated use of oils in deep-frying.

Dietary Recommendations

The requirement for vitamin E is dependent on the quantity of polyunsaturated fatty acids consumed, with the ratio of 0.4 mg d-α-tocopherol to each gram of polyunsaturated lipids being recommended as adequate. The 1989 RDA for vitamin E for men and women is 10 and 8 mg α-TE (α-tocopherol equivalents), respectively. The various tocopherols and tocotrienols have different vitamin E potencies. Median intakes for adult men and women, 20 to 59 years, reported in NHANES III were 8.63 and 6.26 mg α-TE, respectively. Median intakes of vitamin E were below 1989 RDA values for all population subgroups of people one year of age and older. Serum levels of vitamin E were measured in this survey, but accepted criteria for their interpretation have not been agreed upon. Many individuals, particularly older adults, in the United States take supplements containing vitamin E. The *1995 Third Report on Nutrition Monitoring in the United States* classified antioxidant vitamins, including vitamin E, as a "potential public health issue." Studies, both epidemiological and clinical, suggest that antioxidants in food can lower the risk of heart disease, some forms of cancer, cataracts, and mascular degeneration , and many people consume less than recommended levels of vitamin E.

Deficiency

Rats made dietarily deficient of both vitamin E and the trace element selenium are subject to liver necrosis and death from peroxidation. In other animal species, conditions attributed to vitamin E deficiency included muscular myopathies, accumulation of tissue lipofusin pigments, anemia, *in vitro* hemolysis, cataracts, and retinal degeneration. Vitamin E deficiency in humans occurs in PEM and in individuals with lipid malabsorption problems. Vitamin E status is clinically evaluated indirectly by measuring erythrocyte hemolysis. Research laboratories frequently quantitate plasma levels of the individual forms of the vitamin. Newborn infants have low reserves of vitamin E as the vitamin does not cross the placenta. Symptoms of vitamin E deficiency observed in these infants include a hemolytic anemia, thrombocytosis, retinopathy, and occasional edema. Vitamin E deficiency occurs in about half the children with chronic cholestasis and may also be found in children with neuromuscular disorders. Vitamin E deficiency symptoms reported in adults include abnormalities of the nervous system eventually affecting the muscles and the retina. Recently, low-normal vitamin E status has been associated with increased risks of atherosclerosis, cancer, cataract formation, and other aging processes in general.

Pharmacologic Doses

Several diseases have been reported to be responsive to the administration of large doses of vitamin E. Much of the evidence is anecdotal or from poorly controlled as well as short-term studies. Large amounts of vitamin E (200 to 800 IU/day) appears to be beneficial with regard to intermittent claudication and various infectious and chronic diseases in humans. The evidence from epidemiological studies and a limited number of clinical studies, primarily with older people, is considered to be strong that these large doses of vitamin E may be beneficial in decreasing the risk of coronary heart disease, certain cancer, and cataracts as well as perhaps being useful in reducing exercise-induced oxidative stress.

Toxicity

Vitamin E taken orally is relatively nontoxic. Large intakes of vitamin E may exacerbate the coagulation defect of vitamin K deficiency, adversely affect individuals taking anticoagulant therapy, decrease the absorption of vitamin A, and increase the quantity of iron needed for a hematologic response in anemic individuals.

Needs in Exercise

Vitamin E is needed for normal muscle function. Exercise is known to alter skeletal muscle blood flow. Exercise influences oxidative metabolism and vitamin E may lower the oxidative stress associated with exercise (often referred to as *exercise-induced oxidative stress*). Training does increase the capacity of endogenous antioxidants to neutralize reactive oxygen species; however, more antioxidants, particularly vitamin E, may be needed to maintain the oxidant:antioxidant balance. Vitamin E may function along with vitamin C and the carotenoids in this regard. Several studies indicate that animals supplemented with vitamin E have a reduction in oxidative stress from physical activity. This effect has also been shown in a few controlled human studies. Most studies have shown no improvement in exercise performance of humans with vitamin E supplementation. However, individuals, including athletes, who habitually consume low levels of antioxidants may be at high risk for the harmful effects of oxygen radicals. Well-designed, long-term research is needed with regard to the beneficial effects of vitamin E supplementation in lowering oxidative stress as well as perhaps influencing the recovery time from muscle fatigue and stress after heavy training and maybe enhancing performance in extreme environmental conditions.

Vitamin K

Name: Phylloquinone, Menaquinone, Menadione
Active form: Unknown
Function: Cofactor in synthesis of several blood coagulation factors
Note: Form of vitamin synthesized by intestinal microflora

Vitamin K was the first of a series of fat-soluble compounds derived from 2-methyl-1,4-naphthoquinone to be isolated and identified by E. A. Doisy in 1939. The vitamin had earlier been observed as an unidentifiable lipid-soluble factor that produced hemorrhaging in chicks fed a fat-free diet. This lipid-soluble factor present in plants was recognized in 1935 by H. Dam and named vitamin K after the Dutch word koagulation. In 1939, Dam isolated vitamin K from alfalfa.

Forms

Phylloquinone (vitamin K_1) is the form of the vitamin found in green plants. *Menaquinone* (vitamin K_2) is the form of the vitamin synthesized by bacteria in the intestinal microflora. This bacterially synthesized form of vitamin K is absorbed by humans and other monogastric animals excluding chicks. Humans get about half of their vitamin K, ranging from 5 to 95 percent (large individual differences), via synthesis by the intestinal microflora. Foods from animal sources contain both phylloquinone and menaquinones. Dietary vitamin K is absorbed more efficiently in the presence of lipids, bile, and pancreatic secretions.

Menadione (vitamin K_3) is a synthetic form of the vitamin. Menadione is utilized clinically as a coagulant. Menadione is the most potent form of vitamin K, having about twice the vitamin activity of vitamin K_1. Vitamin K_2 has about 75 percent of the vitamin activity of vitamin K_1. Phylloquinone is the form of the vitamin generally utilized in supplements.

Coumarins and their derivatives (such as dicumarol), which are used clinically as anticoagulants, are vitamin K antagonists. The same is true of certain indandiones and their derivatives. Any drugs that function in decreasing the intestinal microflora, also decrease its ability to synthesize vitamin K_2.

Functions

The process of **blood coagulation** (clotting) involves a highly complex and not fully understood process involving cells: thrombocytes, platelets, and erythrocytes, numerous protein factors, and Ca^{2+} ion. The net result of this complex process is the conversion of a highly soluble protein, fibrinogen, into a highly insoluble protein matrix, insoluble fibrin. Vitamin K is known to be needed for the synthesis of four coagulation factors and two protein factors which also function in coagulation. In 1974, prothrombin was found to contain many residues of carboxylated γ-glutamate. In the following two years, it was demonstrated using *in vitro* systems that vitamin K was a necessary cofactor in a γ-carboxylase enzyme system which functions in converting precursor proteins to coagulation factors. Vitamin K functions in the synthesis of prothrombin (factor II), proconvertin (factor VII), the Christmas factor (factor IX), and the Stuart-Prower factor (factor X) as well as that of proteins C and S.

TABLE 7.5

Selected Foods Containing Vitamin K

Broccoli	Cabbage	Cauliflower
Kale	Liver	Spinach

Note: Vitamin K is synthesized by the intestinal microflora and absorbed, but this contribution is variable.

Vitamin K also is required for the synthesis of some of the proteins in bone, kidney, liver, and plasma. Vitamin K metabolism in these tissues may not be as sensitive to the coumarins, which are vitamin K antagonists.

Food Sources

Green leafy vegetables and liver are rich sources of vitamin K (Table 7.5). Limited data indicate that vitamin K is stable to food processing and cooking procedures.

Dietary Recommendations

Humans get much of their vitamin K (~50 percent on the average) from *bacterial synthesis* in the intestines which is absorbed primarily in the ileum. The 1989 RDA for men and women, 25+ years of age, for vitamin K is 80 and 65 µg, respectively.

Deficiency

Hemorrhaging is observed in vitamin K deficiency as there is decreased synthesis of prothrombin and other vitamin K-dependent coagulation factors. Vitamin K deficiency is relatively rare in individuals over the age of about one year and when observed is associated with lipid malabsorption or decreased intestinal microflora generally caused by prolonged use of antibiotics. Due to poor placental transfer of vitamin K and a lack of vitamin K_2-producing intestinal microflora, newborns, particularly those who are pre-term, frequently have inadequate vitamin K status and are hemorrhagic. Vitamin K deficiency is also frequently seen in infants. Vitamin K status is most often evaluated by determining plasma or blood prothrombin concentration.

Pharmacologic Doses

Menadione or phylloquinone is frequently administered clinically to individuals having problems getting the blood to clot. All commercial infant formulas contain added phylloquinone. Phylloquinone is given to individuals who have accidently ingested large quantities of anticoagulants. Phylloquinone or menadione is also given to individuals who have had long-term treatment with broad-spectrum antibiotics or long-term hyperalimentation as well as those with lipid malabsorption and chronic biliary obstruction.

Toxicity

Excessive vitamin K, as menadione not phylloquinone, given to infants results in increased incidence of hemolytic anemia, hyperbilirubinemia, kernicterus, and liver damage, especially in premature infants who have erythroblastosis. A problem with vitamin K overdosing in adults is reduced effectiveness of anticoagulants.

Needs in Exercise

Studies have not been conducted with regard to vitamin K and exercise. It may be that the functioning of the vitamin K-dependent protein osteocalcin is of importance with regard to bone formation, and hence, perhaps to exercise performance. Otherwise, no clear association appears to exist between vitamin K and exercise.

Vitamin C

Name: Ascorbic acid and Hydroascorbic acid
Active form: Reduced ascorbic acid
Function: Aqueous antioxidant, hydroxylations

A deficiency of vitamin C causes *scurvy*. Scurvy was first described by Hippocrates, a Greek physician of the fifth century. Scurvy ravaged the thirteenth-century French (crusaders) in Palestine, and it became perilous for sailors of the sixteenth and seventeenth centuries to be at sea for more than four or five months. A voyage of six months or more meant almost certain death.

Admiral Richard Hawkins of the British Royal Navy wrote in 1662 "that sour oranges and lemons" were effective against the disease, but scurvy continued to be the primary cause of death of sailors at sea. Not until Royal Navy Surgeon James Lind did his human experiments with scorbutic sailors using oranges, lemons, cider, and seawater aboard the Salisbury at sea (May 20, 1747) was the value of citrus fruits appreciated. Published in 1753, Lind's *Treatise on the Scurvy* and other publications led the British admiralty in 1795 to order rations of lemons to sailors at sea. Lemons, often referred to as limes by the British, resulted in future sailors of the Royal Navy being called limeys. This *anti-scorbutic factor* was isolated in 1932 by C. G. King and W. A. Waugh and independently by J. L. Surbely and A. Szent-György, who received the Nobel Prize for this discovery in 1937.

Forms

Vitamin C, *ascorbic acid*, is similar in structure, but functionally different from D-glucose or D-galactose. Vitamin C is dietarily required by humans, other primates, and several other animals such as the guinea pig. The guinea pig is most often employed in vitamin C research as an animal model. Most animals possess the enzyme L-gulono-γ-lactone oxidase, which is needed for the synthesis of vitamin C from glucose or galactose.

Ascorbic acid is a strong reducing agent and upon oxidation, *dehydroascorbic acid* is formed. Dehydroascorbic acid is the most active form of the vitamin. Further oxidation produces diketoglutamic acid, which has no vitamin C activity. The water-soluble vitamin C is absorbed in the small intestine and goes via the circulatory system to the body tissues. Vitamin C is found in the liver, adrenals, kidneys, and spleen, where it apparently is in equilibrium with serum levels. Large amounts are excreted in the urine as ascorbic acid, oxalic acid, and other metabolites.

Functions

One of the major functions of ascorbic acid is that of an *antioxidant*, protecting cells and cellular components from free-radical attack. As a strong reducing agent, vitamin C may facilitate the absorption of the ferric form of *iron* (Fe^{3+}) by its reduction to ferrous iron (Fe^{2+}), and of the cupric form of *copper* (Cu^{2+}) by its reduction to cuprous copper (Cu^+). Vitamin C functions in the cytochrome series in conjunction with iron. Vitamin C also plays a role in transferring iron from its blood carrier transferrin to the storage form *ferritin*. In hydroxylation reactions in which either iron or copper must remain in a reduced state for the function of an enzyme, vitamin C is needed. Vitamin C may also function in oxidation-reduction systems along with other antioxidants.

TABLE 7.6

Selected Good and Rich Sources of Vitamin C

Asparagus	Broccoli	Blackberries
Brussels sprouts	Cantaloupe	Cabbage
Cauliflower	Cranapple juice	Fortified cereals
Grapefruit	Grapefruit juice	Green pepper
Kale	Horseradish	Lemons
Limes	Liver	Oranges
Orange juice	Parsley	Red currants
Red pepper	Spinach	Strawberries
Tomatoes	Tomato juice	Tomato soup
Turnips	Watercress	White potatoes

As a coenzyme, vitamin C functions in the hydroxylation of the amino acids proline and lysine in the formation of *collagen*, of cholesterol to *bile acids*, of tyrosine in the formation of norepinephrine, of tryptophan in the formation of 5-*hydroxy tryptophan*, of histidine in the formation of *histamine*, and in the *detoxification* of certain poisonous compounds. Vitamin C is also involved in the conversion of the *folic acid* found in foods to its active form, in *corticosteroid* synthesis, in *carnitine* synthesis, in enzymatic amidation of *neuropeptides*, in the *immune response*, and possibly in wound healing and allergic reactions. In some manner, the vitamin functions in bone and tooth formation. Recent evidence indicates that vitamin C may regulate protein translation. Vitamin C may reduce the formation of nitrosamines which are weak carcinogens formed from nitrates. Epidemiological studies and some clinical studies indicate that the incidence of coronary heart disease, some cancers, and cataracts may be lower in individuals having high plasma vitamin C levels, though some studies contradict these findings. Vitamin C status is most often evaluated by measuring plasma vitamin C concentrations.

Food Sources

The richest food sources of vitamin C are citrus fruits and juices as well as vegetables and organ meats (Table 7.6). Vitamin C is the most labile nutrient. Considerable quantities of the vitamin are destroyed during common food preparation procedures. If possible, vitamin C-rich foods should be eaten raw. Vegetables retain more vitamin C if microwaved or steamed as opposed to boiled.

Dietary Recommendations

The 1989 RDA for adults is 60 mg daily, and cigarette smokers should ingest at least 100 mg of vitamin C daily. Numerous respected nutritionists indicate that a daily intake, of about 200 mg daily seems to provide for maximal body retention of the nutrient and perhaps optimal immune function. The median vitamin C intakes of men and women, 20 to 59 years, in NHANES III were 85 and 67 mg, respectively. Many individuals in our country report taking vitamin C as a supplement. The *1995 Third Report on Nutrition Monitoring in the United States* classified antioxidant vitamins, including vitamin C, as "potential public health issues." Studies, both epidemiological and clinical, suggest that antioxidants in food can lower the risk of heart disease, some forms of cancer, cataracts, and macular degeneration. The amount of vitamin C needed for maximal antioxidant activity is unknown.

Deficiency

The deficiency disease is *scurvy*. Symptoms include fatigue, perifollicular hyperkeratosis, swollen or bleeding gums, joint pain, ocular hemorrhaging, lethargy, followed by death.

Today in our country, the deficiency appears primarily in alcoholics and elderly men living alone. Scurvy is still found worldwide and is associated with poverty.

Pharmacologic Doses

Higher-than-adequate intakes of vitamin C have been suggested to accelerate healing, increase immunoresistance, prevent or reduce the severity of the common cold, and reduce the risks of cardiovascular disease and cancer. The true effective value of higher-than-recommended dietary intake of vitamin C remains to be elucidated more fully.

Toxicity

Many people take gram levels of ascorbic acid without apparent toxicity. However, reports exist indicating adverse effects when consuming over about 4 g daily on a habitual basis. Reported adverse effects include nausea, diarrhea, development of kidney stones, mobilization of bone minerals, iron overabsorption, increase in serum cholesterol concentrations in atherosclerotic patients, systematic conditioning to high intakes, and abortion. These effects have not been found in all studies. The risk of sustained ingestion of these quantities of the vitamin is unknown.

Needs in Exercise

More research has been done on ascorbic acid as it relates to physical and exercise performance than on any other single nutrient. Vitamin C deficiency is known to affect physical performance. Impaired collagen formation leading to increased ligament and tendon problems is seen in the deficiency state as is decreased synthesis of carnitine, which impairs the use of fatty acids for energy formation. In the deficiency, there is also decreased synthesis of the hormones epinephrine and norepinephrine, which affects metabolic responses to exercise, and impaired folate metabolism, which results in fatigue and anemia. Various physiological stresses (e.g., infections and tobacco usage) affect the body's need for vitamin C. Studies indicate that athletes have daily vitamin C intakes of about 100 to 500 mg, which appears to be an acceptable range of intake. Several studies indicate that vitamin C has an ergogenic effect, while just as many studies report no effect. Vitamin C supplements are frequently consumed by athletes along with vitamin E and perhaps even β-carotene supplements in an effort to alleviate effects of exercise-induced oxidation; research is needed as to the effectiveness of this treatment.

Thiamin

Name: Thiamine, vitamin B_1
Active form: Thiamin pyrophosphate
Function: Oxidative decarboxylations, transketolations

Dietary deficiency of thiamin may lead to a neurological condition known as *beriberi*. The disease sometimes involves atrophy of cardiac muscles and paralysis of involuntary muscles. The Dutch physician C. Eijkman is credited with the 1897 discovery that rice polishings prevented nutritional polyneuritis in chickens fed polished rice and that the disease in chickens was similar to beriberi in humans. The antineuritic factor in rice bran and yeasts was indirectly investigated until its isolation and identification as thiamin by B. C. P. Jansen and W. F. Donath in 1926. Its organic synthesis was completed in 1936 by R. R. Williams and J. K. Cline.

TABLE 7.7

Selected Good and Rich Sources of Thiamin

Almonds	Dried beans	Dried peas
Enriched breads	Enriched cereals	Green peas
Liver	Peanuts	Pork cuts
Soybeans	Sunflower seeds	Watermelon
Wheat germ	Whole grain breads	Whole grain cereals

Forms

Thiamin is comprised of pyrimidine and thiazole rings connected by a methylene ($-CH_2-$) bridge (Figure 5.7). The active form of thiamin as a coenzyme is *thiamin pyrophosphate* (TPP), which is formed by phosphorylation of thiamin with ATP *in vivo*; Mg^{2+} is required for this phosphorylation, which usually takes place in the intestinal mucosa during thiamin absorption. Thiamin is transported in erythrocytes and plasma and is stored primarily in the liver, heart, kidneys, skeletal muscles, and brain. The vitamin is excreted in the urine. Thiamin was formerly known as vitamin B_1.

Functions

The best known coenzyme functions for TPP are the *oxidative decarboxylation* of α-keto acids and the transfer of ketones ($-C \neq O$) from α-keto acids in *transketolase* reactions. The oxidative decarboxylase and transketolase reactions usually require a divalent cation, either magnesium or manganese. The oxidative decarboxylation of pyruvic acid and α-ketoglutaric acid, which are part of the TCA (tricarboxylic acid or Krebs) cycle, are examples of α-keto acid oxidative decarboxylations. These reactions are part of the aerobic metabolism of oxidizable substrate for the generation of energy. Valine, leucine, isoleucine, methionine, and threonine can also undergo oxidative decarboxylations. The transketolase reaction involves the hexose monophosphate shunt or pathway (also referred to as pentose phosphate shunt or pathway and as direct oxidative shunt), which uses TPP to transfer a ketol to an aldose (aldehyde carbohydrate), thereby adding two new carbons to the carbohydrate. In this manner, three-, four-, five-, six-, and seven-carbon sugars are interconvertible. The hexose monophosphate shunt is an alternate pathway for the oxidation of glucose, and is a major source of pentoses for synthesis of nucleic acids and NADPH (contains niacin) for the synthesis of fatty acids. TPP is also concentrated in the nervous tissues, affecting the chloride permeability and functioning in these cells.

Food Sources

Rich sources of thiamin include bakers and brewers yeasts, pork, wheat germ, organ meats, cereal germs, whole grains, nuts, and dried legumes (Table 7.7). Thiamin is the second most labile nutrient and is frequently used as an "index nutrient" in research studies on nutrient retention. Much of the thiamin present in foods is destroyed during the cooking process. Much of the thiamin is lost in the production of polished rice and white flour; rice, flour, and many baked products are frequently *enriched* with thiamin.

Dietary Recommendations

The 1998 RDA for thiamin for men and women, 19 years and above is 1.2 and 1.1 mg/day, respectively. The median thiamin intake of adults 20 to 59 years in the United States according to NHANES III is 1.77 mg for men and 1.23 mg for women. Thiamin deficiency in developed countries is mainly confined to the alcoholic population. Many individuals in the United States report taking multivitamin preparations containing thiamin hydrochloride. The deficiency is still seen in developing countries in populations consuming unen-riched polished rice as their dietary staple.

Deficiency

The deficiency condition is known as *beriberi*. Symptoms observed in beriberi include anorexia, degenerative changes first in the lower extremities followed by multiple periph-eral neuritis, mental confusion, muscular weakness (dry beriberi), edema (wet beriberi), ataxia, tachycardia, enlarged heart, and death. Dry beriberi is associated with both energy deprivation and physical inactivity, whereas wet beriberi is associated with a high carbo-hydrate intake and strenuous physical activity. Thiaminase, an enzyme found in raw fish, is a thiamin antagonist, but is only a problem if about 10 percent and more of the diet is raw fish. Thiamin status is most often evaluated by determining the erythrocyte transketolase activity coefficient.

Pharmacologic Doses

Thiamin is sometimes used in the treatment of alcoholism. Because some individuals are hypersensitive to the vitamin, parenteral administration of the vitamin is used only in spe-cific cases.

Toxicity

No toxic effects other than gastric upset have been reported with high doses (up to 1 g) of thiamin other than in some individuals who are *hypersensitive* to the vitamin. Parenteral administration of thiamin has led to conditions resembling anaphylactic shock in these individuals.

Needs in Exercise

Thiamin is needed for optimal neuromuscular functioning. Vigorous exercise has been reported to lower blood thiamin levels, yet controlled studies indicate that comparatively low intakes of thiamin may be adequate for humans doing some aerobic exercises. Vigor-ous exercise practiced long term may increase the requirement for thiamin. Initial thiamin status was not determined in most studies prior to supplementation trials. Thiamin is needed for the metabolism of carbohydrates and branched-chain amino acids. Currently more emphasis is being placed on the consumption of higher percentages of calories from complex carbohydrates and lower percentages from fats. The greatest demand for thiamin occurs during the course of vigorous physical activity when carbohydrates are the major source of energy expenditure. More research is needed on the thiamin needs of groups con-suming high caloric amounts of carbohydrates and lower caloric amounts of fats. To date, the research findings on thiamin and exercise are equivocal. Available data indicate that thiamin intakes of 1.5 to 3.0 mg/day meet the requirements for this vitamin in healthy adults participating in moderate aerobic physical activity.

Riboflavin

Name: Riboflavine, vitamin B$_2$
Active form: Flavin mononucleotide (FMN), flavin adenine dinucleotide (FAD)
Function: Hydrogen carrier (oxidases, dehydrogenases)

Riboflavin was recognized early as a separate entity often found in the presence of thiamin. As a separate growth factor for animals, it was named vitamin B_2, following the convention established for naming the vitamins by the British, and as vitamin G in the United States. Riboflavin was first isolated in 1934 from egg whites by P. György, and was synthesized by R. K. Khun and P. Karrer in 1935.

Riboflavin is a bright orange-yellow compound. It gives the slight yellow color to egg "whites," where it is found as ovoflavin. One of only two highly colored vitamins, it is strongly fluorescent in solution, and its ability to absorb ultraviolet light causes it to be chemically unstable. Former names of riboflavin include vitamin B_2, vitamin G, lactoflavin, and ovoflavin.

Forms

Riboflavin consists of a conjugated isoalloxazine ring (flavin) and a five-carbon carbohydrate, ribitol. Riboflavin forms part of and is the functional moiety of two larger coenzymes, *flavin mononucleotide* (FMN) and *flavin adenine dinucleotide* (FAD); these two coenzymes are called *flavoproteins*. Riboflavin is absorbed in the small intestine, phosphorylated in the intestinal mucosa to FMN, and sometimes converted in the liver to FAD. Both of these phosphorylation reactions require magnesium. FMN and FAD are easily interconvertible. The vitamin is found primarily in the liver, kidney, and heart, and generally is excreted as riboflavin.

Functions

Riboflavin as FMN or FAD functions in *oxidation-reduction* reactions (particularly as a hydrogen carrier) as a component of oxidases and dehydrogenases. FMN and FAD designate the oxidized forms of the respective riboflavin coenzymes, while $FMNH_2$ and $FADH_2$ designate the reduced forms of the coenzymes. The flavoproteins function in conjunction with amino acid oxidases (catabolism of amino acids), xanthine oxidase (also contains iron and molybdenum), cytochrome reductase (part of electron transport chain), succinic dehydrogenase (part of TCA cycle), acyl-coenzyme A dehydrogenase (needed for catabolism of fatty acids), in fatty acid synthesis, α-glycerophosphate dehydrogenase (part of glycolysis), lactic acid dehydrogenase (needed for conversion of lactic acid), kynurenine 3-hydroxylase (needed for conversion of tryptophan to niacin), and aldehyde oxidases such as those which function in the interconversion of two forms of vitamin B_6. Free riboflavin exists in the retina, but how it functions there is unknown.

Food Sources

Selected good and rich sources of riboflavin are given in Table 7.8. Rich food sources of riboflavin include bakers and brewers yeasts, meats, dairy products, and enriched cereals and breads. Asparagus, broccoli, collard and turnip greens, and spinach are good to rich sources of the vitamin. The vitamin is relatively stable to various food processing and cooking methods, but loss does occur if the food is exposed to light.

Dietary Recommendations

The 1998 RDA for men and women, 19 to 70 years, is 1.3 and 1.1 mg daily, respectively. The median daily intakes of the vitamin for men and women, 20 to 59 years, living in the United States according to NHANES III is 2.11 and 1.49 mg, respectively. Many individuals ingest

TABLE 7.8

Selected Good and Rich Sources of Riboflavin

Asparagus	Banana	Beef cuts
Broccoli	Chicken cuts	Dairy products
Enriched breads	Enriched cereals	"Greens"
Liver	Mushrooms	Peanut butter
Pork cuts	Prunes	Sardines
Spinach	Tuna	White potatoes

riboflavin as part of a multivitamin preparation. The accepted method for evaluating riboflavin status is a determination of erythrocyte glutathione reductase activity coefficient.

Deficiency

Riboflavin deficiency symptoms include seborrheic dermatitis, lacrimation, burning and
itching of the eyes, cheilosis, angular stomatitis, purple swollen tongue (geographic
tongue), normocytic anemia, photophobia, and presenile cataracts. In that riboflavin is
needed for the functioning of vitamin B_6 and niacin, some of the symptoms of the deficiency are actually due to functional insufficiencies of the other two B-vitamins. Clinical
signs of riboflavin deficiency is rarely seen in developed countries, except in chronic alcoholics. Riboflavin deficiency is seen in conjunction with PEM.

Pharmacologic Doses

There are no known pharmacologic effects of riboflavin.

Toxicity

Riboflavin toxicity has not been reported in humans. Riboflavin will precipitate in the kidneys and hearts of rats given high doses of the vitamin.

Needs in Exercise

Riboflavin functions in respiratory metabolism. Exercise in individuals who were previously sedentary or nonathletic seems to alter some of the indices of riboflavin status. It
appears that athletes and physically active individuals have adequate riboflavin status,
perhaps because of long-term training adaptation, or the fact that they may have been consuming more riboflavin. There is no advantage of riboflavin supplementation of athletes
unless these individuals are deficient in this vitamin.

Niacin

Name: Nicotinic acid and nicotinamide
Active form: Nicotinamide adenine dinucleotide (NAD),
            Nicotinamide adenine dinucleotide phosphate (NADP)
Function: Hydrogen carrier (dehydrogenases, reductases)

Niacin is the generic term for ***nicotinic acid*** and ***nicotinamide***. The discovery of nicotinamide as a vitamin was tied to the search for the cause of human ***pellagra*** (meaning
"rough skin") in the southern United States by J. Goldberger just prior to World War I.
Believing that pellagra was an infectious disease, Goldberger and associates failed at
attempts to transfer pellagra to healthy individuals. In dogs, a disease comparable to

human pellagra, black tongue, developed when animals were fed human diets that knowingly caused the disease. Meanwhile, C. A. Elvehjem and associates were feeding nicotinic acid and nicotinamide to dogs with black tongue. Nicotinic acid, then packaged in bottles with a skull and crossbones, and nicotinamide isolated from liver both cured black tongue in dogs and were later found to prevent human pellagra.

Forms

Nicotinic acid is known to be converted to nicotinamide (also known as niacinamide) by the liver in a series of reactions involving ATP, ADP, and glutamine, which provides the amine in the conversion of nicotinic acid to nicotinamide. *Tryptophan*, an essential amino acid, in a series of biochemical transformations, is also capable of being transformed by liver into nicotinamide, as first demonstrated in rats; however, vitamin B_6, copper, riboflavin, iron, magnesium, and niacin itself are required for this conversion.

Niacin, or more specifically, nicotinamide-like riboflavin forms a portion of two larger redox coenzymes *nicotinamide adenine dinucleotide* (NAD^+) and *nicotinamide adenine dinucleotide phosphate* ($NADP^+$). These two coenzyme molecules differ only by the addition of the phosphate ester supplied by ATP to the 2'-hydroxyl of ribose.

Niacin and its precursor tryptophan are absorbed in the small intestine. Tissue stores of the vitamin are small. Niacin is excreted as N'-methyl-nicotinamide and its pyridones.

Functions

NAD and NADP are present and function in all cells in *oxidation-reduction* reactions primarily as hydrogen carriers. NAD^+ is utilized in most catabolic (oxidation) reactions, while $NADPH_2$ is the coenzyme for most anabolic (reduction) reactions . These coenzymes are components of dehydrogenases and reductases. NAD is a component of the electron transport chain and functions in the TCA cycle and glycolysis. NADP functions in fatty acid and steroid synthesis. Niacin functions in the vitamin A visual cycle and in the interconversion of choline and betaine.

Food Sources

Rich sources of niacin include bakers and brewers yeasts, organ meats, lean meats, poultry, fish, nuts, and enriched products such as cereals and grains (Table 7.9). The amino acid tryptophan can be converted to niacin; rich sources of tryptophan include lean meats, fish, poultry, and nuts. Little niacin or tryptophan is lost during the cooking of foods.

Dietary Recommendations

In that tryptophan can be converted to niacin, recommendations are given as *niacin equivalents* (NE). Approximately 60 mg tryptophan is converted to 1 mg niacin. The 1998 RDA for men and women 19 years and above is 16 and 14 mg NE, respectively. The median niacin intakes for men and women 20 to 59 years in the United States according to NHANES III are 26.2 and 17.5 mg daily not counting the tryptophan. Many people ingest the vitamin as part of a multivitamin preparation.

TABLE 7.9

Selected Good and Rich Sources of Niacin

Almonds	Beef cuts	Chicken cuts
Enriched breads	Enriched cereals	Fish
Liver	Mushrooms	Peanuts
Pork cuts	Tuna	White potatoes

Deficiency

The niacin deficiency disease is known as *pellagra* or the three or four D's (diarrhea, symmetric dermatitis, dementia, and death). Early symptoms include insomnia, anorexia, anemia, weight loss, muscle loss, numbness, and nervousness. The nervous system becomes malfunctional in the advanced stages. Pellagra is a wasting disease slow in its development. The deficiency is rare in developed countries, being seen only in malnourished alcoholics and in individuals having disorders of tryptophan metabolism. Pellagra is still seen in individuals in the Near East and Africa. Niacin status most often is evaluated by determining the urinary excretion of N'-methyl-nicotinamide (and sometimes also its pyridones) following a tryptophan test dose.

Pharmacologic Doses

Pharmacologically nicotinic acid and nicotinamide are dissimilar. Large doses (<3 g daily) of nicotinic acid can reduce serum cholesterol, free fatty acids, and total lipid levels. Large doses of nicotinic acid may improve vascular tone and decrease fatty acid mobilization from adipose tissue during exercise. Side effects of these large doses include acute flushing of the skin with a concomitant itching and feeling of heat and possible liver damage. If choline or another methyl group donor is given along with nicotinic acid, there is decreased incidence of fatty liver. Nicotinic acid was thought for years to be useful in the treatment of mental disorders, but evidence now indicates that this is not true. A Tolerable Upper Intake Level of 35 mg NE has been established for adults; this level was based upon the adverse effect of flushing.

Toxicity

Both nicotinic acid and nicotinamide can be toxic when 3 to 9 g are consumed. Hypertension, gastrointestinal problems, and hepatic toxicity are among the problems associated with nicotinic acid toxicity, while individuals chronically taking excessive quantities of nicotinamide are unable to focus their eyes.

Needs in Exercise

Niacin functions in respiratory metabolism. Niacin deficiency does impair glycolysis and respiratory metabolism. Although experimental data are lacking, a *10 percent increase* in the niacin requirement has been recommended by the panel that prepared the 1998 Dietary Reference Intakes to adjust for increased energy utilization and physical sizes of individuals who exercise vigorously. There is no evidence of inadequate niacin status in athletes or physically active individuals, and there is no need for niacin supplementation in exercise or sport. Supplementation with nicotinic acid reduces the availability of free fatty acids and potentiates the use of carbohydrates as sources of energy.

Vitamin B$_6$

Name: Pyridoxal, pyridoxol, pyridoxamine, pyridoxal phosphate, pyridoxol phosphate, pyridoxamine phosphate

Active form: Pyridoxal phosphate

Function: Transaminations, nonoxidative deaminations, desulfhydrations, decarboxylations, dehydrations

Vitamin B_6 was initially recognized as an antidermatitis factor in rats by J. Goldberger and R. Lillie in 1926 and was again recognized as the same antidermatitis factor by P. György, who in 1934 proposed the vitamin's name. Independently isolated by three research teams in 1938, vitamin B_6 was then synthesized in 1939.

Forms

Since 1945 it has been known that vitamin B_6 could be isolated in three different forms: two in animal tissues, *pyridoxal* and *pyridoxamine*, and from plants, *pyridoxol* (also known as pyridoxine; *pyridoxine is not another name for vitamin B_6*, but is the name of one of the forms of the vitamin). The three forms also exist as 5'-phosphorylated vitamers: pyridoxal phosphate, pyridoxol phosphate, and pyridoxamine phosphate. ATP is needed for the formation of the phosphorylated forms of the vitamin. Riboflavin, as FMN, functions in the conversion of pyridoxal phosphate to pyridoxol phosphate and pyridoxamine phosphate. The vitamin is absorbed in the small intestine and may be phosphorylated in the intestinal mucosa. The liver and muscle are where most of the reserves are located; even so, very little vitamin B_6 is stored in the body. The major excretion product of the vitamin is urinary 4-pyridoxic acid.

Function

Vitamin B_6, like other B vitamins, participates in enzymatic reactions as a coenzyme. Its coenzyme functions in the metabolism of predominantly *amino acids*. Pyridoxal phosphate participates as a coenzyme in several enzymatic reactions in the metabolism of the essential and nonessential amino acids. The enzymatic reactions in which pyridoxal phosphate participates are transamination reactions, in which α-amino acids are converted to α-keto acids with the concurrent transfer of the amino moiety to a different α-keto acid, forming a second and usually different amino acid. Such transamination reactions are responsible for the synthesis of the nonessential amino acids from the α-keto acids. These α-keto acid substrates exist as metabolic intermediates of carbohydrate and lipid catabolism. Other vitamin B_6-requiring reactions add hydrocarbons or cleave the side chain (R) of amino acids, providing for the racemization, deamination, or desulfhydration of amino acids. Vitamin B_6 is needed in hemoglobin formation. The vitamin also functions in the conversion of glycogen to glucose (actually glucose-1-phosphate), the synthesis of the fatty acid arachidonic acid from linoleic acid, the formation of spingolipids for the myelin sheath, the synthesis of niacin from tryptophan, the synthesis of norepinephrine and epinephrine, and the synthesis of nucleic acids. The vitamin is required for the synthesis of the neurotransmitter γ-amino-butyric acid (γABA or GABA), dopamine, serotonin, taurine, and histamine. The vitamin is also needed for the functioning of the immune system.

Food Sources

Good and rich sources of vitamin B_6 are given in Table 7.10. Rich sources of vitamin B_6 include bakers and brewers yeasts, organ meats, bananas, most legumes, seeds, rice polishings, and egg yolks. Beef, pork, poultry, and fish are either rich or good sources of the vitamin. Much of the vitamin is destroyed by some food processing and common cooking techniques.

Dietary Recommendations

According to many researchers involved in vitamin B_6 research, the requirement for vitamin B_6 is related to the protein intake with the need for vitamin B_6 being higher when

TABLE 7.10

Selected Good and Rich Sources of Vitamin B$_6$

Banana	Beef cuts	Chicken cuts
Dried beans	Dried peas	Egg yolks
Fish	Fortified cereals	Liver
Peanuts	Pork cuts	Prunes
Spinach	Tuna	White potatoes

the protein intake is higher. The 1998 RDA for adults 19 to 50 years is 1.3 mg while that for men and women 51 years and above is 1.7 and 1.5 mg, respectively. The median intake of men and women 20 to 59 years in the United States according to NHANES III is 1.97 and 1.31 mg, respectively. Women in the United States frequently consume less vitamin B$_6$ than is recommended. Many individuals in the United States ingest pyridoxine hydrochloride as part of a multivitamin preparation. The *1995 Third Report on Nutrition Monitoring in the United States* classified vitamin B$_6$ as being a "potential public health issue." This is because of the high prevalence of inadequate vitamin B$_6$ intakes and the health effects of consuming too little or too much of the vitamin. Many methods exist for evaluation of vitamin B$_6$ status, yet no one method is the best.

Deficiency

Vitamin B$_6$ deficiency due to inadequate intake of the vitamin is relatively rare; however, many drugs and medications are known to interfere with the functioning of the vitamin. Symptoms include dermatitis, dental caries, microcytic anemia, stomatitis, abdominal distress, irritability, depression, decreased immune function, epileptiform seizures, and convulsions. Infants fed a milk formula which had been subjected to moist heat developed irritability followed by epileptiform seizures. The infants recovered when pyridoxine hydrochloride was administered. Abnormal electroencephalograms have been reported in infants and adults who are deficient in vitamin B$_6$. Most individuals who are deficient in vitamin B$_6$ are also deficient in other nutrients, and frequently are also alcoholics. Vitamin B$_6$ status most commonly is evaluated by determining the plasma pyridoxal phosphate content using a radioenzymatic method.

Pharmacologic Doses

Vitamin B$_6$ metabolism is altered in several diseases and disorders. Pyridoxine hydrochloride has been utilized pharmacologically (25 to 50 or 100 mg doses daily) in treating several of these diseases and disorders including Down's syndrome, premenstrual syndrome, gestational diabetes, morning sickness, carpal tunnel syndrome, hyperoxaluria, autism, radiation sickness, diabetic neuropathy, various kidney disorders, depression, coronary heart disease, and alcoholism. Researchers have reported variable success in treating individuals with these diseases and disorders with the vitamin. Patients taking isoniazid, cycloserine, and penicillamine are often given vitamin B$_6$ as these drugs interfere with metabolism of the vitamin. A Tolerable Upper Intake Level for vitamin B$_6$ for adults is 100 mg daily.

Toxicity

Neuropathies and ataxias have been reported in individuals who have self-dosed with pyridoxine hydrochloride at intakes of 400 and perhaps even 200 mg daily for over eight months. Vitamin B$_6$-dependency has also been reported in normal adults who took 200 mg of pyridoxine hydrochloride daily for 33 days.

Needs in Exercise

Vitamin B_6 functions in several metabolic pathways including some involving proteins, carbohydrates, and fats during exercise. Several studies have shown that exercise alters vitamin B_6 metabolism. Vitamin B_6 deficiency may compromise exercise performance. Conflicting reports exist as to whether sustained aerobic exercise produces short-term alterations of several of the indices of vitamin B_6 status. The current thinking is that vitamin B_6 supplementation has no beneficial effect on exercise performance; the supplementation could possibly have adverse effects such as increasing lipid peroxidation. Vitamin B_6 is involved in the protective effect of exercise on cardiovascular disease.

Folic Acid

Name: Folate, Folacin
Active form: Tetrahydrofolic acid
Function: 1-carbon metabolism

Folic acid or *folate*, also known as *folacin*, is chemically named *pteroylmonoglutamic acid*. It is composed of pteridine, p-aminobenzoic acid, and glutamic acid. Biermer, in 1872, called an anemia observed in a group of pregnant women a "progressive pernicious anemia." L. Wills and coworkers during the early 1930s observed that females, usually pregnant ones, having a severe type of megaloblastic anemia, improved when given yeast extracts (Wills factor). Monkeys fed diets similar to that consumed by the women developed macrocytic anemia, which was cured by yeast or wheat germ extract (vitamin M). This substance was also shown to be a growth factor for chicks (vitamin B_c) as well as for the lactic acid bacteria *Lactobacillus casei* (*L. casei* or lactic acid factor). The name *folic acid* was coined in 1941 by Mitchell and coworkers. By the late 1940s, it was found that all the above-mentioned factors and vitamins were the same compound. Found in plants, folic acid was both identified as an animal and bacterial nutrient factor and was synthesized in 1946.

Forms

Most of the folic acid found in foods is in the form of *pteroylpolyglutamates*, which contain a pteridine, p-aminobenzoic acid, and 3 to 7 or even 11 glutamic acid molecules. *Vitamin B_{12}* functions as part of a deconjugase in converting the pteroylpolyglutamates to pteroylmonoglutamates, the active form. *Vitamin C* and *niacin* (as NAD) function in reducing folate. During or following absorption primarily in the jejunum, pteroylmonoglutamate in its reduced form is converted to methyl-tetrahydrofolic acid. Small stores of folic acid exist primarily in the liver, cerebrospinal fluid, bone marrow, spleen, and kidneys. Folic acid acquires 1-carbon units at the N^5 or N^{10} or between these two positions. The 1-carbon units can be formyl, methyl, hydroxymethyl, methenyl, and formimino moieties, and form various tetrahydrofolic acid compounds. These tetrahydrofolic acid compounds are interconvertible. The different forms of the vitamin vary in nutritional effectiveness and stability. Bile contains folate due to *enterohepatic circulation* of the vitamin. Absorbed folate is also excreted in the urine.

Function

Folic acid functions as a *1-carbon donor and recipient*. The vitamin is needed for the synthesis of the purines adenine and guanine and the pyrimidine thymine, and thus functions in DNA and RNA synthesis and growth in general. Folic acid functions in amino acid

TABLE 7.11

Selected Good and Rich Sources of Folic Acid

Asparagus	Banana	Beets
Broccoli	Dried beans	Dried peas
Egg yolks	Enriched grain products	"Greens"
Lettuce	Liver	Orange juice
Peanuts	Spinach	Wheat bran/germ

metabolism in the interconversion of serine and glycine (vitamin B_6 also needed), the oxidation of glycine, and the synthesis of methionine from homocysteine (vitamins B_6 and B_{12} also needed) and of glutamic acid from histidine. Folate is needed for the conversion of ethanolamine to choline and of nicotinamide to N'-methyl-nicotinamide. Folate also functions as a nonspecific 1-carbon donor/recipient in reactions in which no specific 1-carbon donor/recipient is required. Folate is needed for the synthesis and maturation of both red and white blood cells.

Food Sources

Rich sources of folic acid include the dark green leafy vegetables, organ meats, legumes, wheat germ and bran, and orange juice (Table 7.11). Good sources include bananas, egg yolks, nuts, and whole grain products. Approximately 20 to 75 percent of the folates found in foods are lost during food storage and preparation (including cooking). Some of the folates are present in the liquid in which food is cooked. Foods such as cabbage and legumes contain conjugase inhibitors that decrease the availability of the folates. Between 25 and 50 percent of the dietary folates are thought to be nutritionally available for metabolism. Older tables of folacin content of foods were inaccurate in that precautions were not taken to preserve the folate derivatives.

Dietary Recommendations

The 1998 RDA for folate is 400 µg *dietary folate equivalents* (DFE) daily for both men and women. This is higher than the previous RDA of 1989 which was 200 µg for men and 180 µg for women. Many nutrition researchers believed that the recommended intakes should be raised to 300 to 400 µg daily in order to provide a more adequate safety allowance for populations at risk, particularly premenopausal women. Women of childbearing age should consume 400 µg of folate according to 1992 recommendations of the United States Public Health Service. The Panel on Folate, Other B Vitamins, and Choline, Food and Nutrition Board, in 1998 stated that *"to reduce the risk of neural tube defects for women capable of becoming pregnant, the recommendation is to take 400 µg of synthetic folic acid daily, from fortified foods and/or supplements, in addition to consuming food folate from a varied diet."* The median daily intakes of men and women 20 to 59 years in the United States according to NHANES III are 280 and 189 µg, respectively. Folate status is most often evaluated by determining plasma or erythrocyte folic acid levels radiometrically. Many individuals, particularly premenopausal and pregnant women in the United States and western Europe, have low plasma or erythrocyte folic acid levels. Many individuals in the United States ingest folate as part of a multivitamin preparation. The *1995 Third Report on Nutrition Monitoring in the United States* classified folic acid as being a "potential public health issue." This is because of the relatively high prevalence of inadequate folic acid status and its relationship to health and disease. Folate is also added to foods in the bread group in the United States.

Deficiency

Folate deficiency is probably the most common vitamin deficiency in humans, at least in western countries. Deficiency symptoms include apathy, irritability, poor growth, *megaloblastic macrocytic anemia*, leukopenia, thrombocytopenia, glossitis, and gastrointestinal disturbances. Women who consume inadequate quantities of folic acid at conception are more likely to have infants with *neural tube syndrome* than those consuming adequate amounts. The folic acid nutriture of the woman for about two months prior to and about one month following conception is critical in reducing the incidence of neural tube syndrome in their newborns.

Folic acid deficiency is commonly caused by malabsorption of folate or of vitamin B_{12}. Alcoholics are frequently folate deficient in that alcohol impairs folate absorption and also appears to block methyl-tetrahydrofolate release from the liver. Individuals taking anticonvulsants, oral contraceptives, and folate antagonists (aminopterin, amethopterin) frequently are folate deficient due to absorption and metabolic impairments. Protein malnutrition may impair folate utilization.

Pharmacologic Doses

Supplements exceeding 400 µg daily are considered to be pharmacologic. Folate may partially reverse the antiepileptic effects of phenobarbital and other anticonvulsants. Folate acid antagonists are generally used in treating malignancies with these drugs being used in massive amounts, and then "rescue therapy" is undertaken giving folates. Folate supplements are also being given to decrease the risk of cardiovascular disease as they may lower plasma homocysteine levels.

Since January 1, 1998 specified amounts of folic acid must be added to every 100 g of enriched flour, bread, pasta, and other grain products according to Food and Drug Administration regulations. This mandate was in recognition of the importance of adequate intakes of folic acid with regard to protection against neural tube defects in infants at birth and atherosclerosis later in life. The upper limit of daily folic acid intake should be 1 mg according to a 1992 recommendation of the U.S. Public Health Service. The Tolerable Upper Intake Level for folic acid for adults is 1,000 µg daily of folic acid, exclusive of folate from foods.

Toxicity

Large doses of folates may obscure diagnosis of vitamin B_{12} deficiency in that it relieves the megaloblastic anemia caused by vitamin B_{12} deficiency, but the irreversible damage to the central nervous system continues. Doses of 5 mg/day can prevent the hematologic relapse in individuals with pernicious anemia. Otherwise, daily doses up to 15 mg of folate to adults seem to be without toxic effects. Rats given massive doses (~500 mg/kg body weight) of folate develop renal toxicity because of folate precipitation. Convulsant effects have been observed in rats given 45 to 125 mg folate intravenously.

Needs in Exercise

Many individuals do not consume adequate quantities of folate. Deficiency symptoms include fatigue and anemia. The use of folate supplements has decreased the prevalence of inadequate status in athletes and nonathletes. The consumption of added quantities of folate by athletes having adequate status seems to have little if any effect on endurance or athletic ability.

Vitamin B_{12}

Name: Cobalamin
Active form: Methylcobalamin, adenosylcobalamin (including 5'-deoxyadenosylcobal-
amin), hydroxocobalamin
Function: 1-carbon metabolism

Vitamin $B1_2$ is a group of *cobalamins* or cobalt-containing corrinoids which have the biological activity of cyanocobalamin. The vitamin is also known as the *anti-pernicious anemia
factor*, the extrinsic factor of Castle, and the animal protein factor. Vitamin B_{12} is very different from all other water-soluble vitamins in that it possesses the mineral cobalt. Vitamin B_{12}
has the largest molecular weight of the vitamins.

As early as the 1820s J. S. Combe described a fatal anemia due to "some disorder of the
digestive and assimilative organs." This anemia was fatal for at least another century, and
therefore, was known as pernicious anemia. G. R. Minot and W. P. Murphy received the
Nobel Prize for finding, in the 1920s, that the disease could be treated by eating liver. W. B.
Castle, in 1929, found that the liver extrinsic factor required an intrinsic factor secreted by
the stomach for absorption. The active component present in liver was later found to be
vitamin B_{12}. Vitamin B_{12} was the last of the vitamins to be isolated in crystalline form. It was
first isolated in 1947 by K. Folkers and E. Rickers from a fermentation process using *Lactobacillus lactis*. From a blood-red solution formed dark-red crystals of the long sought anti-
pernicious anemia factor named vitamin B_{12}, also isolated by Folkers. The synthesis of
vitamin B_{12} was completed in 1973 by R. B. Woodward and coworkers. In 1975, the Nobel
Prize in Chemistry was awarded for the synthesis of the vitamin.

Forms

The vitamin B_{12} found in foods usually is attached to polypeptides which are hydrolyzed
in the stomach and duodenum. *Intrinsic factor*, a glycoprotein produced by the parietal
cells of the gastric mucosa, binds with vitamin B_{12}. The intrinsic factor delivers the vitamin
to receptor sites in the ileum. Calcium is needed for attachment of the intrinsic
factor–vitamin B_{12} complex to the receptor sites. Once absorbed through the ileal mucosa,
the vitamin is bound to transport proteins, the transcobalamins I, II, and III. The major form
of the vitamin in plasma is methylcobalamin, but there is also adenylcobalamin (sometimes
as 5'-deoxyadenylcobalamin). The body also contains hydroxocobalamin. Vitamin B_{12} is
secreted in the bile and participates in *enterohepatic circulation*. Absorbed vitamin B_{12}
may also be excreted in the urine.

Functions

There are only two reactions in humans that have been unequivocally shown to require
vitamin B_{12} as a coenzyme. Methylcobalamin is an intermediate in the transfer of the
methyl group from N^5-methyl-tetrahydrofolate to homocysteine to form methionine; if
vitamin B_{12} is not available, N^5-methyl-tetrahydrofolate is trapped (called the folate or
methyl trap) and can not be converted to tetrahydrofolate, and then to other folates. Vitamin B_{12} enables the tetrahydrofolates to perform their functions. These folates function in
DNA and RNA synthesis. Hence, both folic acid and vitamin B_{12} are needed for the synthesis of nucleic acid and growth in general. A decrease in DNA synthesis results in megalo-
blastosis. Methylcobalamin is also needed for the conversion of homocysteine to
methionine along with folic acid and vitamin B_6. Adenosylcobalamin (actually 5'-deoxyad-
enosylcobalamin) is needed for the interconversion of methyl-malonyl-coenzyme A and

TABLE 7.12

Selected Good and Rich Sources of Vitamin B_{12}

Beef cuts	Chicken cuts	Clams
Dairy products	Egg yolks	Fermented products
Fortified cereals	Liver	Oysters
Pork cuts	Salmon	Sardines
Shrimp	Tofu	Tuna

succinyl-coenzyme A. This reaction is involved in energy metabolism of both carbohydrate and lipid metabolites. This reaction is also involved in the catabolism of odd-chain fatty acids and certain amino acids. If adequate vitamin B_{12} is not available, methyl-malonyl-coenzyme A accumulation may inhibit myelin sheath formation. Vitamin B_{12} may also function in reactions in which no specific *1-carbon donor/recipient* is required.

Food Sources

Vitamin B_{12} is present in foods containing animal proteins. Rich sources of the vitamin include organ meats, beef, pork, lamb, seafood, eggs, some sea vegetables, and fermented foods (Table 7.12). A variety of fermented products are available which contain varying quantities of the vitamin. Vitamin B_{12} is relatively stable to dry heat, but is lost when foods are cooked at an alkaline pH or by prolonged exposure to high temperature.

Dietary Recommendations

The 1998 RDA for vitamin B_{12} was estimated as follows. The minimum quantity of vitamin B_{12} required for maintenance of individuals with pernicious anemia is 1.5 µg daily as judged by maintenance of adequate hematologic and serum vitamin B_{12} values, while the estimate of loss due to lack of reabsorption of biliary vitamin B_{12} is 0.5 µg daily; so, 1.5 µg minus 0.5 µg is 1.0 µg daily. Vitamin B_{12} in foods is approximately 50 percent bio-available, so the requirement of normal individuals for vitamin B_{12} from food is 2.0 µg, and the 1998 RDA is 2.4 µg daily for adults. The 1998 RDA publication advises *"individuals over the age of 50 years to meet their RDA primarily via foods fortified with vitamin B_{12} or a vitamin B_{12}-containing supplement."* Older individuals have malabsorption of protein-bound vitamin B_{12}, which is the major form of the vitamin in whole foods. The median vitamin B_{12} intakes of adults 20 to 59 years according to NHANES III are 4.83 and 3.03 µg daily. Many people ingest the vitamin in the form of cyanocobalamin as part of a multivitamin supplement. Many middle-aged and even more elderly individuals are unable to absorb sufficient vitamin B_{12} from foods or oral supplements, and are given the vitamin by intramuscular injections. The *1995 Third Report on Nutrition Monitoring in the United States* classified vitamin B_{12} as being a "potential public health issue." This is because of the relatively high prevalence of compromised absorption of the vitamin, particularly in the elderly.

Deficiency

The most common cause of vitamin B_{12} deficiency is an inadequacy of **intrinsic factor** secretion rather than an inadequate dietary intake of the vitamin. Individuals can not absorb vitamin B_{12} if sufficient intrinsic factor is not available. Most of the symptoms of vitamin B_{12} deficiency are similar to those of folate deficiency. These include weakness, tiredness, dyspnea, poor growth, glossitis, **megaloblastic macrocytic anemia,** leukopenia, thrombocytopenia, and gastrointestinal abnormalities. These symptoms are primarily caused by a secondary deficiency of reduced folate. There is also irreversible degeneration of the central nervous system in vitamin B_{12} deficiency; early symptoms include paresthesia, numbness and tingling sensations of the hands and feet, moodiness, confusion, and depression. The *neuropathy* is due to a generalized demyelinization of nervous tissue.

Clinical signs of pernicious anemia are not evident until five to seven years after cessation of intrinsic factor secretion primarily because of the enterohepatic circulation of the vitamin. The ability to synthesize and secrete intrinsic factor is inherited as an autosomal dominant trait mainly affecting individuals past middle age, though pernicious anemia has been observed in children. Vitamin B_{12} deficiencies due to low dietary intakes have been reported in vegans who do not consume fermented products as well as in infants of lactating vegan mothers. Also, impairment of gastrointestinal function for an extended period is concern with regard to malabsorption and resulting deficiency of vitamin B_{12}.

Nutritional status with regard to vitamin B_{12} is most often evaluated by determining plasma or erythrocyte vitamin B_{12} concentration by radioassay. All radiodilution kits used in assessment of vitamin B_{12} in the United States must contain purified intrinsic factor as the cobalamin-binding protein.

Pharmacologic Doses

Individuals with pernicious anemia typically are treated with *vitamin B_{12} injections* given intramuscularly, thus bypassing the defective absorption; 1 µg daily by injection seems to be adequate. Frequently 15 to 100 µg of the vitamin are injected following diagnosis of the deficiency; then, after recovery, about 1 µg is injected intramuscularly daily or more often, 30 to 100 µg (or even 1 mg) at monthly intervals. Individuals with gastric atrophy are treated with 25 µg to 1 mg of the vitamin. No success has been reported in treating neural disorders not caused by the deficiency with large doses of the vitamin.

Toxicity

Rare allergic reactions probably due to impurities in the vitamin B_{12} preparation have been reported. There is some evidence that large doses of vitamin B_{12} may obscure diagnosis of folic acid deficiency in that it relieves the megaloblastic macrocytic anemia caused by folic acid deficiency. No toxicity symptoms have been observed in animals given several times their requirement of the vitamin.

Needs in Exercise

Hematopoietic defects are seen in vitamin B_{12} deficiency. The use of vitamin B_{12} supplements does decrease the prevalence of inadequate status in athletes and nonathletes. The consumption of added quantities of vitamin B_{12} by athletes having adequate status seems to have little if any effect on endurance or athletic ability.

Biotin

Name: Biotin
Active form: Biocytin
Function: Carboxylations
Note: Synthesized by intestinal microflora

Biotin, one of only two vitamins to contain sulfur, contains a ureido ring and a valeric acid side chain. Around 1900, F. Wildiers found that some yeasts required a factor found in yeast and wort for their growth; the factor was called "bios." Bios later was found to contain what is now known as biotin, pantothenic acid, and myo-inositol. M. Bias, in 1927, noted that "egg white injury" was cured by "protective factor X," which is now known as biotin. P. György, in 1931, also discovered this factor and named it vitamin H (Haut is German for skin). This vitamin was first isolated from egg yolks by F. Kögl and B. Tönnis in 1936. The chemical synthesis of biotin was first accomplished by S. A. Harris and coworkers in 1945.

Forms

Biotin has been isolated or chemically synthesized in eight isomeric forms. Only D-biotin is biologically active as a coenzyme. In tissues, D-biotin is covalently attached to enzymes by an amide bond linking the vitamin to a lysine residue of the enzyme. This conjugation is facilitated by ATP and magnesium, and the vitamin-enzyme conjugate is known as *biocytin*. D-biotin and biocytin are absorbed in the proximal small intestine, and likely transported by a biotin-binding protein. Biotin-producing microorganisms and fungi exist in the intestinal tract; some of the biotin produced by this microflora is absorbed and utilized by humans, but not enough is obtained to meet dietary requirements for the vitamin. Careful balance studies in men have shown that urinary excretion of biotin normally exceeds intake.

Functions

Biotin as biocytin functions in *carboxylation* reactions. Major carboxylation reactions involving biocytin permit the conversion of odd-numbered hydrocarbons into even-numbered hydrocarbons which are then metabolized in the major metabolic pathways. Both odd-numbered amino acids and fatty acids are converted to even-numbered hydrocarbons by carboxybiocytin. Major carboxylase reactions include the conversion of pyruvate into oxaloacetate, acetyl-coenzyme A into malonyl-coenzyme A, and propionyl-coenzyme A into methylmalonyl-coenzyme A. The biotin containing 3-methylcrotonyl-coenzyme A carboxylase is needed in the catabolism of branched-chain amino acids. Biocytin is additionally important in the synthesis of carbamyl-phosphate, used in the synthesis of the pyrimidines and in the formation of urea. Thus, biotin is needed for the synthesis and degradation of fatty acids and gluconeogenesis as well as protein degradation.

Food Sources

Rich sources of biotin include organ meats, egg yolks, soybeans, and bakers and brewers yeasts (Table 7.13). A relatively small percentage of biotin is lost during normal cooking procedures. Not all of the biotin present in foods is bioavailable. Many individuals in the United States ingest biotin as part of a multivitamin preparation.

TABLE 7.13

Selected Good and Rich Sources of Biotin

Almonds	Chicken cuts	Egg yolks
Liver	Mackerel	Peanuts
Sardines	Soybeans	Salmon

Note: Biotin is synthesized by the intestinal microflora and absorbed, but this contribution is variable.

Dietary Recommendations

The body gets considerable amounts of the vitamin from the absorption of the biotin synthesized by the *intestinal microflora*; its contribution varies greatly from individual to individual. The 1998 Adequate Intake for adults of all ages for biotin is 30 µg daily. Most individuals consume adequate quantities of the vitamin.

Deficiency

In humans, biotin deficiency may be induced by the consumption of large amounts of raw egg whites (about 10 percent of diet). Egg whites contain the glycoprotein *avidin,* which can bind to biotin and prevent its absorption. Avidin is denatured when the egg white is cooked. Biotin deficiency symptoms include anorexia, nausea, pallor, scaly dermatitis, atrophy of lingual papillae, graying of mucous membranes, lassitude, depression, muscle pains, hypercholesterolemia, and electrocardiographic abnormalities. Seborrheic dermatitis of infants less than six months of age may be due to biotin deficiency as the condition reverses promptly when infants are given biotin (~5 mg) intramuscularly or intravenously. Erythematous rash has been observed in adults on total parenteral nutrition (TPN). Biotin deficiency is rare. However, some inborn errors of metabolism exist with regard to biotin. Biotin status is most often evaluated by determining plasma levels of the vitamin using microbiological methods.

Pharmacologic Doses

Biotin (~5 mg) given orally, intramuscularly, or intravenously has been shown to heal skin lesions in the vast majority of infants with seborrheic dermatitis. Patients with biotin-responsive inborn errors of metabolism have improved when given large doses (~10 mg) of biotin.

Toxicity

No toxicity symptoms have been reported in adults taking as much as 10 mg of the vitamin daily. Controversial reports exist as to whether large doses of biotin affect the reproductive performance of female rats.

Needs in Exercise

Biotin is involved in energy metabolism. Biotin deficiency is rare. Controlled research relating biotin supplementation on exercise performance is not available.

Pantothenic Acid

Name: Pantothenic acid
Active form: Forms portion of coenzyme A
Function: 2-carbon metabolism

Pantothenic acid, discovered by R. J. Williams in 1933, is one of the B-complex vitamins. The Greek word "pantos" means everywhere, and it was and is found in a variety of biological materials. T. H. Jukes, in 1939, identified the factor as the "antidermatitis factor" in chicks. Pantothenic acid is composed of pantoic acid and β-alanine.

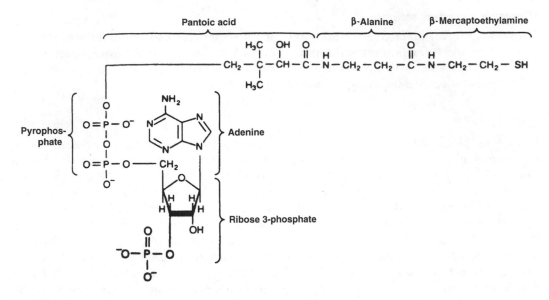

FIGURE 7.1
Structure of coenzyme A. Reprinted with permission from CRC Press. Spallholz, J.E., Boylan, L.M., and Driskell, J.A., Nutrition: Chemistry and Biology, © 1999 by CRC Press, Boca Raton, FL.

Forms

Unlike the other B vitamins, pantothenic acid does not function independently as a coenzyme; rather it forms a portion of a much larger coenzyme, *coenzyme A* (Figure 7.1), often abbreviated CoA or CoASH. The remaining components comprising coenzyme A are β-mercaptoethylamine and adenosine diphosphate (ADP).

Functions

Pantothenic acid as a component of coenzyme A functions in the synthesis of fatty acids, sterols, membrane phospholipids, choline, and acetylcholine as well as the oxidative degradation of fatty acids and amino acids. Coenzyme A also functions in the tricarboxylic acid (TCA) cycle, and thus functions in energy metabolism. Coenzyme A is needed for the synthesis of the porphyrin ring found in hemoglobin and myoglobin. Coenzyme A is needed for acylation reactions in general and can function as a nonspecific acetate (2-carbon) donor/recipient.

Food Sources

Pantothenic acid is widely distributed in foods. Rich sources include all meats, egg yolks, whole grains, and molasses (Table 7.14). About a third of the pantothenic acid present in foods is lost during ordinary cooking.

TABLE 7.14

Selected Good and Rich Sources of Pantothenic Acid

Beef cuts	Chicken cuts	Egg yolks
Fish	Molasses	Peanuts
Pork cuts	Whole grain breads	Whole grain cereals

Dietary Recommendations

Usual pantothenic acid intakes of adults in the United States are 5 to 10 mg daily. The 1998 Adequate Intake for pantothenic acid for adults is 5 mg daily. Many individuals ingest pantothenic acid as a component of multivitamin preparations.

Deficiency

Pantothenic acid deficiency has not been observed in humans except in those who are chronically malnourished. Pantothenic acid deficiency has been reported to cause the "burning foot syndrome" during World War II among prisoners fed only small amounts of watery potato soup as well as in malnourished individuals in the Far East. Deficiency symptoms include numbness and tingling of the extremities, gastric distress and nausea, insomnia, irritability and emotional instability, and muscular weakness. Administration of large doses of the vitamin reportedly reversed these symptoms. Pantothenic acid utilization may be impaired in alcoholics. Pantothenic acid status is most often evaluated by determining plasma or urinary levels of the vitamin using microbiological techniques.

Pharmacologic Doses

Pantothenic acid administration appears to have no pharmacologic effects in humans. A study with rats indicates that pantothenic acid may have a protective effect against radiation sickness.

Toxicity

No toxic effects were reported when 10 g calcium pantothenate were given to young men for six weeks. Occasional diarrhea and water retention has been observed in several studies when humans took 10 to 20 mg of the vitamin daily.

Needs in Exercise

Pantothenic acid is involved in energy metabolism. Deficiency of pantothenic acid is rare. Currently, there is no clear evidence of a beneficial effect of pharmacological doses of pantothenic acid on exercise performance.

Choline

Name: Choline
Active forms: Acetylcholine, phosphatidylcholine
Function: Neurotransmission, membrane integrity, methyl donor precursor

Choline, a water-soluble substance, was discovered in 1862 by A. Strecker. The pathway for synthesis of choline was described in 1941 by V. duVigneaud et al. Choline can be synthesized in humans from ethanolamine and a methyl group donor such as methionine, folate, or vitamin B_{12}. The ability of humans to synthesize choline is variable. Limited data exist as to whether choline is a dietary essential during all stages of the life cycle. Perhaps the choline requirement can be met by synthesis within the body during some of the life stages. Human culture cells do require choline.

TABLE 7.15

Selected Foods Containing Choline

Beef cuts	Chicken cuts	Dried beans
Dried peas	Egg yolks	Fish
Ham	Liver	Peanuts
Pork cuts	Rolled oats	Soybeans

Form

Choline in foods is primarily in the forms of phosphatides. Pancreatic and intestinal secretions contain phospholipases that hydrolyze the phosphatidylcholine consumed as part of the diet. Intestinal microflora convert some of the ingested choline to betaine and methylamines before the choline is absorbed. However, some of the dietary choline is absorbed in all portions of the small intestine as choline. Estimates of choline bioavailability are not available. Choline is found in high concentrations in the brain and nerves, liver, kidneys, mammary glands, and placenta. Choline may be oxidized in the kidney and excreted as betaine, though some is also excreted as choline.

Function

Choline functions as a component of acetylcholine and phosphatidylcholine or lecithin. Acetylcholine is a neurotransmitter, and phosphatidylcholine is a major component of membranes, plasma lipoproteins, and sphingomyelins. Choline, as a component of phospholipids, including phosphatidylcholine and sphingomyelin has cell signaling functions. Choline also functions as a precursor for the methyl group donor betaine.

Food Sources

Rich sources of choline include meats, whole grains, egg yolks, peanuts, and legumes (Table 7.15). In that choline is found in a wide variety of foods, it is unlikely that an individual could consume a diet low in choline that is not lacking in several other nutrients. Lecithin, or phosphatidylcholine, is frequently added to foods during processing by the food industry.

Dietary Recommendations

Although choline intakes have not been reported in national surveys, adults have been estimated to consume 700 to 1,100 mg choline daily. The Panel on Folate, Other B Vitamins, and Choline, Food and Nutrition Board, in 1998 stated that *"sufficient human data are not available to determine if choline is essential in the human diet and how much is required if essential."* However, this panel did recommend an Adequate Intake of choline for men and women 19 years of age and older of 550 and 425 mg/day, respectively.

The young of all animal species, perhaps even humans, appear to be susceptible to choline deficiency. It is likely that *newborns* need dietary choline. The American Academy of Pediatrics recommends that infant formula contain 7 mg choline/100 kcal, an amount approximating that found in milk.

Deficiency

Decreased choline stores and sometimes liver damage have been reported in men fed diets deficient in choline, but adequate in methionine, folate, and vitamin B_{12}. Patients on total parenteral nutrition (TPN) solutions devoid of choline, but adequate in methionine and folate have been reported to develop fatty liver and liver damage. In many cases, this abnormal liver functioning has been successfully treated with choline or lecithin. Serum alanine aminotransferase activities are elevated in choline deficient humans and other animals; this parameter is utilized in assessing choline adequacy.

Pharmacologic Doses

Choline may be beneficial to patients with diseases related to cholinergic neurotransmission deficiency. The Tolerable Upper Intake Level of choline for adults is 3.5 g/day.

Toxicity

Large quantities (~20 g) of choline or lecithin given orally have been reported to result in several adverse effects including nausea, diarrhea, sweating, dizziness, hypotension, fishy body odor (from excessive excretion of the choline metabolite trimethylamine), depression, excessive cholinergic stimulation, and electrocardiographic abnormalities.

Needs in Exercise

Conflicting reports are available from early research on the effects of choline supplementation on muscular power endurance and performance. Decreased plasma choline concentrations have been reported in marathon runners. No increase in grip strength was observed following 30 mg lecithin for two weeks.

8

Minerals

Minerals are inorganic catalysts that function as regulators of metabolic activities in the body. Minerals are *elements*. The periodic table of the elements is given in Figure 8.1. When food is completely combusted, what is left is called *ash*, which is composed of various minerals. About 4 percent of our body weight is minerals. Minerals are found in the body in combination with organic compounds and as free ionized ions.

Our bodies contain and require several minerals. *Essential minerals* are those with which a demonstrable improvement in the health and growth of humans is observed; these provide for normal development and health maintenance. Minerals are frequently separated into macrominerals and microminerals. *Macrominerals* are minerals that are required at levels of 100 mg or more daily. Sometimes macrominerals are defined as being the minerals that are present in the body in larger quantities (5+ g). The macrominerals include calcium (Ca), phosphorus (P), potassium (K), sulfur (S), sodium (Na), chloride (Cl), and magnesium (Mg). Sodium, chloride, and potassium are also classified as *electrolytes* in that they function in their ionic forms. *Microminerals* are required by the body at levels of less than 100 mg daily. Sometimes microminerals are defined as being those present in the body in smaller quantities (5– g). Microminerals sometimes are referred to as *trace elements*. There are a number of trace elements including iron (Fe), manganese (Mn), copper (Cu), iodine (I), zinc (Zn), fluoride (F), selenium (Se), chromium (Cr), cobalt (Co), molybdenum (Mo), vanadium (V), boron (B), tin (Sn), and nickel (Ni). Not all of these trace minerals have been demonstrated to be essential.

Minerals are components of body tissues. Minerals also function as components of many enzymes. Enzymes that contain minerals are referred to as *metalloenzymes*. The metalloenzymes catalyze many reactions in the body. Several of the minerals exist in the body as ions or electrolytes. Minerals are components of some hormones. Some of the metabolic reactions in which minerals are involved include nerve impulse conduction, muscle contraction and relaxation, oxygen transport, maintenance of acid-base balance, maintenance of fluid balance, and blood clotting. Minerals are not a source of energy, though some of the minerals do function as regulators in some of the reactions involving energy.

Minerals are found in the soil, and eventually are incorporated into the plant and animal foods that are eaten by humans. Thus, foods produced in one area may have a very different content of some minerals than foods produced elsewhere. Minerals may also be obtained from drinking water. Good and rich sources of the minerals are given in tabular form in this chapter. *Good sources* of nutrients contain 10 to 19 percent of the Daily Value for the nutrient per serving and *rich sources* contain 20+ percent of the Daily Value.

The essential minerals are listed in Table 8.1. There is some evidence, though not considered conclusive, that other minerals might also be essential for humans. As more people are consuming formula-type diets for several months to years, researchers are finding that some of the minerals present in foods are missing from the formulas, and that these minerals are essential for good health.

PERIODIC TABLE OF THE ELEMENTS

New Notation / Previous IUPAC Form / CAS Version

Key to Chart: Atomic Number (50), Symbol (Sn), 1995 Atomic Weight (118.710), Oxidation States (+2 +4), Electron Configuration (-18-18-4)

1 Group IA	2 IIA	3 IIIA IIIB	4 IVA IVB	5 VA VB	6 VIA VIB	7 VIIA VIIB	8 VIIIA VIII	9 VIIIA VIII	10 VIIIA VIII	11 IB IB	12 IIB IIB	13 IIIB IIIA	14 IVB IVA	15 VB VA	16 VIB VIA	17 VIIB VIIA	18 VIIIA	Shell
1 H +1 -1 1.00794 1																	2 He 0 4.002602 2	K
3 Li +1 6.941 2-1	4 Be +2 9.012182 2-2											5 B +3 10.811 2-3	6 C +2 +4 -4 12.0107 2-4	7 N +1 +2 +3 +4 +5 -1 -2 -3 14.00674 2-5	8 O -2 15.9994 2-6	9 F -1 18.9984032 2-7	10 Ne 0 20.1797 2-8	K-L
11 Na +1 22.989770 2-8-1	12 Mg +2 24.3050 2-8-2											13 Al +3 26.981538 2-8-3	14 Si +2 +4 -4 28.0855 2-8-4	15 P +3 +5 -3 30.973761 2-8-5	16 S +4 +6 -2 32.066 2-8-6	17 Cl +1 +5 +7 -1 35.4527 2-8-7	18 Ar 0 39.948 2-8-8	K-L-M
19 K +1 39.0983 -8-8-1	20 Ca +2 40.078 -8-8-2	21 Sc +3 44.955910 -8-9-2	22 Ti +2 +3 +4 47.867 -8-10-2	23 V +2 +3 +4 +5 50.9415 -8-11-2	24 Cr +2 +3 +6 51.9961 -8-13-1	25 Mn +2 +3 +4 +7 54.938049 -8-13-2	26 Fe +2 +3 55.845 -8-13-2	27 Co +2 +3 58.933200 -8-15-2	28 Ni +2 +3 58.6934 -8-16-2	29 Cu +1 +2 63.546 -8-18-1	30 Zn +2 65.39 -8-18-2	31 Ga +3 69.723 -8-18-3	32 Ge +2 +4 72.61 -8-18-4	33 As +3 +5 -3 74.92160 -8-18-5	34 Se +4 +6 -2 78.96 -8-18-6	35 Br +1 +5 -1 79.904 -8-18-7	36 Kr 0 83.80 -8-18-8	-L-M-N
37 Rb +1 85.4678 -18-8-1	38 Sr +2 87.62 -18-8-2	39 Y +3 88.90585 -18-9-2	40 Zr +4 91.224 -18-10-2	41 Nb +3 +5 92.90638 -18-12-1	42 Mo +6 95.94 -18-13-1	43 Tc +4 +6 +7 (98) -18-13-2	44 Ru +3 101.07 -18-15-1	45 Rh +3 102.90550 -18-16-1	46 Pd +2 +3 106.42 -18-18-0	47 Ag +1 107.8682 -18-18-1	48 Cd +2 112.411 -18-18-2	49 In +3 114.818 -18-18-3	50 Sn +2 +4 118.710 -18-18 -4	51 Sb +3 +5 -3 121.760 -18-18-5	52 Te +4 +6 -2 127.60 -18-18-6	53 I +1 +5 +7 -1 126.90447 -18-18-7	54 Xe 0 131.29 -18-18-8	-M-N-O
55 Cs +1 132.90545 -18-8-1	56 Ba +2 137.327 -18-8-2	57* La +3 138.9055 -18-9-2	72 Hf +4 178.49 -32-10-2	73 Ta +5 180.9479 -32-11-2	74 W +6 183.84 -32-12-2	75 Re +4 +6 +7 186.207 -32-13-2	76 Os +3 +4 190.23 -32-14-2	77 Ir +3 +4 192.217 -32-15-2	78 Pt +2 +4 195.078 -32-17-1	79 Au +1 +3 196.96655 -32-18-1	80 Hg +1 +2 200.59 -32-18-2	81 Tl +1 +3 204.3833 -32-18-3	82 Pb +2 +4 207.2 -32-18-4	83 Bi +3 +5 208.98038 -32-18-5	84 Po +2 +4 (209) -32-18-6	85 At (210) -32-18-7	86 Rn 0 (222) -32-18-8	-N-O-P
87 Fr +1 (223) -18-8-1	88 Ra +2 (226) -18-8-2	89** Ac +3 (227) -18-9-2	104 Rf +4 (261) -32-10-2	105 Db (262) -32-11-2	106 Sg (263) -32-12-2	107 Bh (262) -32-13-2	108 Hs (265) -32-14-2	109 Mt (266) -32-15-2	110 Uun (269) -32-16-2	111 Uuu (272)	112 Uub							-O-P-Q

* Lanthanides	58 Ce +3 +4 140.116 -19-9-2	59 Pr +3 140.90765 -21-8-2	60 Nd +3 144.24 -22-8-2	61 Pm +3 (145) -23-8-2	62 Sm +2 +3 150.36 -24-8-2	63 Eu +2 +3 151.964 -25-8-2	64 Gd +3 157 .25 -25-9-2	65 Tb +3 158.92534 -27-8-2	66 Dy +3 162.50 -28-8-2	67 Ho +3 164.93032 -29-8-2	68 Er +3 167.26 -30-8-2	69 Tm +3 168.93421 -31-8-2	70 Yb +2 +3 173.04 -32-8-2	71 Lu +3 174.967 -32-9-2	-N-O-P
** Actinides	90 Th +4 232.0381 -18-10-2	91 Pa +5 +4 231.03588 -20-9-2	92 U +3 +4 +5 +6 238.0289 -21-9-2	93 Np +3 +4 +5 +6 (237) -22-9-2	94 Pu +3 +4 +5 +6 (244) -24-8-2	95 Am +3 +4 +5 +6 (243) -25-8-2	96 Cm +3 (247) -25-9-2	97 Bk +3 +4 (247) -27-8-2	98 Cf +3 (251) -28-8-2	99 Es +3 (252) -29-8-2	100 Fm +3 (257) -30-8-2	101 Md +2 +3 (258) -31-8-2	102 No +2 +3 (259) -32-8-2	103 Lr +3 (262) -32-9-2	-O-P-Q

The new IUPAC format numbers the groups from 1 to 18. The previous IUPAC numbering system and the system used by Chemical Abstracts Service (CAS) are also shown. For radioactive elements that do not occur in nature, the mass number of the most stable isotope is given in parentheses.

FIGURE 8.1
Periodic table of the elements.

TABLE 8.1

Essential Minerals

Macrominerals	Microminerals	
Calcium	Iron	Fluoride
Phosphorus	Copper	Manganese
Magnesium	Zinc	Chromium
Potassium	Iodine	Molybdenum
Sodium	Selenium	
Chloride		

Subclinical mineral malnutrition may not influence physical performance in any measurable manner. However, physical performance has been demonstrated to be affected in the severe deficiency state, characterized by the presence of clinically manifested symptoms, for several of the minerals.

Calcium

Symbol: Ca
Function: Bone strength

Calcium (*Ca*) is the most abundant mineral in the body, accounting for 1 to 2 percent of adult body weight. Calcium is a divalent cation. Over 99 percent of the body's calcium is found in the bones and teeth. Small quantities of calcium are found in the soft tissues including liver, muscles, and brain.

Absorption and Metabolism

Calcium is absorbed across the intestinal mucosa, primarily that of the ileum, by both active transport and passive diffusion. *Vitamin D* (as 1,25-dihydroxycholcalciferol) and ATP is needed for the active transport of calcium across the intestinal mucosa. Calcium consumed at low and moderate levels is absorbed mostly by active transport, and by primarily passive diffusion at high intake levels. The amount of calcium consumed is positively related to the amount absorbed at a wide range of intake levels. Blood calcium levels are regulated by vitamin D (as 1,25(OH)$_2$D, *calcitonin*, and *parathyroid hormone* (also known as parathormone). Parathyroid hormone also acts on the bones as well as the kidneys, where calcium can be reabsorbed. Vitamin D enhances parathyroid hormone function, whereas calcitonin counteracts parathyroid hormone functioning. Absorbed calcium may be excreted in the urine, while unabsorbed calcium and that secreted into the small intestine is excreted in the feces.

Many individuals in the United States are lactose intolerant, lacking sufficient amounts of the enzyme lactase to digest lactose (milk sugar). Lactose intolerance is more common in individuals of color than in Whites. Lactose intolerant individuals experience diarrhea, bloating, and stomach cramps after consuming large amounts of lactose. Many lactose-intolerant individuals are able to tolerate small amounts of lactose. A wide variety of lactose-free dairy products are commercially available as are products that digest the lactose.

The quantity of calcium that is absorbed varies depending on the physiological status of a person, the food source, and the mixture of food substances available for absorption at the same time. Absorption efficiency is greater in individuals with low calcium stores than those with high calcium stores. Absorption efficiency is greater in young, growing individuals.

Post-menopausal women have lower calcium absorption efficiency than those that are pre-menopausal. *Estrogen* enhances calcium absorption. Treating post-menopausal women with estrogen increases calcium absorption. *Testosterone* enhances calcium absorption even more so than estrogen. Lactose increases calcium absorption in infants. Fiber may decrease calcium absorption. Calcium from foods rich in phytic acid (legumes, seeds, nuts, grains, soy isolates), oxalic acid (spinach, "greens," sweet potatoes, rhubarb, cocoa), and perhaps caffeine may be poorly absorbed. Phytic and oxalic acids bind calcium, making calcium insoluble and not as easily absorbable. Recent research has shown that the oxalate present in the cocoa of chocolate milk is not enough to interfere with calcium absorption to any significant extent. Caffeine may modestly decrease calcium absorption. The levels of phytates, oxalates, and caffeine typically consumed in the United States is believed to have little effect of importance on calcium absorption.

Calcium can be reabsorbed in the renal tubules or excreted in the urine. High sodium intakes may result in increased obligatory losses of calcium because of interactions between these two minerals in the proximal renal tubules. Protein intake also affects calcium excretion, but may or may not affect the retention of calcium. Poor recovery from osteoporotic hip fractures has been observed in elderly individuals with low (34 g daily) protein intakes; also, the risk of hip fractures seems to be inversely related to serum albumin concentrations.

Functions

Calcium is present in bones and teeth as *hydroxyapatite* [$3Ca_3(PO_4)_2 \cdot Ca(OH)_2$] which has been embedded in collagen. The hydroxyapatite provides strength and rigidity to bones, and helps the bones support the weight of the body. Other minerals are absorbed on the surface of the hydroxyapatite crystalline lattice (magnesium, iron, sodium, chloride), while others (fluoride, strontium) are incorporated into the lattice. Fluoride can displace the "hydroxy" of the hydroxyapatite in bones and teeth, producing fluorapatite, which is resistant to decay and also resists being dissolved back into the fluids of the body.

Bone undergoes constant turnover, with synthesis and breakdown of osteocytes (bone cells) always occurring. In the young, osteoblastic (bone-forming) activity exceeds osteoclastic (bone-resorbing) activity, while the reverse is true in the elderly and in many disease states. A positive calcium balance is required during bone growth. *Peak bone mass* or the highest obtainable bone density is obtained when individuals are in their third decade of life. In the typical adult about 600 to 800 mg of calcium is exchanged daily. Parathyroid hormone, calcitonin, and vitamin D (as 1,25-dihydroxycholcalciferol) function in maintaining *calcium homeostasis*. Bone loss occurs in individuals during about their third decade of life. This loss results in decreased bone strength and increased risk of fractures.

Skeletal calcium exists in nonexchangeable and exchangeable pools. The exchangeable pool, which is about 1 percent of skeletal calcium, can be readily mobilized to meet other body needs for calcium. Bone provides a readily available source of calcium for the maintenance of fluid calcium levels when diet is inadequate in the nutrient. The calcium ion is an integral part of cell signaling or the systems that handle communication between the various cells of the body. The movement of calcium from one cell to another is facilitated by the calcium-binding protein calmodulin. The reactions or reaction sequences activated by calcium include fatty acid oxidation, tricarboxylic acid cycle, mitochondrial carrier for ATP (also requires magnesium), glucose-stimulated insulin release, stimulation of olfactory (smell) neurons, conversions of trypsinogen to trypsin (in digestion), pancreatic amylase and phospholipase A_2 activities (in digestion), hydrolysis of troponin to tropomyosin (in muscle metabolism), and conversion of prothrombin to thrombin (in blood clotting). Calcium also plays a role in the death of cells.

TABLE 8.2

Selected Good and Rich Sources of Calcium

Beans	Broccoli	Calcium-set tofu
Cacium-fortified orange juice	Chinese cabbage	Dairy products
"Greens"	Kale	Salmon

Calcium is stored in the sarcoplasmic reticulum of muscle cells until needed for *muscular contraction*. Calcium plays a role in contraction of skeletal, cardiac, and smooth muscles. Sodium, potassium, and magnesium also function in the maintenance of muscle tone.

Food Sources

Dairy products are rich sources of calcium. Chinese cabbage, kale, broccoli, "greens," bony fish and calcium-set tofu are good to rich sources of calcium (Table 8.2). In recent years, the food industry also has produced calcium-fortified orange juices and other beverages.

Dietary Recommendations

The 1997 Adequate Intake (AI) for men and women, aged 19 to 50 years, is 1,000 mg daily, while that for those 51+ years is 1,200 mg. In 1994, the Consensus Development Panel on Optimal Calcium Intake of the National Institutes of Health recommended that women, aged 25 to 50 years, and men, aged 25 to 65 years, consume 1,000 mg of calcium daily; women 51 to 65 years taking estrogen consume 1,000 mg and those not taking estrogen consume 1,500 mg daily; and men and women over 65 years consume 1,500 mg daily. Commercial calcium supplements are used fairly extensively by individuals, particularly women, in the United States. According to NHANES III data, the median daily calcium intakes of men and women, 20 to 59 years, in the United States were 847 and 617 mg, respectively. These intakes, particularly those of women, are below the newly released 1997 AIs for calcium.

The *1995 Third Report on Nutrition Monitoring in the United States* classified calcium as being a "current public health issue." This is because of the possible associations of low calcium intakes and the ability to attain optimal peak adult bone mass and to prevent age-related loss of bone mass as well as increased risk of hypertension.

Deficiency

Calcium deficiency can result in the bone abnormalities rickets, osteomalacia, and osteoporosis. Rickets and osteomalacia àre classically associated with vitamin D deficiency in that vitamin D is essential for most, if not all, of the reactions related to the functioning of calcium. *Osteoporosis* is a disorder in which the quantity of bone is decreased, but its composition is maintained and the bones become porotic, resulting in less skeletal strength. Bone fractures occur in osteoporosis with only minimal stress. Calcium deficiency is not the only cause of osteoporosis. Osteoporosis due to calcium deficiency is frequently observed in the elderly, particularly elderly women.

Low levels of calcium in the blood result in *tetany*; however, calcium deficiency is not the only cause of tetany. In tetany, increased irritability of neural fibers causing muscle spasms is observed. Tetany, due to calcium deficiency, is frequently observed in pregnant women and newborn infants.

Some evidence, though inconclusive, exists that low calcium intakes may play a role in the development of hypertension, particularly gestational hypertension. However, other factors also have been associated with the development of hypertension. Some epidemio-logical evidence exists which tends to indicate that high intakes of calcium are associated with lower incidence of heart disease and colon and rectal cancer; the evidence for these associations is inconsistent.

Calcium status is best measured by determining bone mineral mass or bone density. Plasma/serum levels of calcium are also useful as an indicator of calcium status.

Pharmacologic Doses

Though many individuals in the United States take calcium supplements, the author is not aware of any research involving pharmacologic doses of calcium.

Toxicity

Calcium toxicity, to date, has only been reported in individuals taking nutrient supple-ments. Hypercalcemia has been reported to result in increased kidney stone formation, adverse interactions with other essential minerals (iron, zinc, magnesium, phosphorus), myopathy, excessive calcification of bone and soft tissues, and the so called "milk-alkali syndrome." The "milk-alkali syndrome" is when hypercalcemia and renal insufficiency both occur with and without alkalosis. At one time, higher milk and absorbable antacid intakes were used in treating peptic ulcers. In 1997, the Tolerable Upper Intake Level (UL) for calcium for adults was set at 2.5 g daily as part of the Dietary Reference Intakes.

Needs in Exercise

Research has shown that men and women who are physically active have greater bone mass than sedentary people. The bones of active people have greater bone mineral content than those of their sedentary counterparts.

Calcium intake and exercise both influence bone mass. In children, the effects of calcium intake and exercise on bone mineralization appear to be independent. However, other studies conducted with women and one with men indicate that calcium intakes over 1,000 mg daily enhanced the exercise benefit as measured by bone mineral density (some-times referred to as bone density) at the lumbar spine, but little change was observed at the radius. So, calcium intake and exercise may function independently or synergistically with regard to increasing bone mineral density.

Long-term low intake levels of calcium are detrimental to exercise performance. Calcium deficiency affects both bone density and muscle contraction, both of which definitely affect exercise performance. Approximately 75 percent of adults, particularly women including young women, consume less calcium than is recommended. Estrogen also affects bone density. Premenopausal women who train intensely and reduce their body fat and body mass frequently have athletic amenorrhea. These individuals secrete less estrogen. Athletic amenorrhea is often associated with low bone density or bone mineral content, particularly of the spine and femur. A higher than usual incidence of bone fractures and muscular inju-ries during exercise has been observed in amenorrheic athletes. Evidence exists that when menses returns in the formerly amenorrheic athlete the bone density increases; other reports indicate that the bone mineral loss is partially irreversible. Women with athletic amenorrhea are more likely than usual to develop osteoporosis at an early age. Eating dis-orders and amenorrhea frequently are observed in young female athletes involved in some of the sports where low body weights are desirable. Spinal bone density reportedly is influ-enced by low testosterone levels in male athletes. Treatment for osteoporosis frequently involves calcium supplements, hormone replacement, and exercise. Vitamin D supplements may also be of benefit in treating the osteoporotic athlete. Some evidence exists that weight-bearing and resistance exercises may be of benefit in the treatment of osteoporosis.

Phosphorus

Symbol: P
Function: Bone ossification, energy transfer

Phosphorus (*P*), an anion, is the second most abundant mineral in the body, consisting of 0.65 to 1.1 percent of adult body weight. Most (~85 percent) of the phosphorus in the body is found in combination with calcium in the bones and teeth. Phosphorus is also distributed into the soft tissues, blood, and extracellular fluid. In the body, phosphorus is found bound to carbohydrates, lipids, and proteins as well as being present as inorganic phosphorus (P_i).

Absorption and Metabolism

Foods contain both inorganic and organic (usually bound to protein) forms of phosphorus. Phosphatases (primarily alkaline phosphatase) in the small intestine hydrolyzes the organic forms. Phosphorus is absorbed primarily as inorganic phosphorus, by passive diffusion and by active transport facilitated by *vitamin D* (as $1,25(OH)_2D$); the mechanism is dependent upon the body's need for the mineral. Absorption is reduced by the ingestion of phytates (high in cereals, legumes, and nuts), pharmacologic doses of calcium carbonate, and antacids containing aluminum. Endogenous phosphorus is filtered by the glomerulus of the kidneys and may be *reabsorbed* or excreted in the urine. Phosphorus reabsorption is enhanced by the presence of vitamin D (as $1,25(OH)_2D$), somatotrophin (also called growth hormone) and glucocorticoids, but decreased by the presence of thyroid hormones, parathyroid hormone, estrogen, and elevated blood calcium levels. Optimal calcium:phosphorus levels of 1:2 to 2:1 was previously recommended. The recently released *1997 Dietary Reference Intakes* for these nutrients cites several studies in which no adverse effects on phosphorus retention were observed at calcium:phosphorus ratios of 0.6 to 1.4:1; also, calcium:phosphorus ratios of 0.08:1 to 2.40:1 had no effect on calcium absorption and balance.

Functions

Phosphorus, like calcium, is present in bones and teeth as *hydroxyapatite* and fluorapatite. Phosphorus is continually needed for bone turnover.

Phosphorus, as phospholipids, are components of the various membranes of the body. Phosphorus is also a component of DNA, RNA, and other nucleotides (including ATP, ADP, AMP, GTP, GDP, GMP, NAD, NADP, FAD, and FMN).

The body's "energy currency" *ATP* contains phosphorus as does *creatine phosphate* (also known as phosphocreatine), another high-energy compound. Phosphorus also functions in the activation and deactivation of many of the body's catabolic and anabolic pathways by phosphorylation and dephosphorylation.

Phosphorus helps in maintaining normal pH in various parts of the body by functioning as a *phosphate buffer*. Phosphate buffers are components of the body's fluids.

Food Sources

Foods that are good sources of protein are most often also good to rich sources of phosphorus (Table 8.3). Rich sources include meat, poultry, fish, and eggs. Soft drinks or cola beverages

TABLE 8.3

Selected Good and Rich Sources of Phosphorus

Beef cuts	Chicken cuts	Dairy products
Eggs	Peanut butter	Pork cuts
Salmon	Tuna	Whole grain cereals

are also rich sources of phosphorus as are the processed foods in which phosphate additives were utilized. Foods containing phytates also contain phosphorus; however, there is decreased absorption of this phosphorus.

Dietary Recommendations

The 1997 RDA for phosphorus for individuals 19+ years is 700 mg daily. Few individuals in the United States take phosphorus as an individual supplement; however, an estimated 10 percent or so get supplemental phosphorus as part of a multivitamin/multimineral preparation. According to NHANES III data, the median daily phosphorus intakes of men and women, 20 to 59 years, in the United States were 1,466 and 1,026 mg, respectively. Most people in our country consume adequate quantities of phosphorus.

The *1995 Third Report on Nutrition Monitoring in the United States* classified phosphorus as being a "potential public health issue." In that calcium intakes are low for many adolescents and adults living in the United States, there is concern that interactions between high phosphorus and low calcium intakes may result in adverse effects on the metabolism of calcium.

Deficiency

Symptoms of phosphorus deficiency include anorexia, neuromuscular disorders including muscular weakness, rickets and osteomalacia, increased susceptibility to infection, renal abnormalities, and ataxia. Phosphorus deficiency is rare as phosphorus is found in many foods. The deficiency has been reported in premature infants fed low-phosphorus milk. Long-term parenteral nutrition with insufficient phosphorus results in hypophosphatemia as does the long-term consumption of aluminum-containing antacids. Phosphorus status is usually evaluated by measuring plasma/serum levels of the mineral.

Pharmacologic Doses

Reports were not found on pharmacologic doses of phosphorus.

Toxicity

Hyperphosphatemia is rare. In hyperphosphatemia, effects on the hormonal control system of calcium, soft tissue calcification (kidney especially), possible calcium absorption problems, and increased porosity of the skeleton in animals (rabbits and beef bulls) have been noted. The influence of high phosphorus intakes on calcium metabolism is effectively negated if calcium intake is adequate according to the Panel on Calcium and Related Nutrients, which prepared the *1997 Dietary Reference Intakes* for these nutrients. The 1997 Tolerable Upper Intake Level (UL) for phosphorus for individuals 9 to 70 years is 4 g daily, while that for those over 70 years is 3 g.

Needs in Exercise

Phosphorus is involved in a number of reactions associated with exercise performance. Both phosphorus deficiency and toxicity are rare, and most people eat adequate amounts of phosphorus. ***Phosphate loading*** (with calcium, sodium, or potassium phosphate) may be of benefit to the athlete. Theoretically, the extra phosphate may improve athletic performance by minimizing the effects of excess hydrogens that build up during exhaustive anaerobic exercise. Researchers have reported no effects of phosphate supplements on $\dot{V}O_2$ max and lactic acid production. On the other hand, other researchers have reported decreased lactic acid production during a standard exercise, increased $\dot{V}O_2$ max, and enhanced myocardial efficiency. If one phosphate loads, it should be at about 1 g phosphate several times a day for up to a week. Rather similar findings have been reported using creatine phosphate. Several research groups have reported that creatine phosphate supplements increase body mass; increased body mass can enhance power performance; however, the extra weight may be detrimental with regard to endurance performance in a sport where running is of importance. The findings of supplementation studies using different forms of phosphorus are not in agreement with each other. Well controlled studies are needed regarding the effects of the different forms of phosphorus when taken as a supplement on physical performance.

Magnesium

Symbol: Mg
Function: Bone component, enzyme activity regulator

Magnesium (*Mg*), a cation, is the body's fourth most abundant mineral. Slightly over half of the body's magnesium is found in bone and about 27 percent in muscle, with the remainder being found in other cells and extracellular fluid.

Absorption and Metabolism

Although magnesium can be absorbed by either passive diffusion or active transport along the entire small intestine, most absorption is in the jejunum and ileum. Absorption of magnesium from a typical diet is about 50 percent. Absorption is enhanced to a small extent by the presence of vitamin D (as 25(OH)D or 1,25(OH)$_2$D) and decreased by high levels of dietary fiber. Magnesium circulates throughout the body as free magnesium, bound to protein, and as magnesium salts (citrate or phosphate). The movement of magnesium into and out of cells requires sodium and energy. Magnesium is a predominantly intracellular ion. Magnesium may be ***reabsorbed*** in the kidney tubules or excreted in the urine.

Function

Magnesium is incorporated into ***hydroxyapitite*** crystals in the skeletal system. A portion of skeletal magnesium functions as a reserve.

Magnesium is needed for the functioning of over 300 enzymes, including those involved in anaerobic and aerobic energy generation and the synthesis of fatty acids and proteins. Magnesium can function with ATP as well as ADP. Magnesium also functions in the formation of cyclic adenosine monophosphate (cAMP).

Calcium functions as a stimulator of muscular contraction, while magnesium functions as a relaxer. Magnesium also functions in neural transmission.

Magnesium is found complexed to phospholipids in the various body membranes as with calcium. Magnesium and calcium tend to have a stabilizing effect on these membranes.

Food Sources

Magnesium is widely distributed in the food supply (Table 8.4). Green leafy vegetables, unpolished grains, nuts, and seeds are particularly rich sources of magnesium. Refined

TABLE 8.4

Selected Good and Rich Sources of Magnesium

Dairy products	"Greens"	Oysters
Peanuts	Salmon	Shrimp
Spinach	Sunflower seeds	Walnuts
White potatoes	Whole grain breads	Whole grain cereals

foods are low in magnesium. Magnesium is also found in "hard" water, the amount depending upon the soil content from which the water comes.

Dietary Recommendations

The 1997 RDA for magnesium is 310 and 400 mg for men and women aged 19 to 30 years, and 320 and 420 for men and women 31+ years, respectively. Approximately 15 percent of adults take supplements that contain magnesium. According to NHANES III data (1988-91), the median daily magnesium intakes of men and women, 20 to 59 years, in the United States were 326 and 230 mg, respectively. Many people in our country consume less than recommended quantities of magnesium.

The *1995 Third Report on Nutrition Monitoring in the United States* classified magnesium as being a "potential public health issue." This is because of the possible association of low magnesium intakes with increased risk of hypertension.

Deficiency

The neuromuscular hyperexcitability that is observed in the early stages of the deficiency becomes more severe as the deficiency progresses. Other manifestations of the deficiency include *tetany*, personality changes, and convulsions. Severe deficiencies of magnesium lead to hypocalcemia and disorders in vitamin D metabolism and/or action. Postmenopausal women who are magnesium deficient are more likely to develop osteoporosis than those who are not. The deficiency also increases urinary thomboxane levels and blood pressure. Elevated blood lipid concentrations have been reported in magnesium deficient rats. Magnesium status is most commonly evaluated by measuring plasma/serum magnesium levels.

Pharmacologic Doses

High-dose magnesium sulfate is frequently used in treating eclamptic convulsions that occur with hypertension in late pregnancy and parturition, as well as being used to prevent premature labor. In the elderly, magnesium supplements have been reported to improve glucose tolerance as well as improving insulin response in individuals with noninsulin-dependent diabetes.

Toxicity

Excessive intakes of magnesium from magnesium salts, but not food sources, have been reported to have toxic effects. Toxicity symptoms include diarrhea, dehydration, metabolic alkalosis, hypotension, bradycardia, respiratory depression, and asystolic cardiac arrest. These symptoms are seen more in individuals who have kidney problems and take magnesium salts than in those that don't. The 1997 Tolerable Upper Intake Level (UL) for non-food magnesium for individuals 9+ years of age is 350 mg daily; however, a UL does not exist for magnesium from foods.

Needs in Exercise

Plasma/serum levels of magnesium have been demonstrated to decrease while levels in erythrocytes increase, though slightly, with chronic endurance exercise. Perhaps magnesium is entering the other body tissues, particularly the muscles, during exercise. A non-replicated study indicates that a correlation exists between $\dot{V}O_2$ max and plasma magnesium concentration. A few studies indicate that magnesium supplements positively influenced some exercise measurements, while no effects were observed in other studies. Magnesium status was not evaluated before supplementation was initiated in many of these studies; hence, it is not known whether or not the subjects initially had adequate magnesium status.

Sulfur

Symbol: S
Function: Nonessential mineral

Sulfur (S) is not an essential mineral for humans. Sulfur is a constituent of the sulfur-containing amino acids (methionine, cysteine, and cystine), three vitamins (thiamin, biotin, and pantothenic acid), glutathione, and insulin. Sulfur is found in high concentrations in the keratin of hair, nails, and skin.

Potassium

Symbol: K
Function: Predominant intracellular cation

Potassium (K) is also known as kalium. Potassium is a cation, and is the major intracellular *electrolyte*. Potassium is classified as both a macromineral and an electrolyte. Potassium is the third most abundant mineral in the body. Potassium is a component of muscle.

Absorption and Metabolism

Potassium is absorbed in the upper small intestine. Potassium is distributed in response to sodium redistribution. Potassium balance, like that of sodium and chloride, is regulated by the hormone *aldosterone*. Although potassium may be reabsorbed in the kidneys, about 85 percent of ingested potassium is excreted in the urine of healthy individuals. Minimal quantities of potassium are lost in sweat.

Functions

Potassium is needed for the maintenance of *fluid balance*. Essentially all the potassium in the body is exchangeable except for the small amounts found in bone. Potassium seems to perform many of its functions as *sodium-potassium ATPase*, frequently called the *Na^+K^+ pump* or sodium pump, as it pumps sodium out of the cell with potassium returning to the interior of the cells. This pump is utilized in active transport. Potassium functions in the transport of glucose into muscle cells, glycogen storage, and the synthesis of high-energy compounds. Potassium also functions in the generation of electrical impulses in the muscles and nerves, once again functioning as part of the Na^+K^+ pump. Potassium may play a role in the prevention and treatment of hypertension.

TABLE 8.5

Selected Foods Containing Potassium

Banana	Beef cuts	Cantaloupe
Chicken cuts	Dairy products	Dill pickles
Dried beans	Dried peas	Fish
Orange juice	Pork cuts	Raisins
White potatoes	Whole grain breads	Whole grain cereals

Food Sources

Potassium is found in all whole foods (Table 8.5). Fruits and vegetables are generally rich in potassium. Dairy products, whole grains, legumes, and meats are good sources of potassium.

Dietary Recommendations

The Estimated Minimum Requirement of Healthy Persons for potassium, as listed in the *1989 Recommended Dietary Allowances* publication, for individuals 18+ years of age is 2,000 mg. According to NHANES III data, the median daily potassium intakes of men and women, 20 to 59 years, in the United States were 3,060 and 2,230 mg, respectively. Findings from epidemiologic studies suggest that diets high in potassium and low in sodium may be beneficial in lowering blood pressure, and that diets high in potassium may be protective against death from stroke. The Committee on Diet and Health, National Research Council, in 1989 recommended a daily intake of 3.5 g and above for potassium. Median intakes of Americans for potassium are below 3.5 g.

The *1995 Third Report on Nutrition Monitoring in the United States* classified potassium as being a "potential public health issue." This is because low intakes of potassium may be associated with increased risk of hypertension.

Deficiency

Potassium deficiency symptoms include weakness, anorexia, nausea, listlessness, muscle cramps, constipation, irrational behavior, and even cardiac dysrhythmias. Disturbances in acid-base balance are also seen in potassium deficiency. Potassium deficiency occurs because of excessive losses of potassium through the gastrointestinal tract or kidneys. Prolonged vomiting, chronic diarrhea, and *laxative abuse* may cause increased potassium losses via the gastrointestinal tract. *Diuretics* may increase potassium losses via the kidneys. The evaluation of potassium status by the determination of plasma/serum levels is not accurate, but other methods of evaluation are not commonly available.

Pharmacologic Doses

Potassium chloride tablets are available over the counter. Potassium supplements should only be used when advised by a physician, as potassium does have toxic effects. Potassium supplementation may have vasculoprotective properties. Potassium supplementation tends to decrease blood pressure in normotensive and hypertensive individuals.

Toxicity

Hyperkalemia results in muscle contractility disorders, including cardiac arrest. Hyperkalemia may result from sudden increases in potassium intakes or may be caused by chronic renal failure.

Needs in Exercise

The total amount of potassium lost in sweat is small in proportion to total body stores. Athletes do not seem to need more potassium than other individuals.

Sodium

Symbol: Na
Function: Predominant extracellular cation

Sodium (*Na*) is also known as natrium. Sodium is a cation that is found primarily in the extracellular fluids of the body. Sodium is classified as both a macromineral and an electrolyte.

Absorption and Metabolism

Sodium is absorbed in the upper small intestine. Although sodium can be *reabsorbed* by the tubules of the kidneys, some sodium is lost daily in sweat and feces. The hormone *aldosterone* helps in the maintenance of sodium homeostasis by increasing sodium resorption by the kidney. *Angiotensin* II aids in the conservation of sodium at low serum sodium concentrations, but has the reverse effect at high concentrations. Actually, the control of sodium, potassium, and chloride levels and water balance are all interrelated. In healthy individuals, consuming typical Western diets, over 90 percent of ingested sodium is excreted in the urine. Individuals with renal disorders and diseases are not able to eliminate sodium as well as healthy persons.

Sodium is the major extracellular electrolyte. Sodium plays a role in the maintenance of fluid balance and osmotic pressure in the body. Sodium also functions in nerve impulse transmission, muscle contraction, and in the formation of the bone mineral apatite. Sodium seems to perform its functions as *sodium-potassium ATPase*, frequently called the *Na^+K^+ pump* or sodium pump, as it pumps sodium out of the cell with potassium returning into the cells. This pump is utilized in active transport. In muscle, there is the Na^+K^+ pump as well as a *Na^+Ca^{2+} pump*, which pumps sodium out of the cell while calcium enters the cell, and thus, calcium initiates muscle contraction.

Food Sources

Selected foods containing sodium are given in Table 8.6. The major source of dietary sodium is common table salt, or sodium chloride (NaCl). Soy sauce, catsup, mustard, and monosodium glutamate (MSG) are also high in sodium. Sodium chloride is used by the food processing industry as a preservative, so sodium is found in processed foods. Currently, food manufacturers are adding less salt in processing foods. Sodium-free (contains <5 mg sodium per serving), very-low-sodium (contains no more than 35 mg per serving), and low-sodium (contains no more than 140 mg sodium per serving) processed foods are available commercially. The sodium content of all processed foods must be listed on the label.

TABLE 8.6

Selected Foods Containing Sodium

Catsup	Dill pickles	Monosodium glutamate
Mustard	Soy sauce	Table salt
Most processed foods		

Note: The consumption of high quantities of sodium may be detrimental to one's health.

Dietary Recommendations

The 1989 Estimated Minimum Requirement of Healthy Persons for sodium for individuals 18+ years of age is 500 mg daily. The Committee on Diet and Health, National Research Council, in 1989 recommended that North American adults and children limit their daily intake of salt to 6 g or less, which is equivalent to *≤2400 mg*. One of the Dietary Guidelines for Americans is to "choose a diet moderate in salt and sodium." According to NHANES III data, the median daily sodium intakes of men and women, 20 to 59 years, in the United States were 3,813 and 2,641 mg, respectively. Many Americans consume more sodium than is recommended.

The *1995 Third Report on Nutrition Monitoring in the United States* classified sodium as being "a current public health issue." This is because high intakes of sodium are associated with high prevalences of hypertension.

Deficiency

Symptoms of *hyponatremia* include excessive water intake (polydipsia), edema, diarrhea, heat exhaustion, cachexia, anorexia nervosa, cardiovascular collapse, and congestive heart failure. Conditions of extremely heavy and persistent sweating, chronic diarrhea, trauma, and renal disease can cause the body to be depleted of sodium. Sodium deficiency in its severe form is rare; however, individuals who excrete large quantities of sweat can have low body levels of sodium, if the sodium lost in sweat is not replaced. Sodium status is most commonly evaluated by measuring plasma/serum concentration of the mineral.

Pharmacologic Doses

The blood electrolyte concentrations increase during exercise, thus making body fluids hypertonic. Sweat is hypotonic. *Electrolyte replacement*, especially sodium, during exercise is sometimes recommended.

Toxicity

Many Americans consume too much sodium. *Hypernatremia* results in dehydration, edema, hypertension, and brain stem injury. Increased urinary calcium losses which can lead to osteoporosis and bone fractures have been reported due to high sodium intakes.

Some people are salt-sensitive or sodium-sensitive. For these individuals, high sodium intakes contribute to high blood pressure and hypertension. This problem is often alleviated by consumption of diets low in sodium. However, other factors also contribute to high blood pressure.

Needs in Exercise

Electrolyte replacement during exercise is not necessary if the exercise is of only a couple of hours duration. However, small quantities of electrolytes may have positive effects on water and carbohydrate absorption, as from a *sports beverage*. Electrolyte replacement is needed during prolonged bouts (over one hour) of vigorous physical activity, particularly if the activity is repeated for several days and/or is at high environmental temperatures. Also, for fluid losses over 4 kg (about 9 pounds), electrolyte replacement is recommended. Electrolyte supplements should be in liquid form, and generally are consumed along with carbohydrate(s) and water, as in a sports beverage. The American College of Sports Medicine in 1996 recommended that sodium be present in rehydration solutions ingested during exercise lasting longer than one hour at a concentration of 0.5 to 0.7 g/L water. The presence of sodium in rehydration solutions enhances their palatability, promotes fluid retention, and may possibly prevent hyponatremia in individuals who drink excessive quantities of fluid.

Chloride

Symbol: Cl
Function: Predominant extracellular anion

Chloride (*Cl*), an anion, is the major electrolyte in the extracellular fluid. Chloride is also a macromineral. Chloride is a component of gastrointestinal secretions and cerebrospinal fluid.

Absorption and Metabolism

Chloride is absorbed in the upper small intestine. Although chloride may be *reabsorbed* in the kidneys, some chloride is lost daily in sweat and feces. In healthy individuals, over 90 percent of ingested chloride is excreted in the urine. Individuals with renal disorders and diseases are not able to eliminate chloride as well as healthy persons.

Functions

Chloride is utilized to replace anions lost to cells in various reactions. Chloride functions in the maintenance of fluid and acid-base balance in the body. Chlorine is a component of the gastric acid hydrochloric acid as well as being a fluid component of the other digestive secretions. In the so-called *chloride shift*, hydrogen carbonate diffuses out of the erythrocyte in exchange for chloride as hemoglobin exchanges oxygen for carbon dioxide; hence, chloride contributes to the ability of the blood to carry large quantities of carbon dioxide.

Food Sources

Chloride is distributed in a wide variety of foods. Dietary intake of chloride is associated with that of sodium. Chloride is found in common table salt and processed foods (Table 8.7). Some dietary chloride is also present as potassium chloride. Chloride is also found in most natural waters and municipalities frequently add chloride in the form of chlorine (Cl_2) to the water supply.

Dietary Recommendations

The Estimated Minimum Requirement of Healthy Persons for chloride for individuals 18+ years of age is 750 mg daily. Daily intakes of chloride for Americans were not estimated in the recent NHANES III survey. Dietary problems with regard to chloride are rare.

TABLE 8.7

Selected Foods Containing Chloride

Catsup	Dill pickles	Mustard
Soy sauce	Table salt	Most processed foods

Deficiency

Deficiency of chloride is unlikely, but does result in hypochloremic metabolic alkalosis. Conditions associated with sodium depletion will also cause chloride loss. Chloride status is commonly evaluated by determining plasma/serum concentrations of the mineral.

Pharmacologic Doses

Chloride is used in conjunction with sodium in *electrolyte replacement* usually in the form of salt in a sports beverage.

Toxicity

Long-term consumption of high levels of chloride (as salt) have been associated with high blood pressure and hypertension in salt-sensitive individuals. Water-deficiency dehydration can cause hyperchloremia.

Needs in Exercise

Fluid replacement is recommended during repeated exposures to exercise, especially in high-temperature environments and ultradistance events, in which individuals perform physical activity for a prolonged period of time (over one hour). Chloride is part of the fluid replacement supplement, and it should be in liquid form. Also, for fluid losses of over 4 kg (about 9 pounds), electrolyte replacement is recommended. As with sodium, suggestions for the chloride concentration for fluid replacement varies from 0.5 to 0.7 g/L water.

Iron

Symbol: Fe
Function: Oxygen carrier, electron carrier

Iron (*Fe*) is the most abundant micromineral or trace mineral (also trace element) in the body. Iron is found in every cell of the body. The body of an adult contains 3 to 5 g of iron. Iron is present in both the ferrous (Fe^{+2}) and ferric (Fe^{+3}) forms. Iron is a component of hemoglobin, myoglobin, and several enzymes. Iron deficiency is the most prevalent nutrient deficiency in the United States, being observed most frequently in women and children, according to recent surveys.

Absorption and Metabolism

Several different mechanisms are utilized by the body for the absorption of iron. Dietary absorption of this mineral varies from 5 to 10 percent in healthy people, and can be as high as 50 percent in iron-deficient individuals. The form of iron in foods influences the absorption efficiency. About 40 percent of the iron in animal flesh (meats including poultry and fish) is in the form of hemoglobin and myoglobin (both are pigments that carry oxygen and carbon dioxide); this *heme iron* is absorbed with about twice the efficiency as nonheme iron. The other 60 percent of the iron in animal tissues and all the iron in milk, eggs, grains, vegetables, and other plant foods is *nonheme iron*, consisting primarily of iron salts. Heme iron is 20 to 30 percent absorbed in the duodenum and upper jejunum as intact porphyrins. Nonheme iron is 2 to 5 percent absorbed in the duodenum and upper duodenum; many factors influence the absorption of nonheme iron. Iron absorption efficiency also depends on the body's need for iron.

Nonheme iron must be in a soluble form before being absorbed. Gastric hydrochloric acid aids in the reduction of ferric compounds, and also creates an acidic pH. Dietary ferric salts are converted to the soluble ferrous salts by ascorbic acid. The presence of heme iron or some other component in meats in the upper small intestine at the same time as nonheme iron enhances the absorption of nonheme iron. The presence of calcium phosphate, phytic acid (legumes, seeds, nuts, grains, soy isolates), oxalic acid (spinach, "greens," sweet potatoes, rhubarb, cocoa), bran, polyphenols (teas and some vegetables), and antacids can substantially decrease nonheme iron absorption depending on their concentrations. Pica, the consumption of nonfood substances (such as red clay, ice, paste, and cornstarch can decrease the absorption of iron from food sources. Some evidence exists that some chemical in coffee, perhaps caffeine, may also decrease nonheme iron absorption. Following absorption iron is transported in the circulatory system primarily by transferrin, with some iron being transported as ferritin. **Transferrin** generally transports about one-third of its carrying capacity, or total iron-binding capacity (TIBC), dependent upon the body's need. Once iron enters the cell, it is chelated by ferrochelatase to a protein called *ferritin*. Iron is stored as ferritin (contains ~20 percent iron) and hemosiderin (contains ~37 percent iron), primarily in the liver, bone marrow, and reticuloendothelial cells. The iron bound to ferritin is more readily mobilized than that bound to **hemosiderin**. Iron turnover in the body is constant. Erythrocytes, with a normal life span of 120 days, contain about two-thirds of the body's iron. When erythrocytes are degraded, most of the iron is recaptured and utilized to once again synthesize hemoglobin. Unabsorbed iron and that from minute blood losses and desquamated cells are excreted in the feces. Small amounts of iron are excreted in sweat and urine. Premenopausal women lose iron via **menstruation**.

Function

Iron participates in many **oxidation-reduction** reactions. In erythrocytes the iron present in hemoglobin plays a critical role in carrying oxygen to the cells and carbon dioxide away from the cells. Iron in myoglobin functions in transporting and storing oxygen with the muscle and releasing this oxygen when needed to meet metabolic needs during muscle contraction. In the cytochrome series of the electron transport chain, iron serves as a carrier of electrons, and thus, is important in converting ADP to ATP in the mitochondria. Iron is a component of cytochrome P450, located in liver and intestinal mucosa cells, which functions in the catabolism of various water-insoluble drugs, toxins, and endogenous compounds by oxidation. NADH dehydrogenase (in the electron transport chain), succinate dehydrogenase, and aconitase (both in the tricarboxylic acid cycle) contain iron and are involved in energy metabolism. Hydrogen peroxidases, containing iron, protect against the accumulation of hydrogen peroxides which are responsible for lipid peroxidative damage. Iron also is needed for normal immune functioning as well as being involved in the synthesis of neurotransmitters important in brain functioning.

Food Sources

Selected good and rich sources of iron are given in Table 8.8. The richest food sources of iron are organ meats (especially liver), oysters, clams, and molasses. Rich to good sources of iron are lean meats, spinach, "greens," egg yolks, legumes, some dried fruits, and whole grain cereals and breads. Many foods, particularly cereals as well as some breads, are fortified with iron.

TABLE 8.8

Selected Good to Rich Sources of Iron

Almonds	Apricots	Beef cuts
Broccoli	Clams	Dried beans
Dried peas	Egg yolks	Fortified cereals
"Greens"	Liver	Molasses
Oysters	Peanut butter	Spinach
Swiss chard	Tofu	Walnuts

Dietary Recommendations

The 1989 RDA for iron is 10 mg for males aged 19+ years, women 51+ years of age, and 15 mg daily for females 11 to 50 years of age. Many women in the United States take supplemental iron. According to NHANES III data, the median daily iron intakes of men 20 to 59 years old is 15.8 mg, and of women 50 to 59 years old is 10.6 mg, while that of women 20 to 49 years old is about 10.8 mg. Many premenopausal women and children in our country consume less than recommended amounts of iron.

The *1995 Third Report on Nutrition Monitoring in the United States* classified iron as being a "current public health issue." This is because low iron intakes may lead to anemia, though some research suggests that high iron intakes may also be a public health concern.

Deficiency

Most likely iron deficiency is the most common nutritional deficiency in the world. Many people consume insufficient amounts of iron. Also, iron, particularly its nonheme form, is also poorly absorbed. Iron deficiency is prevalent in premenopausal women, pregnant women, older infants, children, and early adolescents. Plasma ferritin levels decrease in early iron deficiency, followed by decreased total iron-binding capacity (TIBC) values, and then hypochromic, microcytic anemia. Iron-deficient individuals are more easily fatigued, exhibit pallor and weakness, have lowered immunity, have impaired ability to maintain body temperature in cold environments, have lowered work capacity, and have impaired cognitive ability. Preterm deliveries, low-birth-weight infants, and fetal deaths have also been reported to occur more frequently in women who were iron deficient during early pregnancy.

No single status indicator exists for iron. Iron status indicators which are commonly utilized are serum/plasma ferritin, serum/plasma transferrin saturation, and erythrocyte protoporphyrin, frequently in conjunction with indicators (hemoglobin and hematocrit values) of anemia.

Pharmacologic Doses

Large doses of iron (about 60 mg daily for adults) are utilized in treating iron deficiency. The iron supplements may be in the form of elementary iron, ferrous sulfate (the cheapest and most widely used), ferrous gluconate, and ferrous fumarate.

Toxicity

Iron toxicity was first reported in the Bantu tribe in South Africa. Most of the men, but not the women in the tribe developed polycythemia, followed by siderosis, and even death. The tribe made their maize beer (home-brew) in iron pots; the acid produced by the microorganisms which also produced the alcohol, dissolved some of the iron from the pots. The practices of the tribe were that men, but not women, consumed these alcoholic beverages.

Iron poisoning or toxicity is observed in thousands of young children yearly who have ingested iron supplements formulated for women. Early symptoms are bloody diarrhea, vomiting, shock, metabolic acidosis, sometimes followed by liver damage. The lethal dose is about 200 to 250 mg/kg. Individuals with the genetic disorder hereditary hemochromatosis can easily overload on iron; transferrin saturation measurements are useful in screening for this disorder. Iron overload, particularly in individuals with hereditary hemochromatosis, may also be caused by frequent blood transfusions. Large amounts of iron may interfere with copper and zinc metabolism and perhaps that of vitamin E.

High serum ferritin values have been reported to correlate with an increased risk of myocardial infarction in men, according to one epidemiologic study; however, this was not observed in another epidemiologic study. Evidence exists that chronically high-iron intakes are associated with the development of cancer, particularly that of the colon.

Needs in Exercise

Exercise may increase a person's need for erythrocytes. Individuals that exercise vigorously have more erythrocytes than nonathletes. The body may adapt by increasing iron absorption due to increased need.

Many female athletes and nonathletes consume inadequate amounts of iron. Although no biochemical parameter by itself satisfactorily evaluates iron status, several studies, using various individual status indicators, indicate that about 5 to 10 percent of male and 20 to 50 percent or so of female athletes are iron deficient. Blood indicators are affected by exercise. Expanded plasma volumes and increased erythrocyte destruction have been reported in athletes. These blood parameters influence iron status indicators. Even though there is controversy about how iron deficiency should be assessed in athletes, investigators agree that iron deficiency is a problem in the athletic population, particularly the female.

All athletes, particularly females, need to be sure that they consume sufficient iron. Vegetarian athletes, because of their high dietary intakes of phytates and oxalates, need to pay particular attention to obtaining and maintaining optimal iron status. Athletes who train and compete at high altitudes also need to be sure that they obtain and maintain optimal iron status as there is an increased erythrocyte production at high altitudes. The oxygen concentration of the air is lower at high altitudes than at sea level.

Blood is often observed in the urine, called *hematuria*, in athletes, particularly distance runners and weight lifters. This may be due to physical stress on the feet and mechanical stress in the muscles. Trauma to the bladder perhaps caused by running can also cause hematuria. Blood may also be lost in the feces in small amounts in endurance athletes, though this loss may or may not be due to their increased use of aspirin and such drugs to control pain. Iron is also lost, though in very small amounts, in sweat. Athletes may lose more iron from their bodies than nonathletes.

Sports anemia is often associated with endurance training. Sports anemia frequently occurs in the early stages of intense training and seems to be transient. However, long-term sports anemia is observed in some endurance athletes. Endurance training does increase plasma volume as well as erythrocytes. Many researchers indicate that sports anemia is a misnomer as athletes develop anemia for the same reasons as nonathletes.

Some female athletes are amenorrheic and lose very little iron via menstruation. Exercise-related *amenorrhea* has been associated with low levels of the sex hormones estrogen and progesterone.

Research indicates that "blood doping" (withdrawing blood from individuals several months before competitions and giving the blood back as transfusions just prior to competitions) does not increase athletic performance. Blood doping also may be detrimental to one's health.

Iron deficiency does decrease $\dot{v}O_2$ max and physical work capacity as well as increase post-exercise blood lactic acid concentrations. Iron supplementation of iron-deficient individuals does return these measurement values to normal levels. Several studies have been conducted on female athletes with adequate iron status who were given iron supplements; the vast majority of these studies found no improved performance with regard to various exercise measurements. However, the supplementation apparently may positively influence blood lactic acid metabolism after heavy exercise. This improvement may be due to improved aerobic metabolism in the muscles. Athletes are advised not to take large doses of supplemental iron because of possible iron toxicity. Athletes should be screened for iron deficiency.

Copper

Symbol: Cu
Function: Electron carrier, iron metabolism

Copper (*Cu*), a trace mineral (also trace element), frequently functions in conjunction with iron. About 110 mg of copper is found in the normal adult. Copper is found in highest concentration in kidneys, liver, brain, and heart. About 40 percent of the body's copper is found in muscle. Copper exists in the cuprous (Cu^+) and cupric (Cu^{2+}) forms.

Absorption and Metabolism

Copper is absorbed primarily in the upper small intestine by active transport and passive diffusion, though limited absorption occurs in the stomach. Antagonisms are known to exist between copper and zinc as well as cadmium with regard to absorption. Reports exist that antagonism exists or does not exist between copper and iron with regard to absorption. Some evidence exists that amino acids and citrate may enhance absorption of copper while fiber and bile decrease absorption. Average copper absorption is about 12 percent, but is known to vary greatly depending on the body's need for the mineral. Following absorption copper is transported to the liver via the circulatory system by *transcuprein* and *albumin*. Copper leaves the liver as part of the α-globulin transport protein *ceruloplasmin*. Hair and nails contain high amounts of copper. About 2 mg copper daily is excreted as bile. Copper is excreted primarily in the feces (unabsorbed and biliary), though some is present in the urine.

Functions

As a component of ceruloplasmin copper functions as a ferroxidase (releasing iron from storage to transferrin), an amide oxidase, and a superoxide mutase (scavenger of oxygen radicals). As a component of lysyl oxidase in connective tissue copper functions in the maturation of elastin and collagen; hence, contributing to wound healing and maintenance of blood vessel integrity. Tyrosinase, containing copper, functions in the synthesis of the pigment melanin. Copper-containing enzymes function in the synthesis of the hormones norepinephrine and epinephrine. Copper functions in the inactivation of histamine, tyramine, dopamine, and serotonin.

Copper functions in conjunction with iron in the cytochrome series of the electron transport chain. Copper enzymes also play a role in releasing iron from storage and making it available for hematopoiesis. Copper is found in blood-clotting factors.

TABLE 8.9

Good and Rich Sources of Copper

Almonds	Chocolate	Clams
Molasses	Oysters	Peanuts
Raisins	Shrimp	Sunflower seeds
Whole grain breads	Whole grain cereals	Walnuts

Food Sources

Rich sources of copper include organ meats (especially liver), seafoods, nuts, seeds, dried fruits, molasses, whole grains, and chocolate (Table 8.9). Cow's milk, but not that of humans, has a low content of copper. The copper content of drinking water varies, and is high when copper pipes have been utilized.

Dietary Recommendations

The 1989 Estimated Safe and Adequate Daily Dietary Intake of copper for adults is 1.5 to 3 mg. According to NHANES III data, the median daily copper intakes of men and women, 20 to 59 years, in the United States were 1.45 and 1.02 mg, respectively. Many people in our country consume less-than-recommended quantities of copper.

The 1995 *Third Report on Nutrition Monitoring in the United States* classified copper as being a "potential public health issue." This is because in metabolic studies abnormal electrocardiographs have been found in subjects consuming diets low in copper.

Deficiency

Copper deficiency is rare in individuals that consume a wide variety of foods. Symptoms of copper deficiency include microcytic hemochromic anemia, weakness, diarrhea, aching of the joints, neutropenia, leukopenia, poor wound healing, osteoporosis, reduced immune response, hypercholesteremia, arterial aneurysms, heart hypertrophy, and nervous system degeneration. Bone changes observed in infants on long-term total parenteral nutrition (TPN) improved when given copper supplements. Copper status is most commonly evaluated by measuring serum/plasma copper and occasionally ceruloplasmin levels. Erythrocyte superoxide dismutase activity has been proposed for use as a copper status indicator.

Pharmacologic Doses

Reports are not available as to pharmacologic functions of copper.

Toxicity

No adverse effects were observed in humans consuming 0.5 mg copper/kg body weight daily. Reports exist of children getting symptoms of copper toxicity when they accidentally/intentionally ingested copper sulfate intended for use as a pesticide. Early symptoms of copper toxicity include nausea and vomiting. Damage has been observed in the digestive tract, kidneys, liver, and brain due to copper toxicity. These toxic effects may be due to the production of oxygen radicals by copper chelates.

Needs in Exercise

Generally, adults, including athletes in the United States, consume less than recommended amounts of copper. Copper is part of cytochrome oxidase (in the electron transport chain) and superoxide dismutase (free radical scavenger that helps protect tissues from oxidation). Studies exist which do and do not indicate that athletes have different plasma copper or ceruloplasmin concentrations. Plasma copper and ceruloplasmin concentrations may increase, decrease, or remain unchanged during prolonged exercise.

Although some copper is lost in sweat, the increased food intake of individuals who exercise vigorously tends to prevent negative copper balance. Athletes should consume diets that are adequate in copper.

Zinc

Symbol: Zn
Function: Component of many enzymes and proteins, wound healing

Zinc (**Zn**) is a trace mineral (also trace element) that exists only in the Zn^{2+} valence state. The adult body contains 2 to 3 g of zinc, with highest concentrations being found in the liver, pancreas, kidneys, bone, and muscles. High quantities of Zn are also found in the retina of the eye, sperm, prostate, skin, hair, and nails.

Absorption and Metabolism

Zinc is absorbed by passive diffusion and a carrier-mediated transport primarily in the duodenum and jejunum, with the absorption efficiency (usually 10 to 40 percent) being influenced by need. Factors decreasing zinc absorption include pica, low gastric acid secretion, phytates, phosphates, fiber, and perhaps other minerals, such as large doses of iron and calcium. Following absorption, zinc is carried by albumin to the liver. The zinc-binding protein metallothionein appears to regulate zinc metabolism. Zinc is filtered in the kidneys and may be excreted in the urine or in the feces (unabsorbed and biliary excreted zinc).

Function

Zinc functions as a component of over 100 enzymes. In the cell nuclei, zinc-DNA binding proteins (often called "zinc fingers") are observed. Vitamins A and D and several hormones can bind to the zinc-DNA binding proteins, and thus influence gene expression. These proteins are transcription factors. Zinc also plays a role in metallothionein transcription. Proteins are synthesized, requiring zinc, following trauma and sepsis. Zinc is incorporated into the hormone insulin, which plays a role in blood glucose homeostasis. Zinc also functions in the stabilization of membranes and is a component of the bone mineral apatite. Zinc also functions in the disposal of free radicals, behavior and learning, sperm production, immune functioning, taste perception, vision (activating vitamin A), wound healing, and body growth in general.

Food Sources

Rich sources of zinc include oysters, wheat germ, organ meats (especially liver), and poultry. Dairy products, meats, fish, and nuts are good to rich sources of zinc (Table 8.10).

TABLE 8.10

Selected Good and Rich Sources of Zinc

Beef cuts	Chicken cuts	Dairy products
Fish	Fortified cereals	Liver
Oysters	Peanuts	Wheat germ

Dietary Recommendations

The 1989 RDA for zinc is 15 and 12 mg daily for men and women 11+ years of age, respectively. According to NHANES III data, the median daily zinc intakes of men and women, 20 to 59 years, in the United States were 12.7 and 8.3 mg, respectively. Many people consume less-than-recommended quantities of zinc.

The *1995 Third Report on Nutrition Monitoring in the United States* classified zinc as being a "potential public health issue." This is because of the clinical studies suggesting that zinc deficiency, as manifested by growth retardation, has been observed in otherwise apparently healthy children in the United States.

Deficiency

Symptoms of zinc deficiency include anorexia, growth retardation, skin changes, mild anemia, immunologic abnormalities, poor wound healing, impaired taste acuity, abnormal central nervous system development, dwarfism, and hypogonadism. Marginal zinc deficiency has been observed in segments of the United States population, particularly children, women, pregnant women, and the elderly. Zinc status is commonly evaluated by measuring plasma/serum levels of the mineral.

Pharmacologic Doses

Studies are not available as to the effects of pharmacologic doses of zinc other than their use in reversing zinc inadequacies.

Toxicity

Zinc supplements (80 to 300 mg daily) and the consumption of food or drink from galvanized containers have been reported to cause zinc toxicity. Symptoms include nausea, vomiting, diarrhea, central nervous system abnormalities (light-headedness, difficulty with fine finger movement), decreased HDL-cholesterol levels, anemia, neutropenia, and impairment of immune responses. Impairment of copper absorption has been observed in adults taking 18.5 to 25 mg of zinc daily. Chronic ingestion of supplements exceeding 15 mg daily is not recommended.

Needs in Exercise

Zinc is a component of lactate dehydrogenase; hence, zinc deficiency could affect anaerobic muscle performance. Some evidence indicates that zinc supplementation might increase muscle endurance, but other evidence does not. The initial zinc status of the subjects were not determined in these studies, so it is not known whether the individuals originally had suboptimal zinc status. Many individuals, including athletes, have been found to be marginally deficient in zinc.

Stresses of various types, including exercise, stimulate the uptake of zinc by the liver. Low plasma zinc levels often, but not always, observed in athletes during and after exercise may be due to redistribution of zinc in the body. Zinc supplementation at levels exceeding the RDAs is not recommended.

Iodine

Symbol: I
Function: Thyroid hormones

Iodine (*I*, actually I_2), a trace mineral (also trace element), is the oxidized form of iodide (I^-). At one time iodine deficiency was endemic throughout the world, except for the coastal regions. Iodine is found in high concentration in the thyroid gland.

Absorption and Metabolism

Iodine is converted to iodide and almost completely absorbed. About 80 percent of the iodide is utilized for *thyroxine* synthesis. The thyroid-stimulating hormone (TSH), produced by the pituitary, acts on circulating tyrosine-rich thyroglobin making tyrosine available to interact with iodide via iodide peroxidase. A monoiodothyronine is first produced, followed by diiodothyronine, triiodothyronine, and thyroxine. TSH stimulates the thyroid glands to secrete thyroxine; cruciferous vegetables (like cabbage) contain goitrogens which can, in large quantities, inhibit thyroxine release from the thyroid glands. Thyroxine is carried through the circulatory system by the thyroid-binding protein. Once in the target cell, thyroxine is converted to triiodothyronine by 5'-diodinase, which contains selenium. The iodide that is not utilized or sequestered may be filtered by the kidney and excreted via the urine, though some organic iodine is excreted in the feces.

Functions

Iodine functions as a component of the thyroid hormones thyroxine and triiodothyronine. Thyroid hormones influence growth in general, including that of the nervous and skeletal systems. Thyroid hormones are involved in metabolic energy production in most of the cells of the body. Triiodothyronine functions with regard to the regulation of messenger RNA synthesis, which controls protein synthesis.

Food Sources

Selected good and rich sources of iodine are given in Table 8.11. The iodine content of foods is reflective of the iodine content of the soil where plants were grown or animals grazed. The iodine content of soils is highest in land which was once under the ocean. The food processing industry, beginning in 1978, can add iodine to table salt making iodized salt. The box label states whether the salt has been iodized, as in the United States, but not in Canada. Noniodized salt is available for purchase. The iodine content of iodized salt is 76 µg/g.

TABLE 8.11

Selected Good and Rich Sources of Iodine

Iodized table salt
Processed foods containing iodized table salt
Seafoods of all types

Individuals in developed countries get most of their iodine from iodized salt and from sea-foods. Iodized salt is sometimes used as an additive to milk and bakery products.

Dietary Recommendations

The 1989 RDA for iodine is 150 µg daily for males and females 11+ years of age. Most individuals in the United States consume recommended levels of iodine.

Deficiency

Iodine deficiency is the most common, but not the only, cause of *goiter* or enlargement of the thyroid gland. The goiter may be large enough to obstruct the pharynx and damage laryngeal nerves. Severe iodine deficiency in a pregnant woman may cause the infant to be a cretin, which is characterized by physical and mental retardation. Goiter, caused by iodine deficiency, is prevalent in many developing countries. The *1995 Third Report on Nutrition Monitoring in the United States* classified iodine as not being a current public health issue in the United States. Although plasma/serum iodine levels can be measured, plasma/serum concentrations of thyroxine are more often used in the evaluation of iodine (actually thyroxine) status.

Pharmacologic Doses

Reports are not available as to the effects of pharmacologic doses of iodine other than as treatment for the deficiency.

Toxicity

No adverse effects of intakes up to 1 mg daily in children and 2 mg daily in adults have been reported. In Japan, goiter has been induced by consumption of seaweeds, which are rich in iodine (up to 4.5 mg/g dry weight), that are commonly consumed by segments of the population. Thyrotoxicosis has been observed in long-term iodine deficient individuals, having goiters in nodular or paranodular locations, who were given iodine supplements.

Needs in Exercise

Published studies are not available as to the use of iodine as an ergogenic aid.

Selenium

Symbol: Se
Function: Antioxidant

Selenium (*Se*), a trace mineral (also trace element), was first demonstrated to be essential for humans in 1979. Selenium is concentrated in the liver, spleen, and muscles. Selenium exists in the valence states Se^{2+}, Se^{4+}, and Se^{6+}.

Absorption and Metabolism

Selenium is absorbed in the upper small intestine, with the absorption efficiency being dependent upon need. Selenium is transported by VLDLs and LDLs. Selenium is known to exist in tissues as the selenoproteins selenomethionine and selenocysteine. Vitamin B_6

TABLE 8.12

Selected Foods Containing Selenium

Fortified cereals	Liver	Lean meats of all types
Seafood of all types	Whole grain breads	Whole grain cereals

Note: The selenium content of grains and animals is dependent on the selenium content of the soil where the food was grown or the animals grazed.

functions in the joining of selenium and the sulfur-containing amino acids methionine and cysteine. Selenium is excreted primarily in the liver.

Functions

The selenoprotein glutathione peroxidase catalyzes the reduction of hydrogen peroxide and various organic peroxides to water and alcohols. Glutathione peroxidase functions together with other antioxidants and free radical scavengers. Vitamin E also functions in suppressing free radical production, but its site of action is different from that of selenium. Selenium functions in the cytosol and mitochondrial matrix, while vitamin E is present in the membranes. However, selenium functions with vitamin E to protect cell membranes from oxidative damage and aids in the synthesis of immunoglobulins and ubiquinone.

The selenoprotein iodothyronine deiodinase functions in removing iodide from thyroxine producing triiodothyronine. Selenomethionine seems to perform metabolically as methionine. Other selenoproteins which have been isolated from the body include Selenoprotein W (in muscle), Selenoprotein P (in plasma), and sperm capsule selenoprotein; the functions of these selenoproteins have not been elucidated.

Food Sources

Selected foods containing selenium are given in Table 8.12. The selenium content of food varies greatly depending on the content of the soil where plants were grown or animals grazed. Rich sources of selenium are organ meats (especially liver) and seafoods. Lean meats, cereals, and grains are good to rich sources of selenium.

Dietary Recommendations

A RDA for selenium was defined for the first time in 1989, and is 70 and 55 µg for men and women, respectively. The well-balanced North American diet appears to contain adequate amounts of selenium.

The *1995 Third Report on Nutrition Monitoring in the United States* classified selenium as being a "potential public health issue." This is because of several epidemiologic studies which have suggested that selenium status is associated with risk of heart disease and cancer.

Deficiency

Selenium deficiency has been observed in the United States in premature infants and in individuals sustained for months on enteral and parenteral solutions lacking in selenium. Symptoms of selenium deficiency include fragile erythrocytes, cardiomyopathy, growth retardation, decreased spermatogenesis, and skeletal muscle degeneration. In China, selenium deficiency has been associated with Keshan disease. Although selenium supplementation has been demonstrated to control the disease, some features of the disease can not be completely explained on the basis of selenium deficiency. Erythrocyte gluthathione peroxidase activity is commonly utilized in the evaluation of selenium status.

Pharmacologic Doses

Some adverse reactions have been observed when selenium was used in large µg levels in treating selenium deficient individuals.

Toxicity

Selenium toxicity has been observed in individuals having intakes above 750 µg daily as well as those exposed to certain industrial conditions. Hair loss and fingernail changes have been reported in individuals consuming 5 mg of selenium daily from food sources. Thirteen people in the United States developed selenium intoxication after consuming improperly manufactured supplements containing 27.3 mg of selenium per tablet. Fatigue, nausea, diarrhea, nail and hair changes, irritability, and peripheral neuropathy were observed in these individuals. Excessive intakes of selenium are known to interfere with iron, copper, and zinc metabolism.

Needs in Exercise

No significant difference in pre- and 120-h post-race erythrocyte glutathione peroxidase activities were observed in trained athletes; however, the erythrocytes were more suscep- tible to hydrogen peroxide-induced peroxidation after the race than before. Athletes given 100 to 240 µg selenium daily had decreased oxidative damage after exercise as reported in several studies; however, another study indicated that time to exhaustion on a treadmill was not influenced by the supplementation. Selenium supplementation is not recom- mended at levels much above the RDAs because of the toxicities that have been observed at relatively low intake levels.

Fluoride

Symbol: F
Function: Contributes to hardness of teeth and bones

Fluoride (*F*), a trace mineral (also trace element), is the ionized form of fluorine (F_2). Flu- oride is primarily deposited in the skeletal system, particularly the teeth. Some controversy exists as to whether fluoride is an essential mineral for humans; it is definitely a beneficial element for humans because of its positive effects on dental health.

Absorption and Metabolism

Fluoride is readily absorbed in the small intestine at about 80 percent efficiency. From the plasma, fluoride is incorporated into bones and teeth forming *fluorapatite* from hydroxya- patite by substituting for the hydroxyl or the bicarbonate ions. Fluoride is filtered by the kidneys and may be *reabsorbed* or excreted in the urine.

Food Sources

Foods containing high levels of fluoride include seafoods, fish, chicken, and teas (Table 8.13). Many municipalities *fluoridate* their water supply such that the fluoride con- centration is 0.7 to 1.2 mg/L. Fluoride may also be obtained from toothpastes and fluoride supplements and dental topical treatments.

TABLE 8.13

Selected Foods Containing Fluoride

Chicken cuts	Fish	Fluoridated water
Liver	Seafoods of all types	Teas

Functions

Fluoride, as a component of fluorapatite, functions in the prevention of ***dental caries***. Fluoride has been used in the treatment of osteoporosis; however, the vast majority of research studies indicate that there is no correlation between osteoporosis or bone fractures and fluoride intake.

Dietary Recommendations

The 1989 Estimated Safe and Adequate Daily Dietary Intake of fluoride is 1.5 to 4 mg for adults. In 1989, The Food and Nutrition Board National Research Council recommended that public water be fluoridated if the fluoride content of the water is substantially lower than 0.7 mg/L.

The *1995 Third Report on Nutrition Monitoring in the United States* classified fluoride as being a "potential public health issue." This is because of concerns that intakes might be so low as to not provide maximal benefits to some groups, and also that others may be getting enough excessive fluoride to cause mild dental fluorosis.

Deficiency

Individuals lacking sufficient fluoride during their tooth-forming years are more susceptible to dental caries. Serum/plasma levels of fluoride may be utilized in evaluating fluoride status.

Pharmacologic Doses

Pharmacologic doses of fluoride are not recommended because of toxicity problems occurring at relatively low levels. Topical application of some fluorides by dentists to the teeth of children does result in more fluoride being incorporated into tooth enamel, which decreases the incidence of dental caries.

Toxicity

Fluorosis, or chronic fluoride toxicity, affects the functioning of bones and kidneys and perhaps muscles and nerves. *Mottling* of the teeth in children has been observed when as little as 2 mg/kg (or 2 mg/L) concentrations have been consumed from food and drinking water for a period of time. This dental fluorosis is due to hypomineralization of the tooth enamel from excess fluoride reaching the developing teeth.

Needs in Exercise

Fluoride should not be used as an ergogenic aid in that it has adverse effects at relatively low intake levels.

Manganese

Symbol: Mn
Function: Growth, lipid metabolism

Manganese (*Mn*), a trace mineral (also trace element), is somewhat similar in function to magnesium. Manganese is found in the skeletal system as well as the liver, pancreas, and kidneys. Manganese can exist in 11 different oxidation states ranging from –3 to +7; in humans manganese is present as Mn^{2+} and Mn^{3+}.

Absorption and Metabolism

Manganese is rather poorly absorbed (1 to 15 percent) in the small intestine, with iron and cobalt competing for absorption-binding sites. Phytates decrease manganese absorption. Manganese is transported bound to a macroglobin or to transferrin. Absorbed manganese is excreted primarily in the feces after being utilized in bile.

Functions

Manganese is part of the mineral *apatite* in bone, with about 25 percent of the body's manganese being in bone. Manganese is also found in tissues that have high concentrations of mitochondria. Manganese is a component of several enzymes and also acts as an enzyme activator. Enzymes containing manganese include arginase (needed for urea synthesis), glucokinase (enables glucose to enter glycolysis), acetyl CoA carboxylase and isocitrate dehydrogenase (part of tricarboxylic acid cycle), pyruvate carboxylase (needed for carbohydrate synthesis from pyruvate), and superoxide dismutase (breakdown of the superoxide radical). There are a number of manganese-activated enzymes including decarboxylases, transferases, hydrolases, and kinases.

Food Sources

Foods containing manganese include whole grains, legumes, nuts, cereals, teas, and leafy vegetables (Table 8.14).

Dietary Recommendations

The 1989 Estimated Safe and Adequate Daily Dietary Intake for manganese is 2 to 5 mg for adults. Most Americans consume recommended levels of manganese according to data from the *1986 Total Diet Study*.

TABLE 8.14

Selected Foods Containing Manganese

Dried beans	Dried peas	Fortified cereals
"Greens"	Kale	Lettuce
Whole grain breads	Whole grain cereals	Teas

Deficiency

Manganese deficiency has not been observed in noninstitutionalized humans. Deficiency symptoms seen in animals (mice, rats, pigs, cattle) include impaired glucose tolerance, abnormal lipid metabolism, growth retardation, skeletal abnormalities, impaired reproductive performance, and ataxia. Serum/plasma levels are lower in individuals on low-manganese diets and higher in those consuming higher amounts of the mineral. Magnetic resonance imaging (MRI) may be a useful method for monitoring manganese toxicity.

Pharmacologic Doses

Studies involving humans being given pharmacologic doses of manganese are not available.

Toxicity

Manganese toxicity has been reported in miners, and in individuals who habitually consumed water with high manganese content. Adverse effects on the nervous system, similar to those of Parkinson's disease, were reported in miners who had inhaled the manganese as dust. Delayed reaction time, impaired motor coordination, and impaired memory were observed in these miners. In domestic animals, manganese toxicity has been demonstrated to induce iron deficiency as well as depress growth, depress appetite, and alter brain function.

Needs in Exercise

Although it is known that manganese does play a role in the detoxification of free radicals, manganese supplementation is not recommended.

Chromium

Symbol: Cr
Function: Optimal insulin action

Chromium (*Cr*), a trace mineral (also trace element), was once called the "glucose tolerance factor." Chromium is present in the body in very low quantities, primarily in the liver, kidneys, testis, bone, and spleen. Chromium has several valence states with Cr^{3+} being the most stable in biological systems.

Absorption and Metabolism

Chromium is absorbed in the small intestine at 1 to 3 percent efficiency. Vitamin C may enhance and phytates may hinder chromium absorption. Chromium is transported by albumin and transferrin. Absorbed chromium is excreted in the urine.

Functions

Chromium is essential for optimal *insulin* action, and thus, influences blood glucose homeostasis. Chromium has been shown to increase growth in mice, rats, and guinea pigs. Studies exist that show chromium increases serum HDL-cholesterol and decreases serum triacyglycerol concentrations of humans, while other studies show no effects.

Chromium has been reported to enhance RNA synthesis in rats and mice. Several studies have indicated that chromium supplementation of cattle following market-transit stress positively influenced specific immune responses.

TABLE 8.15

Foods Containing Chromium

Liver	Meats of all types	Potatoes
Vegetable oils	Whole grain breads	Whole grain cereals

Food Sources

Organ meats (especially liver), brewer's yeast, potatoes, and whole grains are rich sources of chromium (Table 8.15). The refining of foods, as in milling, decreases the chromium content; however, the processing of foods and beverages in stainless steel containers may add chromium to the food product.

Dietary Recommendations

The Estimated Safe and Adequate Daily Dietary Intake for chromium is 50 to 200 µg for adults. The average chromium content of self-selected diets of adults according to a 1985 study is 25 to 33 µg daily.

Deficiency

Chromium deficiency has been reported in a few patients on long-term total parenteral nutrition (TPN); insulin resistance was observed in these patients. Deficiency symptoms in animals include impaired glucose tolerance, impaired growth, elevated serum cholesterol and triglyceride levels, increased aortic plaque formation, and decreased fertility (especially in males). Serum/plasma chromium levels, though near nondetectable levels in healthy individuals, are utilized in evaluating status.

Pharmacologic Doses

Chromium supplements (100 to 200 µg daily) have been found to be beneficial only to those who are deficient in chromium. Supplementation at this level seem to have no adverse effects.

Toxicity

Chromium toxicity has been reported due to chronic exposure of humans to airborne chromium compounds. Toxicity systems include allergic dermatitis, skin lesions, and increased incidence of lung cancer. Chromium toxicity due to diet or supplement intakes has not been reported.

Needs in Exercise

Individuals who exercise strenuously have been reported to have higher urinary levels of chromium than those not exercising. Theoretically, chromium could improve insulin action, and thus, enhance carbohydrate and amino acid metabolism. Several studies have been conducted on the effects of *chromium picolinate* supplementation on body composition. Early reports suggested that chromium picolinate would favorable increase the loss of body fat; however, these studies had flaws. The findings were not confirmed in subsequent well-controlled research studies. Numerous studies indicate that chromium picolinate supplementation has no effect on percent body fat, lean body mass, or strength.

Molybdenum

Symbol: Mo
Function: Catabolism of purines, aldehydes, and sulfites

Molybdenum (*Mo*) is a trace mineral (also trace element) whose essentiality was first recognized in 1953. Molybdenum is found in the liver, kidneys, bones, and skin. Molybdenum has four valence states ranging from Mo^{3+} to Mo^{6+}.

Absorption and Metabolism

Molybdenum is absorbed primarily in the distal small intestine by carrier-mediated transport and passive diffusion at 40 to 100 percent efficiency. Molybdenum is transported as a protein-bound complex. Molybdenum is excreted in the urine as well as via the bile in the feces.

Functions

Molybdenum functions as a component of the oxidation-reduction enzymes xanthine oxidase (breakdown of purines), aldehyde oxidase (breakdown of aldehydes), and sulfite oxidases (breakdown of sulfites); these three enzymes also contain iron and riboflavin. Molybdenum also activates adenylate cyclase in the brain, cardiac muscle, renal tissues, and erythrocytes, but not in the testis.

Food Sources

Molybdenum is found in legumes, whole grains, dairy products, and dark green leafy vegetables (Table 8.16). Molybdenum is lost during the milling of grains.

Dietary Recommendations

The 1989 Estimated Safe and Adequate Daily Dietary Intake of molybdenum for adults is 75 to 250 µg. Individuals consuming unrefined foods have adequate intakes of molybdenum.

Deficiency

Experimentally produced molybdenum deficiency in goats caused decreased food consumption, retarded weight gain, impaired reproduction, and shortened life expectancy. A patient on long-term total parenteral nutrition (TPN) had hypermethioninemia, increased urinary excretion of sulfite and xanthine, and decreased urinary uric acid levels in addition to amino acid intolerance, irritability, and coma. Treatment with the equivalent of 163 µg molybdenum daily resulted in clinical improvement and normalization of urinary values. A genetic sulfite oxidase deficiency has also been described.

TABLE 8.16

Food Containing Molybdenum

Brussels sprouts	Dairy products	Dried beans
Dried peas	"Greens"	Kale
Spinach	Whole grain breads	Whole grain cereals

Pharmacologic Doses

Studies are not available on the pharmacologic effects of molybdenum.

Toxicity

Excess molybdenum intakes (10 to 15 g daily) may result in an increased incidence of gout-like syndrome associated with elevated blood uric acid level and xanthine oxidase activity. Molybdenum supplements, at doses of 0.54+ mg daily, were antagonistic with regard to copper metabolism.

Needs in Exercise

Studies are not available as to ergogenic effects of molybdenum.

9

Other Substances in Foods and Exercise

Several substances naturally present in foods are dietary requirements of animals or microbes, but their essentiality in humans has not been proven. These substances are referred to as *Other Substances in Foods*. Some of the other substances in foods are categorized as nutrients essential for some higher animals, but not proven to be required by normal humans. Substances in this category include taurine, carnitine, myo-inositol, arsenic, nickel, silicon, boron, cadmium, lead, lithium, tin, vanadium, and cobalt. The other two categories are Growth Factors and Coenzymes as well as Substances with No Known Essentiality in Animals and Humans.

Several of these Other Substances in Foods may have exercise-related functions. These substances are often thought to function as ergogenic aids. Ergon means to increase work or potential for work. This chapter includes information regarding the more common Other Substances in Foods that are often utilized as ergogenic aids. Most of these substances have not been proven to benefit physical performance.

Nutrients Essential for Some Higher Animals That May Be Related to Athletic Performance in Humans

Taurine

Taurine, a water-soluble substance, is also known as β-aminoethanesulfonic acid. Taurine has long been considered an end-product of protein metabolism. Taurine can be synthesized in humans from dietary cysteine or methionine with vitamin B_6 also being needed. Taurine is a vitamin for cats and laboratory animals. Taurine is abundant in muscle foods of all types including shellfish.

Taurine is found in high concentrations in muscles, the nervous system, and platelets. Taurine is needed for the formation of bile salts in humans. Reports exists, though controversial, that taurine may have other functions.

Plasma and urinary levels of taurine are lower in pre-term and full-term infants fed synthetic formulas without added taurine and in infants maintained by parenteral nutrition than in breast-fed infants. Cow's milk is much lower in taurine than in human milk. However, taurine supplementation of infant formulas has failed to have an impact on growth, nitrogen retention, or serum protein levels. Dietary essentialness of taurine has not been demonstrated in humans.

Carnitine

Carnitine, a water-soluble substance, is known chemically as β-hydroxy-[γ-N-trimethyl-ammonia] butyrate. In 1947, G. S. Fraenkel found that the meal worm *Tenebrio molitor* required a growth factor present in the charcoal filtrate of yeast. In 1948, G. S. Fraenkel and H. E. Carter found that vitamin B_T and carnitine were the same.

Carnitine is found primarily in muscle. Rich food sources of carnitine are those of animal origin (particularly meats and dairy products).

Carnitine functions in the transport of long-chain fatty acids into the mitochondrial matrix for energy production. Carnitine can also function as a nonspecific methyl group donor, thus sparing other methyl group donors such as methionine. Carnitine may be needed for fatty acid synthesis.

The first case of carnitine deficiency in humans was reported in 1973 by A. G. Engel and C. Angelini; a young woman had progressively worsening muscular weakness. A muscle biopsy showed that there were lipid droplets in abnormal spaces in the muscle fibers. By 1975, six cases of carnitine deficiency had been reported in humans, and two of the patients were treated with oral carnitine and showed improvement. Over 100 individuals have been diagnosed as having a genetic carnitine deficiency. Symptoms of the deficiency include muscular weakness, lipid infiltration of skeletal muscle, cardiomyopathy, severe hypoglycemia, lower than normal ability to increase ketogenesis during fasting, and lower than normal concentrations of muscle and plasma carnitine. The deficiency has been reported in individuals on long-term total parenteral nutrition (TPN) and those with some kidney conditions. Improvement in the symptoms has been reported in some, but not all patients given oral carnitine. Some studies indicate that oral carnitine increases oxygen consumption levels in endurance athletes while other studies report no effects. Occasional diarrhea has been reported in individuals given large amounts of carnitine.

Carnitine deficiency has also been reported in fetal calves, neonatal rats, and guinea pigs. Symptoms include depressed long-chain fatty acid oxidation and excessive triglyceride synthesis. Well-nourished adults can synthesize sufficient quantities of carnitine in their livers and kidneys from the amino acids lysine and methionine. Newborns seem to have reduced reserves of carnitine and a low capacity for synthesizing carnitine. Human milk has been reported to contain enough carnitine to meet the needs of infants. Infants fed soy-based formulas or those on total parenteral nutrition (TPN) receive no exogenous carnitine and have low plasma carnitine levels. Some researchers believe that carnitine is a vitamin for the newborn, particularly the pre-term. Currently, carnitine is not considered to be a vitamin for humans.

Carnitine transports long-chain fatty acids into the mitochrondria. No effect was observed on free fatty acid utilization, $\dot{v}O_2$ max, anaerobic threshold, exercise time to exhaustion, or work output on a cycle ergometer (60 min) of subjects given 500 mg carnitine supplements daily for four months. Daily consumption of 6 g carnitine for 10 days had little effect on resting oxygen consumption. Supplementation of endurance athletes increased $\dot{v}O_2$ max and reduced the respiratory quotient in some studies, but not in others. Conflicting reports have been published as to the effects of carnitine on exercise performance; however, most reports indicate that carnitine supplementation had no beneficial effects.

Myo-inositol

Myo-inositol, or cyclohexanehexol, is a water-soluble substance having a formula similar to glucose. Myo-inositol is sometimes called meso-inositol. There are nine isomers of inositol, but only myo-inositol is biologically effective. Myo-inositol is found in foods usually as inositol phospholipids. Foods particularly rich in myo-inositol include fruits, meats, milk, nuts, vegetables, whole grains, and yeasts. In plants, myo-inositol is part of phytic acid or inositol hexaphosphate, and in animals it is part of membrane phospholipids. Myo-inositol is sometimes referred to as muscle sugar.

Myo-inositol functions as a component of phosphatidylinositol and polyphosphoinositides (cephalins) in cellular and subcellular membranes. Myo-inositol apparently has a lipotropic action via its effects of lipoproteins. Phosphatidylinositol appears to function as cellular mediators of signal transduction, metabolic regulation, and growth. Myo-inositol triphosphate seems to function in mobilizing intracellular calcium.

Myo-inositol deficiency has been demonstrated in mice, gerbils, and chicks where symptoms include intestinal lipodystrophy, alopecia, poor growth and lactation, encephalomalacia, triglyceride accumulation, and abnormal fatty acid metabolism. Deficiency of myo-inositol has not been demonstrated in humans. Myo-inositol is found in many foods. Myo-inositol can be synthesized from glucose by many of the tissues in the body. The kidney seems to be the main regulator of inositol concentrations in humans as it can synthesize as well as breakdown myo-inositol. The intestinal microflora can synthesize inositol and contribute to the metabolic pool. Human breast milk and colostrum are rich in myo-inositol. The American Academy of Pediatrics has recommended that myo-inositol be included in infant formulas at levels equal to or greater than those of human milk.

The metabolism of myo-inositol appears to be altered in individuals with diabetes mellitus, chronic renal diseases, respiratory distress syndrome, galactosemia, and multiple sclerosis. Large amounts of myo-inositol given orally seems to be nontoxic, although its use in situations where inositol metabolism is impaired has been questioned. Excess dietary myo-inositol has been shown to reduce motor conduction velocities in rats.

Research linking myo-inositol supplementation and exercise performance has not been published.

Arsenic

Arsenic (As) is found in tissues, fluids, hair, and nails of humans. Most tissues in adults contain 0.04 to 0.09 µg/g dry weight of arsenic. Arsenic, as arsenobetaine, is readily absorbed and rapidly excreted by humans.

Arsenic deficiency has been observed in rats, chicks, goats, and minipigs where it has been demonstrated to influence reproductive performance and growth in general. Most human foods contain <0.3 µg/g dry weight of arsenic. Seafoods contain more arsenic than other foods. The suggested adult human requirement for arsenic is 12 to 25 µg daily as extrapolated from data from animals.

Nausea, vomiting, diarrhea, and severe abdominal pains have been attributed to acute arsenic poisoning in humans. Chronic toxicity of arsenic causes muscular aching, skin and mucosal changes, peripheral neuropathy, confusion, and convulsions.

Nickel

Nickel (Ni) is found in all animal tissues, fluids, and hair. Most nickel is not absorbed by the intestinal tract and is excreted in the feces; however, some nickel is absorbed and excreted in the urine.

Nickel deficiency has been produced in rats, chickens, goats, sheep, cattle, and minipigs; decreased growth and depressed hematopoiesis are among the changes observed in the deficiency state. Some evidence indicates that nickel may function in specific metalloenzymes such as urease. Nickel may facilitate the absorption of iron.

Foods that are high in nickel include nuts, cocoa, legumes, spinach, and hydrogenated solid shortening. The canning of some fruits and vegetables increases their nickel content. Reports exist that the nickel intake of adults in the United States is 200 to 600 µg daily. The estimated nickel requirement for humans, as calculated using data from chicks, is about 35 µg daily.

Nickel dermatitis is a common symptom of nickel toxicity in humans. Some individuals may be sensitive to nickel. Nickel toxicity has been observed in individuals on total parenteral nutrition (TPN) solutions contaminated with nickel; symptoms included cardiac and uterine malfunction and allergic reactions. Deficiencies of other nutrients (iron, copper, zinc) may be exacerbated by high nickel intakes in animals.

Silicon

Silicon (Si), a trace element, can form organosilicon compounds. Silicon is found in the body almost entirely as monosilicic acid and is freely diffusible throughout tissue fluid. The highest silicon concentrations are found in the aorta, trachea, tendons, bones, skin, and hair. Most of the small portion of silicon that is absorbed is excreted in the urine.

Rats and chicks have been observed to have larger increases in growth when silicon was added to the diet. Skeletal development has been reported to be retarded in silicon-deficient chicks and rats. The importance of silicon in bone, articular cartilage, and connective tissue activities has been demonstrated in chicks.

Silicon is found in unrefined whole grains, root vegetables, and beer. The daily human requirement for silicon, as estimated using animal data, is 2 to 5 mg.

Silicon toxicity has been reported in miners. Silica particles stimulate a fibrogenic reaction in the lungs as well as the rest of the body. Asbestos is a complex fibrous silicate. Prolonged exposure to asbestos causes lung problems and peritoneal cancer. In domestic animals, silicon can be deposited as calculi in the kidneys, bladder, and urethra, but whether this also occurs in humans is not known.

Boron

Boron (B), a trace element, may be of importance in bone metabolism. The boron that is present in foods is rapidly and efficiently absorbed (about 90 percent efficiency). Boron is found in highest concentrations in bone, spleen, and the thyroid glands. Boron is excreted primarily in the liver.

Boron deprivation depresses growth and elevates plasma alkaline phosphatase activity (needed for conversion of organic to inorganic phosphorus) in chicks, particularly those fed inadequate amounts of vitamin D. In chicks, boron has been shown to normalize the abnormalities associated with magnesium deficiency. Boron has been suggested to alter parathormone activity in rats. Therefore, boron may influence calcium, phosphorus, magnesium, and vitamin D metabolism.

Plant-derived foods are high in boron content, as are beer, wine, and drinking water in some locations. Humans likely obtain adequate amounts of boron. The development of problems similar to those observed in boron-deficient animals has been observed in individuals that received long-term total parenteral nutrition. Some evidence exists that boron may enhance or even mimic some of the positive effects seen with estrogen repletion in postmenopausal women.

Boron toxicity signs include nausea, diarrhea, dermatitis, lethargy, and riboflavinurea. Teratogenic abnormalities of the skeletal system have also been reported due to boron toxicity.

Boron supplementation has been associated with optimizing bone mineralization, which is of importance to the athlete. Boron has been advertised as an anabolic steroid, which it is not. Boron supplementation of male body builders has been shown not to affect lean body mass or muscle strength.

Other Trace Elements

Evidence exists that cadmium (Cd), lead (Pb), lithium (Li), tin (Sn), and vanadium (V) may be of importance to growth and reproductive performance in rats; however, insufficient data are available to draw conclusions with regard to humans. Cadmium, lead, lithium, tin, and vanadium are found in many foods and frequently in drinking water, so low intakes would be observed infrequently. The concentrations of these elements in foods is dependent on that of the soil where the plants were grown or the animals grazed. Vanadium has been advertised as being an anabolic steroid, which it is not. Otherwise, research is not available as to the ergogenic effects of these five trace elements.

Cobalt (Co) is of importance to humans as a component of vitamin B_{12}. Unlike some higher animals, particularly ruminants, humans are unable to synthesize vitamin B_{12} utilizing cobalt.

Cadmium, lead, lithium, tin, vanadium, and cobalt are generally toxic at relatively low levels. Hence, the taking of supplements containing these six trace elements is not recommended.

Coenzymes, Growth Factors, Amino Acids, and Buffers That May Be Related to Athletic Performance in Humans

Several coenzymes, growth factors, amino acids, and buffers have been suggested to improve athletic performance in humans. These include Coenzyme Q_{10}, creatine, arginine and its metabolic derivatives, aspartate and asparagine, branched-chain amino acids, inosine, and bicarbonate, phosphate, and citrate salts (buffers).

Coenzyme Q_{10}

Coenzyme Q_{10} (CoQ_{10}), ubiquinone, is a lipid found in the mitochondria of cells where ATP is produced. CoQ_{10} functions in oxidative phosphorylation and as a reduction-oxidation carrier. CoQ_{10} is an antioxidant. CoQ_{10} is actually a form of CoQ. Foods that are rich in CoQ_{10} include soybeans, animal tissues, and many of the vegetable oils.

High concentrations of CoQ_{10} are found in the heart. CoQ_{10} has been used therapeutically for treatment of cardiovascular disease. CoQ_{10} has been suggested for use by endurance athletes because of the increased oxygen uptake and physical performance observed in cardiac patients.

Some studies have reported positive effects of taking CoQ_{10} supplements on exercise performance, while others reported no effects. Different exercise measurements were utilized in the various studies. Daily doses of 60 to 100 mg have been associated with enhancement of exercise performance after aerobic endurance exercise in trained and untrained adults. Most studies were not "blind" and had low subject numbers. Additional well-designed studies are needed on the effects of CoQ_{10} supplementation on athletic performance.

Creatine

Creatine exists as free creatine and as *creatine phosphate* (also called phosphocreatine), a high-energy compound, in skeletal muscle. Creatine phosphate is converted to ATP plus creatine by the enzyme creatine phosphokinase.

The creatine reserve in muscle represents a combination of that from diet and from synthesis within the body. Meats, fish, and animal products contain creatine. Creatine can be synthesized from the amino acids glycine, arginine, and methionine primarily in the liver, kidneys, and pancreas. During short-term muscular contractions (up to about 15 seconds) creatine phosphate restores rapidly diminishing ATP levels before the majority of the energy is generated from the energy-yielding stores of carbohydrates and fats.

In that creatine serves as a short-term high-energy compound with phosphate, increased stores of creatine may help prolong exercise performance. Twelve studies have reported positive effects of *creatine supplementation* on short-term, intense exercise performance, while six studies report no effects. Creatine supplementation tends to increase lean body mass by 1 to 2 kg in adults. Creatine supplementation, particularly along with resistance training, seems to be beneficial with regard to increased muscle strength and hypertrophy; this finding has been observed in many studies. It is important that individuals taking any protein including creatine increase their water consumption. Creatine appears to be relatively nontoxic. Several research studies have been conducted the last few years on creatine's effects on exercise performance and additional findings are forthcoming. Creatine, taken with additional water, appears to be beneficial with regard to exercise performance.

Arginine, Ornithine, and Citrulline

The amino acid arginine and its metabolites ornithine and citrulline are sometimes advocated by the media as ergogenic aids that stimulate the release of growth hormone (or somatotrophin) which enhances muscle growth. Humans obtain sufficient arginine and ornithine from protein-containing foods.

Arginine and ornithine infusion has been shown to release significant amounts of growth hormone, though research finding no effects has also been reported. Arginine supplementation has been shown to increase creatine synthesis and to reduce ammonia levels in subjects induced to high ammonia concentrations. The reduction of ammonia toxicity in the muscle may reduce fatigue. Side effects of stomach cramping and diarrhea have been reported by some subjects. Daily doses of 200 to 500 mg/kg body weight seem to be nontoxic. Conflicting results have been reported on the effects of arginine, ornithine, and citrulline on body composition and muscular strength.

Aspartate and Asparagine

The nonessential amino acid *aspartate*, as its potassium or magnesium salt, has been reported to lower the accumulation of ammonia in the blood during exercise, and thus, serve as an antifatigue agent. However, this usage has been refuted.

Aspartic acid and its amide *asparagine* can be synthesized in the body. Glutamic acid is transaminated, forming aspartic acid. Aspartic acid is involved in urea synthesis. It is this function that has been suggested to lower blood ammonia concentration. Asparagine, via its involvement with intracellular magnesium metabolism, may interact with ATP stability. Studies have indicated conflicting results on the effects of aspartic acid as well as asparagine on athletic performance, particularly muscular fatigue.

Branched-Chain Amino Acids

Leucine, isoleucine, and *valine* are branched-chain amino acids which have been proposed to improve exercise performance with regard to endurance by preventing the increase of free tryptophan in the plasma during exercise. Free tryptophan elevates brain serotonin and fatigue. Conflicting reports have been published regarding the effects of branched-chain amino acids on exercise performance.

Inosine

The nucleoside *inosine* is a DNA and RNA precursor. Inosine has been advocated to increase adenosine synthesis, and thus, provide more ATP.

Inosine, given parenterally, has been shown to have therapeutic benefits in some cardiac conditions. Human supplementation studies indicate that inosine does not have ergogenic effects. Excess inosine is metabolized to uric acid and can, thus, contribute to the development of gout.

Bicarbonate, Phosphate, and Citrate Salts (Buffers)

The body has a buffering system controlled chiefly by *bicarbonates* which functions in keeping the blood slightly alkaline, even in exercise. Lactic acid, formed during anaerobic glycolysis during exercise, leads to muscle fatigue and even acidosis. Bicarbonate salts are buffering agents which can increase alkaline reserves in exercising subjects.

Several studies have reported beneficial effects on physical performance with sodium bicarbonate loading, while other studies showed no effect. Some subjects had nausea, bloating, and diarrhea after consumption of sodium bicarbonate. *Sodium citrate*, at 0.5 g/kg body weight, does not seem to cause gastrointestinal distress. Some evidence exists that the positive effects may be due to sodium itself. Large amounts of water should be taken with bicarbonates. Chronic use of bicarbonates may be dangerous.

Phosphates are also body buffers. Phosphate loading was discussed in the section on phosphorus in Chapter 7.

Citrates also function as buffers. Citrates are better tolerated than bicarbonates at high doses.

Bicarbonates, phosphates, and citrates are buffers. These buffers may improve pH balance and improve performance with regard to exercises which are short-term, repetitive, and exhaustive.

Substances Not Determined Essential for Animals or Humans That May Be Related to Athletic Performance in Humans

Several substances not determined essential for animals or humans may affect exercise performance. These substances include dimethylglycine, lecithin, oryzanoles and ferulic acid, octacosanol, gamma hydroxybutyrate and hydroxymethylbutyrate, glandulars, Smilax compounds, yohimbine, ginseng, bioflavonoid derivatives, glutathione, carotenoids, bee pollen, caffeine, and alcohol.

Dimethylglycine

Dimethylglycine originally was isolated from grain germs and plant seeds. *Pangamic acid,* is an ill-defined mixture of dimethylglycine and sorbitol, often referred to as vitamin B_{15} although it is not a true vitamin.

Dimethylglycine is a methyl group donor. Methyl group donors are important in metabolism including that in muscle. Although some studies indicate beneficial effects of dimethylglycine on blood lactic acid levels, most studies report no effect. Large doses of dimethylglycine can be converted to nitrososarcosine, a weak carcinogen.

Lecithin

Lecithin is phosphatidylcholine. The body can easily synthesize lecithin from choline. Choline, a vitamin, was discussed in Chapter 6. Lecithin supplements may be used to increase plasma choline levels.

Oryzanoles and Ferulic Acid

Oryzanoles are plant sterols resulting from the processing of rice bran oil. Oryzanoles occur as esters of *ferulic acid*. Oryzanoles and ferulic acid function as antioxidants. Oryzanoles and ferulic acid are proposed to stimulate growth in humans. Ergogenic effects of oryzanoles and ferulic acid have not been reported.

Octacosanol

Octacosanol is a long-chain (C_{28}) waxy alcohol found in plants, especially wheat germ oil. Improved endurance and reaction times have been reported due to octacosanol supplementation. One study reported no beneficial effects of octacosanol on physical performance.

Gamma Hydroxybutyrate and Hydroxymethylbutyrate

Gamma hydroxybutyrate has been promoted as a potent releaser of growth hormone. Gamma hydroxybutyrate is a known hallucinogenic and has been banned.

Hydroxymethylbutyrate is a metabolite of leucine's ketoacid ketoisocaproate. One study reports that hydroxymethylbutyrate supplementation for four weeks increased bench press strength, lean mass, and body fat loss in men undergoing resistance training.

Glandulars

Glandular extracts from the adrenal, ovary, pancreas, pituitary, prostate, and spleen are used to stimulate the tissues and glands of the body. These extracts have not been reported to be needed by the body. These extracts seem not to function as ergogenic aids.

Smilax Compounds

Smilax products are derived from the herb *Smilax officinalis* that contains steroids similar to testosterone and estrogen. These products include sarsaspogenin, sitosterol, smilagein, and stigmasterol. These products are advocated as boosting existing hormone levels and substituting for anabolic steroids. Research documenting the anabolic effectiveness of these products on physical performance has not been published even though the products are advertised as natural forms of testosterone.

Yohimbine

Yohimbine is an extract of the bark of the Yohimbe tree (*Pausinystalia yohimbe*). Yohimbine is advertised as a natural source of testosterone or a testosterone enhancer. Yohimbine has been utilized in treating impotence. Yohimbine's effectiveness as either an anabolic steroid or an ergogenic aid has not been proven.

Ginsengs

Ginseng supplementation is a revered custom in many Asian countries. The herb ginseng is said to promote vitality and prolong life. A variety of forms of Chinese and Korean (*Panax ginseng*), American (*Panax quinquefolium*), and Siberian (*Eleutherococcus senticosus*) ginsengs are available, including root extracts. These ginsengs have been proposed to spare glycogen and increase fatty acid oxidation. Oral or injected ginsengs have been reported to increase endurance and reduce fatigue in exercised animals. These effects of ginsengs in animals have encouraged the use of ginseng as an ergogenic aid in humans. Human studies have not shown positive effects when subjects were given 200 to 2,000 mg ginseng root or placebo daily for four to nine weeks. Ginseng safety has been well documented; however, possible estrogenic activities of ginseng have been observed in some individuals.

Bioflavonoid Derivatives

Several herbs contain phenolic antioxidants which are bioflavonoid derivatives. These include **green tea** (*Camellia sinensis*) and *Ginkgo biloba*. Studies are lacking as to the effectiveness of these bioflavonoid derivatives on physical performance.

Glutathione

Glutathione functions in oxidation-reduction reactions. Improved and no change in endurance performance has been reported in animals given glutathione intraperitoneally.

Carotenoids

Carotenoids can be converted to vitamin A as discussed in Chapter 6. Carotenoids also function as **antioxidants**. Carotenoids seem to enhance immune function. Epidemiologic studies indicate that high intakes of carotenoid-containing fruits and vegetables are associated with decreased risk of cancer.

Strenuous exercise may raise oxygen consumption with an increase in the production of free radicals. Carotenoids may protect tissues against oxidative damage. In most research involving exercise-induced lipid peroxidation, β-carotene was used along with other antioxidants, making it difficult to ascertain if β-carotene or any other substance was responsible for any observed beneficial results.

Bee Pollen

Bee pollen contains various vitamins and minerals which may participate as cofactors in energy cycles. Several studies have indicated that bee pollen has no effect on physical performance.

Caffeine

Caffeine is a methylxanthine found in coffee, tea, guarana, kola nut, chocolate, and some soft drinks. Caffeine is not an essential nutrient. Effects of caffeine include stimulation of the nervous system, diuresis, lipolysis, and gastric acid secretion. Particularly due to the lipolysis stimulation function, some athletes use caffeine as an ergogenic aid.

Over 30 studies have shown that caffeine enhances exercise performance, while no effect was reported in over 30 studies. Some studies divided subjects into caffeine responders and nonresponders. The general consensus of research indicates that caffeine at doses of 3-6 mg/kg body weight may enhance almost any type of exercise performance in caffeine responders. Central nervous system stimulation by caffeine may also help performance. Generally, the effectiveness of caffeine is accentuated by abstinence for about four days and ingestion three to four hours prior to the event.

The ingestion of over five cups of coffee may produce urinary caffeine levels unacceptable for competition. Side effects of caffeine include diuresis, which can lead to dehydration, and stomach upset. Excess and chronic consumption of caffeine can cause anxiety, nervousness, shaking of the hands, and even heart arrhythmias and memory impairment.

Ethanol

Moderate *ethanol* (frequently referred to as simply *alcohol*) consumption may be associated with reduced risk of coronary heart disease and increased blood HDL-cholesterol concentrations. Ethanol consumption in habitual male exercisers was reported to increase blood HDL–cholesterol levels in one study. In another study involving premenopausal exercising women, no effect on these variables was observed. At the present time, ethanol intake can not be recommended to beneficially alter lipid/lipoprotein profiles.

Ethanol is a mild diuretic and causes dehydration. It is important that an exercising individual remain hydrated. Even moderate ethanol consumption is not recommended without adequate fluid replacement. Ethanol is a poor substrate for energy metabolism during exercise.

Energy Requirements

Energy Requirements

Energy is the capacity to do work. Food energy must be supplied regularly to individuals for their survival and is necessary for the maintenance of human life. Food energy is also needed for muscle contraction. In nutrition, energy expenditure refers to the manner in which the body utilizes the energy obtained via the metabolism of the energy-yielding nutrients carbohydrates, lipids (fats), and proteins. The body is about 40 percent efficient in capturing the energy from the catabolism (breakdown) of the energy-yielding nutrients. The cells of the body do not use the energy-yielding nutrients in the diet for their immediate energy supply. Rather, adenosine triphosphate (*ATP*), a high-energy compound, is the fuel for energy requiring reactions. The potential energy stored in ATP molecules provides the chemical energy for biological work. Energy released during ATP hydrolysis activates other energy-requiring molecules. ATP is the "energy currency" of the cell. *Creatine phosphate*, a high-energy compound, serves as an energy reservoir for the body, functioning in the regeneration of ATP. Adipose tissue is also a long-term energy reserve.

The amount of energy in foodstuffs is generally expressed as *calories* (actually kilocalories). The net caloric yield values are 4 cal/g for carbohydrates, 4 cal/g for proteins, and 9 cal/g for lipids. Most foods contain varying portions of these three energy-yielding nutrients as well as water. The amount of energy stored in ATP is equal to about 7.3 kcal/mol.

Carbohydrates in the typical American diet contribute 51 percent of the total dietary calories consumed; lipids, typically fats and oils, contribute 34 percent of total calories; and protein contributes the remaining 15 percent of calories consumed. In our "Western" American diet, much of the carbohydrate is refined sugars, lipids are animal fats and refined vegetable oils, and protein is usually of high quality, derived primarily from animal sources. In the diets of people in developing countries, most calories are supplied by naturally occurring sugars and complex carbohydrates. Calories supplied by animal fat and refined oils are greatly reduced.

Caloric intakes or energy intakes of an individual can be estimated by adding up the calories of each food item consumed by that person. *Caloric expenditures* or energy expenditures can be estimated utilizing tables based on body size, gender, and physical activity level. *Energy balance* is maintained when energy intake is equal to energy output. When intake is greater than output for a period of time, the individual gains weight and may become overweight or even obese. When an individual's energy output is greater than the intake for a period of time, the individual will lose weight and may become underweight. One of the Dietary Guidelines for Americans is to "balance the food you eat with physical activity." Maintenance of energy balance contributes to health in adults by minimizing the risk for developing many common health problems. Energy balance is an important goal for individuals who want a long, healthy life. Optimal energy intake and output is especially of importance to physically active individuals in that it is necessary for optimal performance.

10

Assessment of Energy Intake

The body gets its energy from foods, beverages, and some types of supplements that are consumed. Dietary intake estimations include the collection of information on the quantity of each food item an individual consumes. Food composition tables, including those that are computerized, listing the energy and nutrient content of each food, are utilized in calculating energy and nutrient intakes. The U.S. Department of Agriculture's *Handbook of Food Composition* (http://www.nal.usda.gov/fnic/foodcomp) is considered to be the gold standard for food composition. However, many nutrient composition tables are available which are more easily utilized by consumers. Great variability exists with regard to the energy and nutrient content of one sample of a food to another sample of the same food. These composition values are estimations at best. Information as to energy and nutrient content is also found in the **Nutrition Facts** portion of *food labels*.

Hunger, Appetite, and Satiety

Hunger, appetite, and satiety affect energy intake as a component of food intake. **Hunger** is the physiological need to eat. Hunger is influence by heredity. **Appetite** is the psychological desire to eat. Appetite is a learned behavior. Appetite is influenced by some of the sensory attributes of foods — thinking about, seeing, and smelling foods. When food is ample, as it is to most individuals in Western countries, appetite triggers eating rather than hunger. Some drugs may suppress appetite. **Satiety** is the sense of feeling full. The **hypothalamus** helps regulate satiety. The hypothalamus responds to blood glucose concentrations as well as other factors such as amino acids and fatty acids in the blood and various hormones. The hypothalamus may also respond to fat cell size and number.

   Social customs and culture also influence food intake. Food selection is influenced by many factors including culture, ethnicity, heredity, family traditions, religion, socioeconomic level, educational level, occupation, rural-urban residence, peer influences, sensory attributes of foods, convenience and availability, health beliefs, current health status, nutritional knowledge, and idiosyncrasies.

Calories

The amount of energy that is consumed by the body is measured in calories. A *calorie* is the amount of heat needed to raise the temperature of one gram of water 1° Celsius. Likewise, one kilocalorie is the amount of heat needed to raise the temperature of 1 kilogram (kg) of water 1° Celsius. In nutrition, Calorie (or calorie, cal) is used to mean a kilocalorie (kcal), so calorie is really a misnomer. The joule (J) is the accepted international unit of

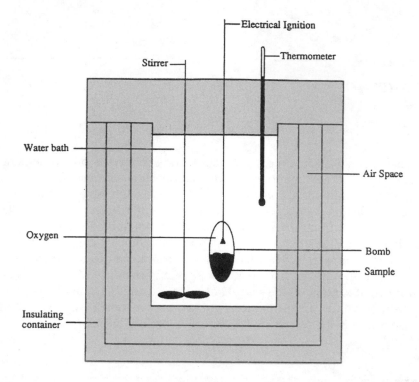

FIGURE 10.1

Cross-section of a bomb calorimeter showing essential features. Reprinted with permission from CRC Press. Berdanier, C.D., Advanced Nutrition: Macronutrients, © 1995 by CRC Press, Boca Raton, FL.

energy. Energy measured in kcal is multiplied by 4.2 (actually 4.184) in converting kcal to kJ (kilojoules). The energy content of diets is generally given in calories (cal) or in megajoules (MJ), which is 1,000 kJ.

Calories may be measured by **direct or indirect calorimetry.** The calories present in foods are measured directly by the amount of heat produced when a food is completely burned in a **bomb calorimeter** (Figure 10.1). The heat that is released as the food is burned (literally exploded) is called the **heat of combustion.** The heat of combustion values for the energy-yielding nutrients are as follows: 1 g carbohydrate yields 4.20 cal, 1 g protein yields 5.65 cal, and 1 g lipid yields 9.45 cal. The body must expend energy in converting the amino groups from amino acids to urea so that amino acids can be used for energy production. Thus, the energy yield from protein is reduced to 4.35 cal/g. Typically, 97 percent of carbohydrates, 92 percent of proteins, and 95 percent of lipids are digested and absorbed. After digestive efficiencies have been taken into consideration, the net caloric yield values are as follows: carbohydrates, 4 cal/g; proteins, 4 cal/g; and lipids, 9 cal/g. Most foods contain varying portions of these three energy-yielding nutrients as well as water. The caloric value of a food can be determined if its composition of energy-yielding nutrients is known by utilizing the net caloric values. For example, cooked oatmeal contains 2 percent protein, 1 percent fat, 10 percent carbohydrate, and 87 percent water. Using these compositional values, the cal in the oatmeal can be calculated as follows for 100 g of cooked oatmeal: 4 cal/g protein times 2 g + 9 cal/g fat times 1 g + 4 cal/g carbohydrate times 10 g = 57 cal. Normally, one does not have to calculate food energy in this manner, as food energy values are given as cal in food composition tables and databases. Alcohol contains calories; the net caloric yield of alcohol is 7 cal/g.

Dietary Intakes

No single dietary intake methodology is suitable for all purposes. Differences exist with regard to precision needed, population group, period of interest (past or present), available resources, and purposes. Dietary intake methodologies are also geared toward determining intakes of individuals or of groups of individuals. Methodologies intended for use in determining intakes of individuals will be discussed in this chapter. Generally, these methods include diet (or food) recalls, records, frequencies, or histories.

Food recalls, usually 24-hour, are used in estimating intakes from foods consumed yesterday. Essentially, an individual is asked to recall and describe the amounts and kinds of food items consumed during the previous 24-hour time period. Recall questionnaires are generally administered by *trained interviewers* in person, by phone, and by automated devices. Interviewees frequently have trouble remembering what and how much they ate. Cross-checking or probing questions are used to increase accuracy. *Food models* or pictures and measuring devices (cups, spoons) are often used in helping to ascertain *serving sizes*. Information is also obtained as to type (as in whole or skim milk), brand name, or cooking method used for some foods and what ingredients were in combination (mixture) foods. The 24-hour recall takes 15 to 30 minutes to administer and it places little burden on the interviewees. Individuals generally are able to remember what and how much of each food item they ate when visual aids for ascertaining serving sizes are utilized. The major limitation of the 24-hour recall is that there usually is large variability in the kinds and amounts of foods eaten by an individual from one day to another. Multiple or repeated 24-hour recalls, particularly those obtained on random days, provide more satisfactory data with regard to typical intakes of an individual. Also, many people eat differently on weekend days as compared to week days, so intakes on both weekend and week days should be recalled.

Food records or food diaries may be collected by individuals or designated persons for a specified time period, generally one to seven days. Individuals are given instructions regarding serving sizes, types of items, brand names, and combination foods prior to their writing down what they ate. They may also actually weigh each food item that they consume. Food records require that an individual or their designate record information about the foods they eat. The individual should eat as usual while keeping food records. Individuals may realize how much (or how little) food they are eating when they keep diet records; this is particularly true when participants actually *weigh* each food. Food records do not rely on memory. A drawback may be that food intakes are atypical for the person during the time that records are being kept.

Individuals may complete *food frequency questionnaires* providing information about their usual intakes of listed food items. Food frequency questionnaires vary as to the foods listed, the time period, and the response formats. Food frequency questionnaires are not generally used in calculating energy intakes.

Diet histories obtain information about dietary habits over the past day, week, month, year, decade, or even lifetime. Diet histories sometimes related to specific dietary constituents rather than total dietary intake. Diet histories are not generally used in calculating energy intakes.

Combinations of two or more of these methods are frequently used in research studies as this provides for greater accuracy. The shortcomings of one method may be counterbalanced by the strengths of a second method.

Caloric Density of Foods

The caloric value of food — carbohydrates, lipids, and proteins — is the amount of potential energy stored in the molecule's covalent bonds. The proportion of hydrocarbon in the molecular structure contributes to the caloric value of foods, as does the proportionate content of water. Foods containing a high proportion of water (also fiber) possess a lower caloric density than that of foods low in moisture and with a proportionately higher content of either fats or oils. Foods high in water content such as lettuce and tomatoes have a low caloric density (~0.20 cal/g), whereas butter, oils, and lard, which have essentially no water, have the maximum caloric density of any food (~9.0 cal/g). Foods with intermediate water content have intermediate caloric densities. The caloric variation between carbohydrates and lipids is seen for dry cereals, white sugar, and the lipids. These foods are all low in water content, but the caloric density of the foods high in lipids (butter, oils, lard) is twice that of sugar and dry cereals owing to the higher proportion of total hydrocarbon.

11

Assessment of Energy Expenditure

The energy expenditure of an individual is usually estimated utilizing tables. Energy expenditures may also be measured in a laboratory setting.

Body Calorimetry

Direct and indirect calorimetry are used to determine the amount of energy expended by the body. A *human calorimeter* is an air-tight chamber with an oxygen supply in which an individual can live and work. The heat produced and radiated by that person can be measured. The human calorimeter is expensive and involves subjects not participating in their regular lives. Generally, human energy expenditure is measured by *indirect calorimetry* in which oxygen utilization is measured either as oxygen consumption or carbon dioxide production or both. Approximately 4.82 kcal of heat is produced when one liter of oxygen is consumed by an individual burning a mixture of carbohydrates, proteins, and lipids. A value of *5 kcal/L* is used for calculations. Indirect calorimetry is simple and quite accurate, yielding reproducible results.

Human indirect calorimetry may be of the open-circuit or closed-circuit variety. In *open-circuit indirect calorimetry* individuals breathe ambient air that has a constant oxygen content. In *closed-circuit indirect calorimetry* individuals breathe again and again from an oxygen tank or chamber. Portable spirometry, the Douglas bag technique, and computerized instrumentation are common indirect calorimetry procedures used to measure oxygen consumption during different physical activities.

Components of Energy Expenditure

The three components of human energy expenditure are basal metabolism, thermic effect of food (also known as specific dynamic effect, specific dynamic action, and diet-induced thermogenesis), and thermic effect of exercise (also known as physical activity). Frequently, resting metabolism is measured rather than basal metabolism. For most individuals, basal or resting metabolism constitutes the largest portion of the *total energy expenditure* (also known as gross energy expenditure).

Basal and Resting Metabolism

Basal metabolism is the minimum amount of energy expenditure needed to maintain the vital activities of life. The *basal metabolic rate* (BMR) is determined by measuring the oxygen intake of a fasting individual (at least 12 hours of fasting) at physiological and psychological rest. The subject arrives at the testing site in the early morning and lies quietly in a dimly lit room (comfortable temperature and humidity) with oxygen uptake being measured after about 30 to 60 minutes. The subject is relaxed but not asleep. The *resting metabolic rate* (RMR) is measured at any time of day, but at three to four hours after the last meal. BMR and RMR generally differ by less than 10 percent in healthy individuals. Frequently, these two terms are used interchangeably.

Several factors affect basal and resting metabolism. On the average, the BMRs of women are 5 to 10 percent lower than those of men. In most cases, women have a larger percent of body fat and smaller proportion of lean body (muscle) mass than men. Body surface area also affects the BMR as it is related to the amount of heat lost via evaporation from the skin. Body composition also affects the BMR as the amount of actively metabolizing tissue correlates with BMR. The BMR decreases as individuals age, perhaps because of the shift in proportion of muscle to fat. Some research suggests that exercise may help maintain a higher BMR. The quantities of thyroxine and norepinephrine in the body affect the metabolic rate. Cortisol, growth hormone, and insulin, to a lesser extent, also affect the metabolic rate. The metabolic rate decreases by about 10 percent during sleep as compared to when a subject is awake but reclining. Physical stresses, such as trauma, burns, and fevers, increase the metabolic rate. Environmental temperature, both hot and cold, increase metabolic rate. As expected, the metabolic rate is also increased during pregnancy and lactation as well as during growth in children.

Thermic Effect of Food

Energy is expended during the digestion, absorption, and metabolism of nutrients. This diet-induced thermogenesis reaches a maximum within about an hour after a meal. The *thermic effect of food* usually accounts for 6 to 10 percent of the total energy expenditure. Some research indicates that exercising after eating increases a person's normal thermic response to food intake.

Thermic Effect of Exercise

The contribution of the *thermic effect of exercise* to the total energy expenditure varies greatly from individual to individual. According to several surveys, about a third of most individuals' time is spent in resting activities and the rest is spent in a wide range of physical activities. Researchers have measured the energy expended in various types of activities by individuals using indirect calorimetry. Tables have been constructed for total energy expenditure and for thermic effect of exercise for various specific or general physical activities; expenditure values are given on a body weight basis (kcal/kg) or a total body basis depending on the tables utilized. Body size affects energy expenditures due to physical activity. The energy expended during weight-bearing activities increases as body mass increases; more energy is required for a man weighing 250 pounds to walk at a given speed than for a 170-pound man to walk at the same speed. Little relationship is observed between body mass and energy expended due to exercise in nonweight-bearing activities,

TABLE 11.1

Equations for Predicting Resting Energy Expenditure (REE) from Body Weight (BW in kg)

Gender	Age Range (y)	Equation to Derive REE in kcal/day
Males	0-3	$(60.9 \times BW) - 54$
	3-10	$(22.7 \times BW) + 495$
	10-18	$(17.5 \times BW) + 651$
	18-30	$(15.3 \times BW) + 679$
	30-60	$(11.6 \times BW) + 879$
	60+	$(13.5 \times BW) + 487$
Females	0-3	$(61.0 \times BW) - 51$
	3-10	$(22.5 \times BW) + 499$
	10-18	$(12.2 \times BW) + 746$
	18-30	$(14.7 \times BW) + 496$
	30-60	$(8.7 \times BW) + 829$
	60+	$(10.5 \times BW) + 596$

Reprinted with permission from National Research Council, *Recommended Dietary Allowances*, 10th ed. © 1989 by the National Academy of Sciences. Courtesy of the National Academy Press, Washington, DC.

such as using a stationary ergometer. The level of fitness also affects the energy expended due to exercise with regard to voluntary activities, most likely due to increased muscle mass.

Estimating Energy Expenditure

Several tables have been developed by various researchers and organizations for estimating *energy expenditures*. Tables suggested for use by a committee of the Food and Nutrition Board, National Research Council, National Academy of Sciences will be given in this book. The first step in estimating total energy expenditure is to calculate the resting energy expenditure using values given in Table 11.1. Table 11.2 lists approximate energy expenditures for various activity categories as multiples of resting energy expenditure. The number of hours that one participates in each activity category should be multiplied by the activity category factor as multiples of REE (resting energy expenditure) accounting for all 24 hours of the day. An example of this multiplication step is shown in Table 11.3. Then the weighted REE factors are added together and the mean weighted REE factor calculated (as shown in the example in Table 11.3). The total energy expenditure is calculated by multiplying the REE by the mean weighed REE factor, and then multiplying the answer by 1.1 (thus accounting for the thermic effect of food).

If details as to the number of hours a person spends doing various physical activities are not available, then the total energy expenditure can be roughly estimated using values given in Table 11.4. Values are given in the table for individuals having light to moderate physical activity levels. Most Americans have light to moderate levels of physical activity.

A committee of the Food and Nutrition Board, National Research Council, National Academy of Sciences has recommended *average energy allowances* for individuals having light to moderate physical activity levels (Table 11.5). These recommended allowances should be adjusted for increased physical activity and larger or smaller body size.

TABLE 11.2

Approximate Energy Expenditure for Various Activities in Relation to Resting Energy Expenditure (REE)

Activity Category	Representative Value for Activity Factor per Hour
Resting	REE × 1.0
Sleeping, reclining	
Very light	REE × 1.5
Seated and standing activities, painting trades, driving, laboratory work, typing, sewing, ironing, cooking, playing cards, playing a musical instrument	
Light	REE × 2.5
Walking on a level surface at 2.5 to 3 mph, garage work, electrical trades, carpentry, restaurant trades, house-cleaning, child care, golf, sailing, table tennis	
Moderate	REE × 5.0
Walking 3.5 to 4 mph, weeding and hoeing, carrying a load, cycling, skiing, tennis, dancing	
Heavy	REE × 7.0
Walking with load uphill, tree felling, heavy manual digging, basketball, climbing, football, soccer	

Reprinted with permission from National Research Council, *Recommended Dietary Allowances,* 10th ed. © 1989 by the National Academy of Sciences. Courtesy of the National Academy Press, Washington, DC.

TABLE 11.3

Example of Calculation of Estimated Daily Energy Allowances for a 20-Year-Old Woman

---

Step 1

Calculate kg body weight by dividing pounds by 2.2.

In this example the woman weighs 130 pounds or 59.1 kg (130 ÷ 2.2)

Step 2

Use appropriate equation from Table 11.1 to derive REE.

(14.7 × 59.1) + 496 = 1364 kcal/day

Step 3

Categorize the day's (24 hour) physical activities to derive mean activity factor.

Activity	Activity Factor	Duration (h)	Weighted Activity Factor (activity factor × duration)
Resting	1.0	11.0	11.0
Very light	1.5	10.0	15.0
Light	2.5	2.0	5.0
Moderate	5.0	0.5	2.5
Heavy	7.0	0.5	3.5
Total		24.0	37.0

Step 4

Calculate mean weighted activity factor.

37 ÷ 24 = 1.54

Step 5

Calculate energy expenditure for REE and physical activity (REE × mean weighted activity factor).

1364.8 × 1.54 = 2101.8 kcal/day

Step 6

Calculate total energy expenditure by multiplying answer of Step 5 above by 1.1 to account for thermic effect of food.

2101.8 × 1.1 = 2312 kcal/day

TABLE 11.4

Factors for Estimating Daily Energy Allowances
at Various Levels of Physical Activity for Men
and Women (Ages 19 to 50 Years)

Level of Activity	Activity Factor (× REE)	Energy Expenditure[a] (kcal/kg BW/day)
Very light		
Men	1.3	31
Women	1.3	30
Light		
Men	1.6	38
Women	1.5	35
Moderate		
Men	1.7	41
Women	1.6	37
Heavy		
Men	2.1	50
Women	1.9	44
Exceptional		
Men	2.4	58
Women	2.2	51

[a] Resting Energy Expenditure was computed from
equations given in Table 11.1.

Reprinted with permission from National Research
Council, *Recommended Dietary Allowances*, 10th ed.
© 1989 by the National Academy of Sciences. Courtesy
of the National Academy Press, Washington, DC.

TABLE 11.5

Median Heights and Weights and Recommended Energy Intake

	Age (y)	Weight		Height		REE[a]	Average Energy Allowance (kcal)[b]		
							Multiples		
Category	Condition	(kg)	(lb)	(cm)	(in)	(kcal/day)	of REE	Per kg	Per day[c]
Infants	0.0-1.5	6	13	60	24	320		108	650
	0.5-1.0	9	20	71	28	500		98	850
Children	1-3	13	29	90	35	740		102	1300
	4-6	20	44	112	44	950		90	1800
	7-10	28	62	132	52	1130		70	2000
Males	11-14	45	99	157	62	1440	1.70	55	2500
	15-18	66	145	176	69	1760	1.67	45	3000
	19-24	72	160	177	70	1780	1.67	40	2900
	25-50	79	174	176	70	1800	1.60	37	2900
	51+	77	170	173	68	1530	1.50	30	2300
Females	11-14	46	101	157	62	1310	1.67	47	2200
	15-18	55	120	163	64	1370	1.60	40	2200
	19-24	58	128	164	65	1350	1.60	38	2200
	25-50	63	138	163	64	1380	1.55	36	2200
	51+	65	143	160	63	1280	1.50	30	1900
Pregnant	1st trimester								+0
	2nd trimester								+300
	3rd trimester								+300
Lactating	1st 6 months								+500
	2nd 6 months								+500

[a] Resting Energy Expenditure.

[b] In the range of light to moderate activity, the coefficient of variation is ±20%.

[c] Figure is rounded.

Reprinted with permission from National Research Council, *Recommended Dietary Allowances,* 10th ed. © 1989 by the National Academy of Sciences. Courtesy of the National Academy Press, Washington, DC.

12

Energy Production in the Body

The ultimate energy source is the sun. Solar energy from the sun is harnessed by plants which utilize carbon, hydrogen, oxygen, and nitrogen to form carbohydrates, fats, and proteins. Foods containing carbohydrates, fats, and proteins have stored energy. Once humans consume foods, digestion and absorption of food components take place and nutrients are transported to the cells (see Chapter 2). The cells of the body are able to transform the energy from carbohydrates, fats, and proteins into substances that can be used for immediate or future energy. Energy from foods (and some types of supplements) enables people to do everything that they do. Adenosine triphosphate (*ATP*), a high-energy compound, is the fuel the body uses immediately. The high-energy compound *creatine phosphate* serves as an energy reservoir for the body, functioning in the regeneration of ATP. The body stores of carbohydrates, fats, and proteins are energy reserves.

Energy Currency

The potential energy stored in ATP molecules provides the chemical energy for biological work. Energy released during ATP hydrolysis activates other energy-requiring molecules. ATP is the "energy currency" of the cell. Slightly over 85 grams of ATP are stored in the adult body at any one time.

Energy Reservoir

Creatine phosphate, a high-energy compound, serves as an energy reservoir for the body. Anaerobic catabolism of creatine phosphate provides energy for the resynthesis of ATP from adenosine diphosphate (ADP) and inorganic phosphate (P_i), forming creatine plus inorganic phosphate (P_i). Both of the above reactions are reversible. The cells of our bodies, particularly those of skeletal muscles, are able to store creatine phosphate in larger quantities than ATP. All-out exercise, such as swimming or running, can be maintained for about six to eight seconds utilizing the energy released from creatine phosphate and ATP. In time, the body can be resupplied with creatine phosphate and ATP. Through appropriate training, individuals can slightly increase their storage capacity for creatine phosphate.

Aerobic and Anaerobic Energy Release

Aerobic means oxygen-requiring. Anaerobic reactions do not require oxygen. Energy can be released by the cell both *aerobically* and *anaerobically*. Energy produced anaerobically can be immediately utilized by the cell, and is important in such activities as sprinting and surviving underwater submersion.

Anaerobic and Aerobic Energy from Foods

Glucose undergoes glycolysis when it is to be used for energy formation. Glycolysis is an anaerobic pathway. Two molecules of net ATP are obtained via *glycolysis* of one molecule of glucose under anaerobic conditions. The by-products of glucose glycolysis can be completely catabolized to CO_2 plus H_2O in subsequent aerobic reactions. The ATP produced in glycolysis provides a rapid source of energy for muscular activity that is particularly useful in short-duration, high-intensity physical activities.

Over 90 percent of the total ATP produced in the body comes from aerobic pathways of the mitochondria. The *tricarboxylic acid cycle* (TCA) (also called Krebs cycle, carboxylic acid cycle, and citric acid cycle) and the *electron transport chain* (ETC) (also called electron transport system, ETS) take place in the mitochondria. If oxygen is not available, the pyruvic acid, produced primarily by glycolysis, is converted to *lactic acid*. Lactic acid may be reconverted to glucose under aerobic cellular conditions.

The cell can utilize carbohydrates, fats, and proteins for energy production. Carbohydrate is primarily present in the body as glucose (though other monosaccharides are present in very small quantities) and as glycogen in the liver and muscles. Fats are present in the body primarily as triglycerides in tissues including adipose tissues, though small amounts of free fatty acids are also present. The major protein reserve in the body is the skeletal muscles, though free amino acids are also present in limited quantities. Optimally, carbohydrates and fats, but not proteins, should be used for energy production. Carbohydrates can be used to produce small quantities of ATP anaerobically. Carbohydrates and fats are the major sources of ATP as produced aerobically. Vitamins and minerals are needed to catalyze many of the reactions necessary for energy production. Water participates in hydrolysis reactions. So, all six classes of nutrients function in energy production.

The amount of oxygen available to the body's cells affects the proportions of carbohydrates and fats that will be used for energy production. The utilization of fat always requires oxygen, but carbohydrate can be utilized for energy production with less oxygen because glycolysis is anaerobic. Examples of anaerobic activities are power lifting and sprints of swimming and running. Examples of aerobic activities are walking, jogging, swimming, and dancing.

During anaerobic activity, lactic acid is produced. The lactic acid builds up in muscles that are strenuously exercised and one then feels fatigued. Hence, one can sustain anaerobic activity for only one to two minutes or so at a time. The lactic acid lowers the pH of the muscle and reduces its ability to contract and one gets muscle fatigue. One gradually recovers as lactic acid is converted to glucose and metabolized aerobically as one rests.

The energy pathways will first be discussed briefly. A more detailed description of the energy pathways follows after brief sections on feasting and fasting as each influences energy metabolism.

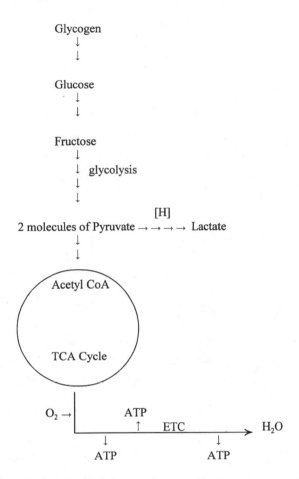

FIGURE 12.1
Energy production from carbohydrates.

Brief Description of Energy Pathways

How is energy produced by the body? Figure 12.1 summarizes the pathways by which the body produces energy from *carbohydrates*. Glucose, the end-product of starch digestion in humans, is stored in muscle (particularly skeletal muscle), heart, and liver as the polysaccharide *glycogen*. Glycogen, a ready store of energy, is broken down to glucose molecules if it is to be used for energy formation. The 6-carbon monosaccharides *glucose* and *fructose* are broken down to two molecules of the 3-carbon monosaccharide pyruvic acid or pyruvate with a small amount of energy being produced. The pathway in which glycogen, glucose, or fructose is broken down to pyruvate is known as *glycolysis* or the Embden-Meyerhof pathway. Glycolysis occurs in either aerobic or anaerobic conditions.

Under aerobic conditions pyruvate enters the *tricarboxylic acid cycle* (TCA cycle), also known as the Krebs cycle or citric acid cycle. Carbon dioxide is produced in the TCA cycle. Other intermediates formed in the TCA cycle go on to the aerobic pathway *electron transport chain* (ETC), also known as electron transport system. ATP and water are produced from TCA cycle intermediates in the ETC.

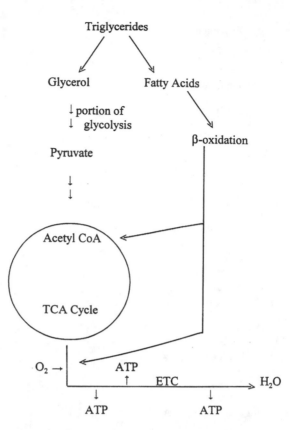

FIGURE 12.2
Energy production from fats.

Under anaerobic conditions pyruvate is converted to *lactic acid* or lactate. The lactic acid, produced primarily in the muscles, goes to the liver, where it is utilized to synthesize glucose via the *Cori cycle*. Then the glucose can be broken down to pyruvate via glycolysis, and if oxygen is available the pyruvate will enter the TCA cycle.

Figure 12.2 summarizes the pathways by which the body produces energy from *fats*. The triglycerides found in body tissues, including adipose tissues, that are to be used for energy formation are hydrolyzed to glycerol and fatty acids. Glycerol, a 3-carbon compound, enters glycolysis at the point where 3-carbon monosaccharides are present in the pathway and it then is broken down to pyruvate. Pyruvate enters the TCA cycle and then the ETC if oxygen is available just as with energy production from carbohydrates. The fatty acids are broken down into 2-carbon units (acetyl coenzyme A or acetyl CoA) by β-*oxidation*; intermediates are formed during β-oxidation which can go into the ETC for energy production. The 2-carbon units enter the TCA cycle (as acetyl CoA past the 3-carbon pyruvate step) and then the ETC just as with energy production from carbohydrates.

Figure 12.3 summarizes the pathways by which the body produces energy from *proteins*. Body proteins, predominantly those in skeletal muscle, are broken down to amino acids if they are to be used for energy formation. The nitrogen-containing amino group of the amino acid is deaminated (removed) or transaminated (transferred). The amino groups are condensed, forming *urea*, which is excreted in the urine. Once the amino group is removed from the amino acid, it becomes an α-keto acid, a type of carbohydrate. Some amino acids are glucogenic and some are ketogenic, so when the amino groups are removed they enter

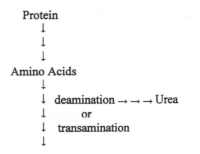

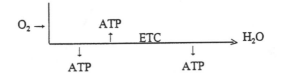

FIGURE 12.3
Energy production from proteins.

the TCA cycle at various points. The intermediates formed in the TCA cycle enter the ETC and are converted to energy and water.

The central pathways of energy metabolism are depicted in Figure 12.4. Energy may be obtained from any or all of the three energy-yielding nutrients. For many people, particularly those in developing countries, carbohydrates supply the majority of energy needs. Lipids as adipose tissues are the major store of body energy and possess more than twice the caloric density (9 cal/g) of carbohydrates or protein (4 cal/g).

Feasting

If one eats too many calories whether from carbohydrates, fats, or proteins, *adipose tissue* will be synthesized. Carbohydrates and proteins will be converted by the body to glycerol and fatty acids. Glycerides, primarily triglycerides, will then be synthesized from the glycerol and fatty acids.

Fasting

If one eats too few calories or fasts, the body draws upon its energy stores of glycogen and adipose tissues. Glucose and short-chain fatty acids are utilized for energy production in the brain. Glycogen and adipose tissue will be used for energy production by the rest of the body's tissues. Body proteins will also be used for energy formation if necessary. Carbohydrates and fats spare proteins from being used for energy production by first being used themselves.

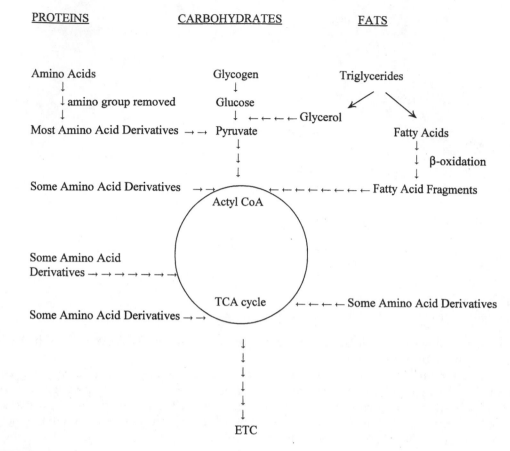

FIGURE 12.4
Central pathways of energy metabolism.

When large quantities of fats and ketogenic amino acids are used for energy formation, *ketone bodies* are produced. The ketone bodies are acetoacetate, acetone, and β-hydroxy-butyrate. The ketone bodies can be used by the skeletal and heart muscles to produce energy. The buildup of ketone bodies causes ketosis. Ketosis leads to ketoacidosis, which affects the acid-base balance of the body and may be fatal if continued.

Detailed Description of Energy Pathways

Catabolic Pathways of Carbohydrates

Glycolysis

Glucose, the end product of starch digestion, is stored in muscle (particularly skeletal muscle), heart, or liver as the polysaccharide glycogen. Glycogen is a ready store of energy and it or glucose can be rapidly degraded to either pyruvate or lactate by the enzymes of the cytoplasm with the concomitant synthesis of ATP. The glycolytic or Embden-Meyerhof pathway is shown in Figure 12.5. *Glycolysis* occurs *in vivo* under either aerobic or anaerobic conditions. Aerobic glycolysis, beginning with the phosphorylation of glucose by ATP,

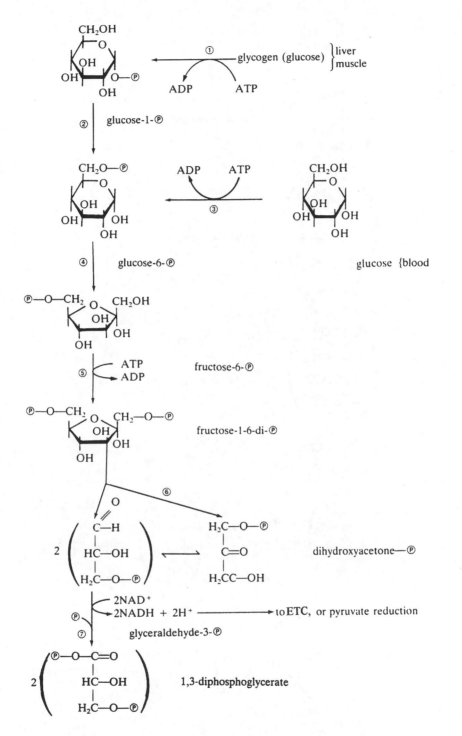

FIGURE 12.5

Glycolytic pathway. 1. Phosphorylase b. 2. Phosphoglucomutase. 3. Glucokinase. 4. Phosphoglucoisomerase. 5. Phosphofructokinase. 6. Aldolase. 7. Glyceraldehyde-3-phosphodehydrogenase. 8. Phosphoglycerolkinase. 9. Phosphoglycerolmutase. 10. Enolase. 11. Pyruvate kinase. 12. Pyruvate decarboxylase. Reprinted with permission from CRC Press. Spallholz, J. E., Boylan, L. M., and Driskell, J. A., *Nutrition: Chemistry and Biology,* © 1999 by CRC Press, Boca Raton, FL.

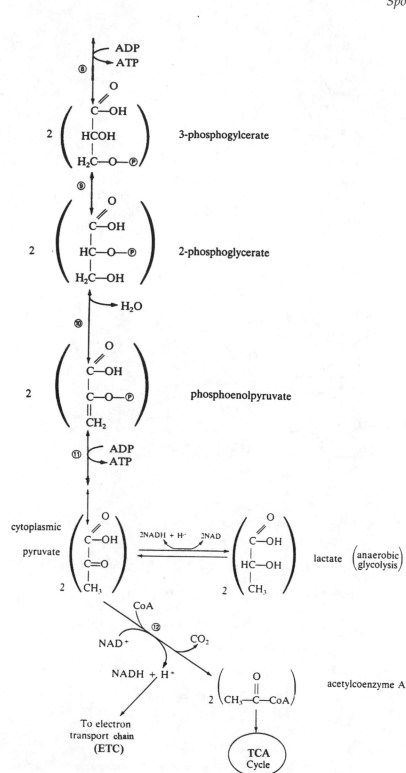

FIGURE 12.5 (Continued)

activates glucose as either glucose-1-℗ (from glycogen) or glucose-6-℗ (from blood). This 6-carbon molecule is isomerized and phosphorylated with a second molecule of ATP to form fructose 1,6-di-℗. This hexose is then divided into two 3-carbon molecules — dihydroxyacetone-℗ and glyceraldehyde-3-℗ — by an aldolase. Both 3-carbon molecules transverse the remaining intermediate steps of glycolysis (one step of which requires niacin as NAD), being transformed into pyruvic acid. Conversion of 1,3-diphosphoglycerate to 3-phosphoglycerate and phosphoenolpyruvate to pyruvate (one-half of the glucose) yields one molecule each of ATP. These steps are repeated again for the remaining one-half of the original glucose molecule, yielding two more ATP molecules. Thus, it is observed that phosphorylation of one molecule of glucose by ATP, forming glucose 6-℗ or glucose-1-℗, results in a net yield of two ATP molecules during glycolysis in the conversion of glucose to two molecules of pyruvate. Such phosphorylations are called substrate-level phosphorylations (SLPs) because ATP is synthesized from phosphorylated metabolites and ADP. The net yield of ATP is shown in Equation 12.1.

EQUATION 12.1
Net Yield of ATP by Substrate-level Phosphorylation
in Glycolysis

1.	Phosphorylation of glucose	=	−1 ATP
2.	Phosphorylation of fructose-6-℗	=	−1 ATP
3.	1,3-Diphosphoglycerate × 2 (SLP)	=	+2 ATP
4.	Phosphoenolpyruvate × 2 (SLP)	=	+2 ATP
	Net yield of ATP from SLP	=	+2 ATP

Reprinted with permission from CRC Press. Spallholz, J. E., Boylan, L. M., and Driskell, J. A., *Nutrition: Chemistry and Biology*, © 1999 by CRC Press, Boca Raton, FL.

Under anaerobic conditions, the two molecules of reduced NADH + H⁺ (produced by the oxidation of glyceraldehyde-3-℗) are used to reduce two molecules of pyruvate to *lactate*. This happens in muscle tissue when muscular contractions are rapid under persistent anaerobic conditions and pyruvate can not enter the tricarboxylic acid cycle (TCA cycle) (Figure 12.6) because of a deficiency of oxaloacetate. Such events cause lactic acid to accumulate and produce a respiratory oxygen debt.

With purely aerobic conditions, pyruvate is oxidatively decarboxylated and transformed into acetyl-coenzyme A (acetyl-CoA), the most important metabolic intermediate common to the catabolism of carbohydrates, fatty acids, and amino acids. Acetyl-coenzyme A condenses with oxaloacetate, forming citric acid in the initial metabolic step of the TCA cycle, whereby the catabolism of glucose is continued.

The Tricarboxylic Acid Cycle

From glycolysis, two molecules of pyruvate are decarboxylated and are condensed with coenzyme A, forming two molecules of acetyl coenzyme A. Thiamin (as thiamin pyrophosphate), lipoic acid, niacin (as NAD), and pantothenic acid (as a component of coenzyme A) function in the conversion of pyruvate to acetyl-coenzyme A as well as later in the cycle in the conversion of α-ketoglutarate to succinyl-coenzyme A. In this reaction, the carboxylic moiety of pyruvate is lost as respiratory CO_2 and the remaining acetyl, a 2-carbon unit, is metabolized through the TCA cycle.

The *TCA cycle*, is also known as the citric acid cycle or Krebs cycle, bearing the name of Sir Hans Krebs, who elucidated the details of this metabolic pathway within the mitochondria. For this remarkable accomplishment, Krebs received the Nobel Prize in Medicine in 1953.

Acetyl coenzyme A (acetyl-CoA), in the first reaction of the TCA cycle, condenses with oxaloacetate, a 4-carbon dicarboxylic acid, forming the 6-carbon tricarboxylic acid, citric acid (Equation 12.2). The complete TCA cycle is shown in Figure 12.6. The 6-carbon atoms of citric acid then pass through a series of TCA cycle metabolic intermediates. Four of citric acid's six carbons are retained throughout the TCA cycle and reappear as oxaloacetate, completing one turn of the cycle. The 2-carbon atoms unaccounted for are lost in thiamin-mediated oxidative decarboxylations of the TCA cycle intermediates, oxalosuccinate and α-ketoglutarate. During each turn of the TCA cycle, one ATP equivalent is made in a SLP of GDP → GTP, guanosine diphosphate to guanosine triphosphate. While glycolysis yields four equivalent ATPs from SLPs of glucose metabolites, the TCA cycle yields only two equivalent ATPs through the synthesis of GTP. The net reactions of one turn of the TCA cycle can be summarized as in Equation 12.3.

EQUATION 12.2
Condensation Reaction of Acetyl-CoA and Oxaloacetate.

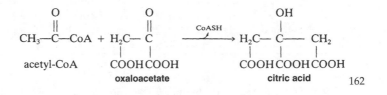

Reprinted with permission from CRC Press. Spallholz, J. E., Boylan, L. M., and Driskell, J. A., *Nutrition: Chemistry and Biology,* © 1999 by CRC Press, Boca Raton, FL.

EQUATION 12.3
Chemical Summary of TCA Cycle

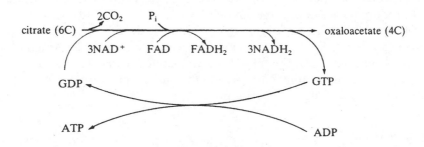

Reprinted with permission from CRC Press. Spallholz, J. E., Boylan, L. M., and Driskell, J. A., *Nutrition: Chemistry and Biology,* © 1999 by CRC Press, Boca Raton, FL.

Two turns of the TCA cycle are necessary to fully oxidize the equivalent of one molecule of glucose (6C). The equivalent of these 6-carbon atoms are lost as CO_2; two are lost in the oxidative decarboxylations of pyruvate and its conversion to acetyl CoA, and four are lost in the oxidative decarboxylations during two turns of the TCA cycle.
Oxidation of one molecule of glucose has now been followed through glycolysis and the TCA cycle. Six molecules of CO_2, equivalent to all the carbon atoms of one glucose molecule,

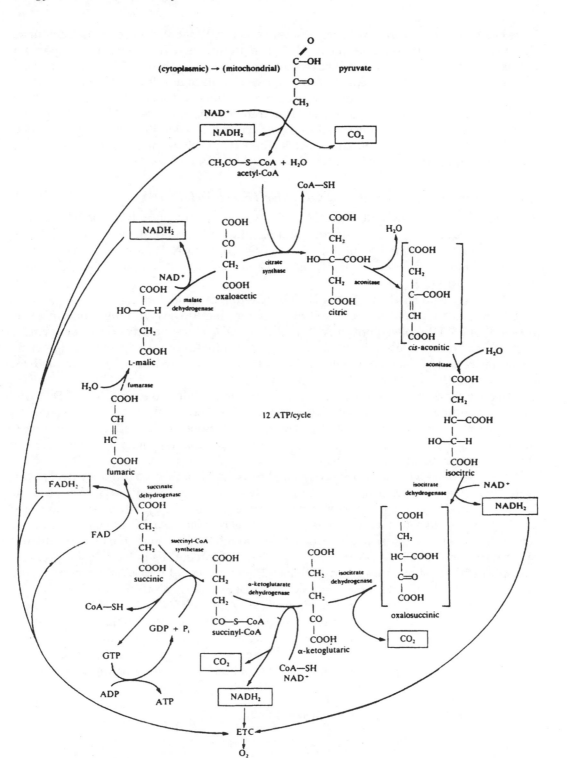

FIGURE 12.6

TCA cycle. Reprinted with permission from CRC Press. Spallholz, J. E., Boylan, L. M., and Driskell, J. A., *Nutrition: Chemistry and Biology*, © 1999 by CRC Press, Boca Raton, FL.

have been lost along with the oxygen atoms of glucose. What remains metabolically unaccounted for in the glucose molecule ($C_6H_{12}O_6$) are the atoms of hydrogen. These hydrogen atoms in glucose were used to reduce NAD^+ (containing niacin) and FAD (containing riboflavin) to $NADH + H^+$ and $FADH_2$, forming reduced niacinamide and flavin coenzymes. These reduced coenzymes are then oxidized in the mitochondrial electron transport chain (ETC). The ETC is also known as the electron transport system. The ETC is the fixed common pathway for the oxidation of reduced coenzymes formed in the catabolic pathways of carbohydrates, fatty acids, and amino acids. The ETC provides the majority of newly synthesized cellular ATP by the oxidative phosphorylation of ADP.

The Electron Transport Chain and Oxidative Phosphorylation

The *ETC* is found, along with the TCA cycle, within the mitochondria. The ETC is composed of a sequential series of enzymes and membrane-bound proteins, the cytochromes, arranged for the enzymatic coupling of P_i to ADP, forming ATP, and for the reduction of oxygen, forming metabolic water. The ETC, the formation of ATP and metabolic water, is shown in Figure 12.7.

In the first reaction of the ETC, $NADH_2$ formed from the oxidation of glucose, fatty acids, and TCA cycle metabolites is oxidized by FAD, forming $FADH_2$ with the concurrent synthesis of one ATP molecule from ADP and P_i. $FADH_2$ is then oxidized by coenzyme Q (CoQ), also known as ubiquinone. $CoQ \cdot H_2$ gives up two protons ($2H^+$) to the mitochondrial matrix and transfers two electrons ($2e^-$) from the two hydrogen atoms to oxidized cytochrome b (Fe^{3+}) . Vitamin C and copper function in conjunction with iron in the ETC. The two electrons, one at a time, are sequentially passed along to each oxidized Fe^{3+} form of the succeeding cytochrome. The final acceptor of the pair of elections is oxygen ($\frac{1}{2} O_2$). Oxygen (O^{2-}) returns the pair of electrons to the two protons discharged from coenzyme Q in combining to form a molecule of water. It is this water that is called metabolic water, for it is formed as a result of metabolism.

In the cascade of the pair of electrons from the discharge of the two protons by coenzyme Q through the sequential array of cytochromes, two molecules of ATP are synthesized from $2ADP + 2P_i$. ATP is synthesized, resulting from the coupling of cytochromes b and c_1 and cytochromes a and a_3 (cytochrome series) with oxygen. From $NADH_2$, arising from the catabolic pathways, hydrogen and electrons flow through the ETC, with the resulting synthesis of ATP. Each $NADH_2$ gives rise to the synthesis of three ATPs in the ETC by oxidative phosphorylation, sometimes referred to as a P/O ratio equal to 3 (ATP formed/oxygen consumed). While $NADH_2$ produces P/O ratios of 3, $FADH_2$ produces a P/O ratio equal to 2. Why this happens can be seen in Figure 12.6. $FADH_2/FMNH_2$ derived from the β-oxidation of fatty acids, TCA cycle intermediate succinate, or other metabolic oxidations bypasses the synthesis of the first ATP in the ETC, and therefore, yields only two ATPs synthesized by the enzymes of cytochromes b and c_1, a and a_3. The net reactions of the ETC from $NADH_2$ and $FADH_2/FMNH_2$ can thus, be summarized as in Equation 12.4.

EQUATION 12.4
Chemical Summary of the Electron Transport Chain.

$$NADH_s + 3\ ADP + 3\ P_i + \tfrac{1}{2}O_2 \rightarrow NAD^+ + 3\ ATP + H_2O \qquad\qquad P/O = 3$$

$$FADH_2/FMNH_2 + 2\ ADP + 2\ P_i + \tfrac{1}{2}O_2 \rightarrow FAD/FMN + 2\ ATP + H_2O \qquad P/O = 2$$

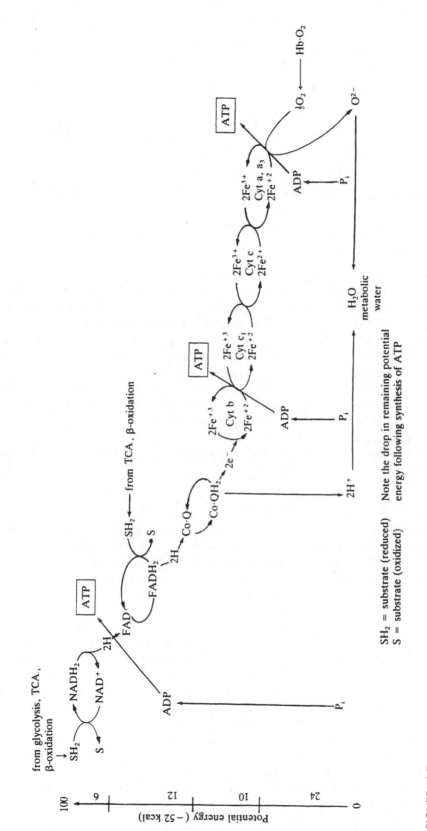

FIGURE 12.7

Electron transport chain and oxidative phosphorylation. Reprinted with permission from CRC Press. Spallholz, J. E., Boylan, L. M., and Driskell, J. A., *Nutrition: Chemistry and Biology*, © 1999 by CRC Press, Boca Raton, FL.

TABLE 12.1

Sequential Summary of ATP Synthesis from the Catabolism of Glucose

1. Phosphorylation of glucose from glycogen (–1 ATP or from glucose –2 ATP)	–1 ATP
2. Phosphorylation of fructose-6-Ⓟ	–1 ATP
3. Oxidation of 2 glutaraldehyde-3-Ⓟ by 2 NAD⁺ (NADH$_s$)	+6 ATP by ETC
4. Phosphorylation by 2 1,3-diphosphoglycerates	+2 ATP by SLP
5. Phosphorylation by 2 phosphoenolpyruvates	+2 ATP by SLP
6. Oxidation of 2 pyruvates by 2 NAD⁺ (NADH$_2$)	+6 ATP by ETC
7. Oxidation of 2 isocitrates by 2 NAD⁺ (NADH$_2$)	+6 ATP by ETC
8. Oxidation of 2 α-ketoglutarates by 2 NAD⁺ (NADH$_2$)	+6 ATP by ETC
9. Phosphorylation of 2 GDP by succinyl-CoA (2 ATP equivalents)	+2 ATP by SLP
10. Oxidation of 2 succinates by 2 FAD (FADH$_2$)	+4 ATP by ETC
11. Oxidation of 2 malates by 2 NAD⁺ (NADH$_2$)	+6 ATP by ETC
Net ATPs from Glycolysis and TCA via ETC	+38 ATP

Reprinted with permission from CRC Press. Spallholz, J. E., Boylan, L. M., and Driskell, J. A., *Nutrition: Chemistry and Biology,* © 1999 by CRC Press, Boca Raton, FL.

Close examination of glycolysis and the TCA cycle reveals that the metabolism of glucose yields a considerable amount of collective reduced coenzymes, NADH$_2$ and FADH$_2$, which are oxidized by the ETC, producing ATP. From a single molecule of glucose it is possible to ascertain the number of ATPs theoretically synthesized. This summary for the synthesis of ATP from glucose is given in Table 12.1. An examination of the source of ATP from the complete oxidation of glucose reveals that most of the net yield of the 38 ATPs arises from the NADH$_2$ and FADH$_2$ formed by the oxidation of TCA cycle intermediates and the single SLP initiated by succinyl-CoA. Fully 24, or 63 percent, of the net ATPs synthesized from the oxidation of glucose is from the metabolic operations of the TCA cycle. When reduced coenzymes are included from the oxidation of pyruvate to acetyl-CoA, 79 percent of the ATP is formed from this reaction and the TCA cycle. Under aerobic conditions, glycolysis accounts for just 21 percent of the ATP formed from the oxidation of reduced coenzymes produced in this pathway.

Thermodynamics of ATP and ATP Synthesis

We have examined how and where ATP is synthesized in the mitochondria by oxidative phosphorylation. Let us turn our attention now to the thermodynamics; the energy considerations of ATP synthesis and the metabolic transfer of energy within cells.

The amount of energy stored in ATP is equal to a free-energy yield of $\Delta G^{\circ\prime}$ = –7.3 kcal/mol under standard conditions. The negative sign signifies that the energy that is "stored" in ATP is released upon hydrolysis as in Equation 12.2.

The reaction in Equation 12.5 can be diagrammed showing the approximate energy content of the reactant (ATP) and products (ADP + P$_i$) (Figure 12.8). In order to "store" the –7.3 kcal/mol of hydrolysis in ATP, the drop in potential energy across the point of ATP synthesis (ADP + P$_i$ → ATP) in the mitochondria in the ETC must be greater than –7.3 kcal/mol. In the ETC, the potential drop in energy across all the electron carriers from NADH$_2$ to O$_2$, is approximately 52 kcal per electron pair. Figure 12.8 demonstrates that approximately 12 kcal of potential energy is used in the synthesis of the first ATP, 10 kcal is used in the synthesis of the second ATP, and 24 kcal is expended in the synthesis of the third and final ATP. The total amount of energy "stored" by oxidative phosphorylation of ADP per NADH$_2$ is 21.9 kcal. From this value an estimate of overall thermodynamic efficiency can be calculated for a P/O ratio of 3. This efficiency is 21.9 kcal/52 kcal × 100, or ~42 percent. The ETC is therefore 42 percent efficient in conserving total potential electron energy as ATP.

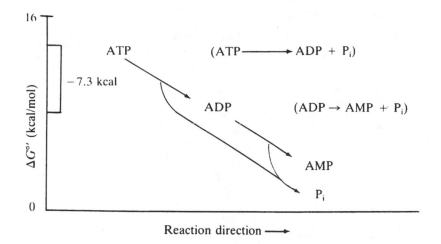

FIGURE 12.8

Free energy of hydrolysis of ATP and ADP. Reprinted with permission from CRC Press. Spallholz, J. E., Boylan, L. M., and Driskell, J. A., *Nutrition: Chemistry and Biology,* © 1999 by CRC Press, Boca Raton, FL.

EQUATION 12.5
Hydrolysis of ATP.

Hydrolysis of ATP.

$$ATP \xrightarrow{\text{Mg2+-ATPase}} ADP + P_i + (-7.3\ \text{kcal/mol})$$

Reprinted with permission from CRC Press. Spallholz, J. E., Boylan, L. M., and Driskell, J. A., *Nutrition: Chemistry and Biology,* © 1999 by CRC Press, Boca Raton, FL.

Why, one may ask, is ATP synthesized and so important as a carrier of free energy? ATP is an unusual carrier of free energy for anabolic reactions, for its $\Delta G^{\circ\prime}$ of hydrolysis is of intermediate value among a variety of energetically active compounds. Table 12.2 provides a list of energy-containing compounds ranging from $\Delta G^{\circ\prime} = -14.8$ kcal/mol to -2.2 kcal/mol. The free energy of hydrolysis for the reaction ATP → ADP + P_i (-7.3 kcal/mol) is intermediate among these compounds. Compounds with $\Delta G^{\circ\prime}$ less than ATP can be phosphorylated by ATP as in Equation 12.6. In this equation, ATP transferred -5.0 kcal/mol of its -7.3 kcal/mol to glucose. This reaction energy transfer was 68 percent efficient. It may be recalled from glycolysis that conversion of phosphoenolpyruvate to pyruvate is a SLP which yields ATP (Equation 12.7). In this reaction phosphoenolpyruvate has a $\Delta G^{\circ\prime}$ of -14.8 kcal/mol and transfers its phosphate to ADP, yielding ATP with a $\Delta G^{\circ\prime}$ of -7.3 kcal/mol. This phosphate transfer shows how ATP is formed only by molecules with a higher $\Delta G^{\circ\prime}$ of hydrolysis than that of ATP. This reaction energy transfer is about 50 percent efficient.

EQUATION 12.6
Phosphorylation of Glucose by ATP.

ATP + glucose → ADP + glucose-1-℗

Reprinted with permission from CRC Press. Spallholz, J. E., Boylan, L. M., and Driskell, J. A., *Nutrition: Chemistry and Biology,* © 1999 by CRC Press, Boca Raton, FL.

TABLE 12.2

Free Energy of Hydrolysis of Energy-Containing Compounds

Name	$\Delta G^{\circ\prime}$ (kcal/mol)	Direction of phosphate or energy transfer
Phosphoenolpyruvate	−14.8	
α-Glycerol phosphate	−11.8	
Creatine phosphate	−10.3	
Acetylphosphate	−10.1	
ATP ($\to$ AMP + PP$_i$)	−8.6	
Acetyl-CoA	−8.2	
ATP ($\to$ ADP + P$_i$)	−7.3	
Aminoacetyl AMP	−7.0	
PP$_i$ ($\to$ 2P$_i$)	−6.7	
Glucose-1-phosphate	−5.0	
Fructose-6-phosphate	−3.8	
Glucose-6-phosphate	−3.3	
3-Phosphoglycerate	−3.1	
Glycerol-1-phosphate	−2.2	

Reprinted with permission from CRC Press. Spallholz, J. E., Boylan, L. M., and Driskell, J. A., *Nutrition: Chemistry and Biology.* © 1999 by CRC Press, Boca Raton, FL.

EQUATION 12.7
Phosphorylation of ADP by Phosphoenolpyruvate.

$$\text{phosphoenolpyruvate} + \text{ADP} \to \text{ATP} + \text{pyruvate}$$

Reprinted with permission from CRC Press. Spallholz, J. E., Boylan, L. M., and Driskell, J. A., *Nutrition: Chemistry and Biology,* © 1999 by CRC Press, Boca Raton, FL.

Creatine phosphate ($\Delta G^{\circ\prime}$ = −10.3 kcal/mol) is a high-energy compound found in muscle used in the phosphorylation of ADP for muscular contraction (Equation 12.8). This equation is thermodynamically permissible. During muscular rest, creatine is phosphorylated by ATP, forming creatine phosphate, which seemingly is thermodynamically impossible. This reaction occurs, however, by expending the energy of two molecules of ATP (Equation 12.9). In this equation, the $\Delta G^{\circ\prime}$ of creatine phosphate is restored in a reaction energy transfer that is 70 percent efficient. These examples of energy transfer from two ATPs between molecules which have both greater and lesser $\Delta G^{\circ\prime}$ than ATP should serve to emphasize why coupling energies for the synthesis of ATP in oxidation phosphorylation must be larger than +7.3 kcal/mol to form ATP.

EQUATION 12.8
Phosphorylation of ADP by Creatine Phosphate.

$$\text{creatine phosphate} + \text{ADP} \to \text{ATP} + \text{creatine}$$

Reprinted with permission from CRC Press. Spallholz, J. E., Boylan, L. M., and Driskell, J. A., *Nutrition: Chemistry and Biology,* © 1999 by CRC Press, Boca Raton, FL.

EQUATION 12.9
Phosphorylation of Creatine by ATP.

$$\text{creatine} + 2 \text{ ATP} \to \text{creatine phosphate} + 2 \text{ ADP} + \text{P}_i$$

Reprinted with permission from CRC Press. Spallholz, J. E., Boylan, L. M., and Driskell, J. A., *Nutrition: Chemistry and Biology,* © 1999 by CRC Press, Boca Raton, FL.

Catabolic Pathways of Lipids

Triglycerides, in comparison to equal anhydrous weights of carbohydrate and protein, contain more calories because they have a higher proportion of total hydrocarbons. Body stores of triglycerides are mobilized in response to low blood glucose and insulin levels by the release of free fatty acids (FFAs) from triglycerides into the blood stream. Bound to serum albumin, FFAs are taken up by the cell's cytoplasm. These cytosolic FFAs undergo an enzymatic activation by ATP and are transferred to carnitine, which acts as a mitochondrial membrane shuttle moving FFAs from the cytoplasm into the mitochondrial matrix, as shown in Equations 12.10 and 12.11. Once transferred by carnitine into the intramitochondrial matrix, the fatty acid is re-esterified with coenzyme A. This coenzyme A, however, is of mitochondrial origin (Equation 12.11) and provides an activated free fatty acid for β-oxidation.

EQUATION 12.10
Activation of Cytoplasmic Fatty Acids.

$$CH_3CH_2(CH_2)_nCOOH$$

$$+ \ ATP \xrightarrow{\text{CoASH (cytoplasmic)}} CH_3CH_2(CH_2)_n\text{—}\overset{\overset{\textstyle O}{\|}}{C}\text{—}S\text{—}CoA \ + \ AMP \ + \ PP_i$$

Transfer of Activated Fatty Acid to Carnitine

$$CH_3CH_2(CH_2)_n\text{—}\overset{\overset{\textstyle O}{\|}}{C}\text{—}CoA \ + \ \underset{\underset{\textstyle OH}{|}}{HOOC\text{—}CH_2\text{—}\overset{\text{Carnitine}}{CH}\text{—}CH_2\text{—}\overset{+}{N}(CH_3)_3} \longrightarrow$$

$$\underset{\underset{\underset{\textstyle O=C\text{—}(CH_2)_nCH_2CH_3}{|}}{O}}{HOOC\text{—}CH_2\text{—}\overset{+}{CH}\text{—}CH_2\text{—}\overset{+}{N}(CH_3)_3} \ + \ CoASH \ \text{(cytoplasmic)}$$

Reprinted with permission from CRC Press. Spallholz, J. E., Boylan, L. M., and Driskell, J. A., *Nutrition: Chemistry and Biology,* © 1999 by CRC Press, Boca Raton, FL.

EQUATION 12.11
Transfer of Acylcarnitine to Mitochondrial Coenzyme A.

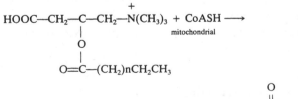

$$\underset{\underset{\underset{\textstyle O=C\text{—}(CH_2)nCH_2CH_3}{|}}{O}}{HOOC\text{—}CH_2\text{—}\overset{+}{C}\text{—}CH_2\text{—}\overset{+}{N}(CH_3)_3} \ + \ \underset{\text{mitochondrial}}{CoASH} \longrightarrow$$

$$CH_3CH_2(CH_2)_n\text{—}\overset{\overset{\textstyle O}{\|}}{C}\text{—}S\text{—}CoA \ + \ carnitine$$

Reprinted with permission from CRC Press. Spallholz, J. E., Boylan, L. M., and Driskell, J. A., *Nutrition: Chemistry and Biology,* © 1999 by CRC Press, Boca Raton, FL.

β-Oxidation

The oxidation of fatty acids was first described by F. Knoop, a German biochemist, in 1904. Oxidation of fatty acids and cleavage of the thioester occurs at the second or β-carbon of the fatty acid, and thus the cyclic process of fatty acid degradation bears the name *β-oxidation*. β-Oxidation, it may be remembered, is initiated by activation of a cytoplasmic free fatty acid by ATP and it exists as a thioester (Figure 12.9). Equation (1) of Figure 12.9 is the dehydrogenation of the activated fatty acid by a flavoprotein containing oxidized FAD, yielding an unsaturated C:2,3 activated fatty acid. Hydration of either a *cis* or *trans* fatty acid [equation (2) or (2′)] produces a stereoisomer which upon dehydrogenation by NAD^+ [equation (3)] produces a (C:3)β-ketoacetyl-CoA fatty acid and $NADH_2$. The β-ketoacetyl-CoA fatty acid is cleaved between C:2 and 3, producing acetyl-coenzyme A. The remaining fatty acid fragment, shortened by the loss of 2-carbon atoms, condenses with another molecule of coenzyme A. This activated free fatty acid [equation (4)] recycles to equation (1) for repetition of the cyclic process. In each repetitive cycle of β-oxidation, the activated fatty acid is shortened by 2-carbon atoms until butryl-CoA is cycled. In the final cycle of β-oxidation, this 4-carbon fatty acid is symmetrically cleaved to yield two acetyl-CoAs [equation (5)].

Inspection of the β-oxidation of fatty acids reveals that any fatty acid of even carbon number n = 6 or greater undergoes (n/2) – 1 cycles, producing (n/2) per molecule of $FADH_2$ and n/2 molecules of acetyl-CoA. β-Oxidation of stearic acid, a saturated C_{18} fatty acid, would go through eight cycles, producing eight molecules of $FADH_2$ and $NADH_2$ and nine molecules of acetyl-CoA. These reactions can be summarized as in Equation 12.12.

EQUATION 12.12
β-Oxidation of Stearic Acid.

$$\text{stearic acid} + ATP + 9\,CoASH + 8\,FAD + 8\,NAD + 8\,H_2O \xrightarrow{\ 8\,cycles\ }$$

$$9\,\text{acetyl-Co-A} + 8\,FADH_2 + 8\,NADH_2 + AMP + PP_i$$

Reprinted with permission from CRC Press. Spallholz, J. E., Boylan, L. M., and Driskell, J. A., *Nutrition: Chemistry and Biology,* © 1999 by CRC Press, Boca Raton, FL.

All the acetyl-CoA produced by β-oxidation of fatty acids enters the TCA cycle. It may be recalled that each turn of the TCA cycle results in the oxidation of two atoms of carbon and the synthesis of reduced coenzymes and GTP equivalent to 12 ATPs per cycle. It should be apparent, therefore, that β-oxidation of cytoplasmic long-chain fatty acids, activated by two ATPs, generates large quantities of $FADH_2$ and $NADH_2$ for ATP synthesis from the ETC and oxidative phosphorylation of ADP. Complete oxidation of the C_{18} fatty acid, stearic acid, by β-oxidation nets 146 ATPs or 1,066 kcal/mol of stearic acid (calculations shown in Table 12.3). The number of kcal/mol for the complete oxidation of stearic acid by O_2 is shown in Equation 12.13.

EQUATION 12.13
Complete Oxidation of Stearic Acid by Oxygen.

$$\text{stearic acid} + 27\,O_2 \rightarrow 18\,CO_2 + 18\,H_2O + (-2596\ \text{kcal/mol})$$

Reprinted with permission from CRC Press. Spallholz, J. E., Boylan, L. M., and Driskell, J. A., *Nutrition: Chemistry and Biology,* © 1999 by CRC Press, Boca Raton, FL.

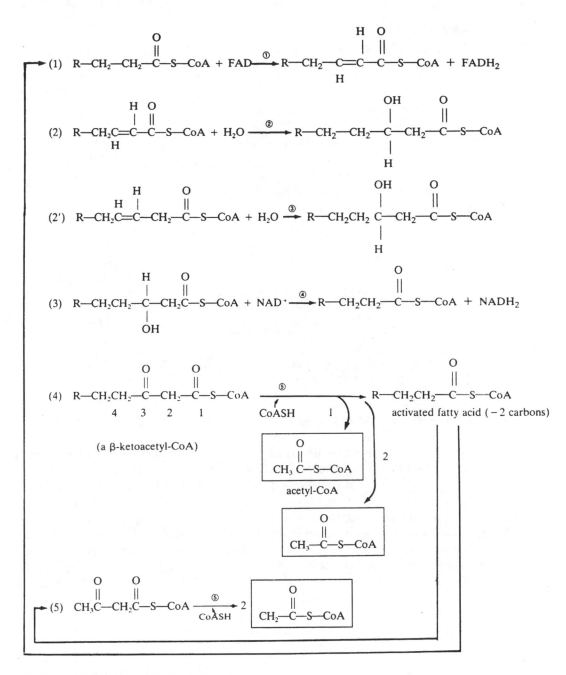

FIGURE 12.9 β-Oxidation of Fatty Acids
1. Acyl-CoA dehydrogenase. 2. Enoyl-CoA hydratase (trans fatty acid). 3. Enoyl-CoA hydratase (cis fatty acid).
4. β-Hydroxyacyl dehydrogenase. 5. Thiolase. Reprinted with permission from CRC Press. Spallholz, J. E., Boylan, L. M., and Driskell, J. A., *Nutrition: Chemistry and Biology,* © 1999 by CRC Press, Boca Raton, FL.

β-Oxidation of stearic acid results in the conservation of 41 percent of the total energy of stearic acid, preserved and transferred as ATP equivalents. The efficiency of recovered energy as ATP is reduced for shorter-chain fatty acids, as each requires activation by the

TABLE 12.3

Energy Yield and Efficiency of the Complete Oxidation of Stearic Acid (C_{18}:O) by β-Oxidation and the TCA Cycle Through Electron Transport

		P/O ratio		Total ATP
From β-oxidation of stearic acid	8 $FADH_2$	× 2	=	16
	8 $NADH_2$	× 3	=	24
	From β-oxidation		=	40 ATP
From TCA	9 GTP	× –	=	9
	9 $FADH_2$	× 2	=	18
	27 $NADH_2$	× 3	=	81
			=	108 ATP
	Gross			
	– (Activation) 2 ATP			148 ATP
	Net yield			146 ATP

β-oxidation of stearic acid $\Delta G^{\circ\prime} = -7.3 \times 146 = 1{,}066$ kcal/mol
Complete oxidation of stearic acid $\Delta G^{\circ\prime}$ by $O_2 = 2{,}596$ kcal/mol

$$\frac{1066}{2596} \times 100 - 41\% \text{ efficient}$$

equivalent of two ATPs, and short-chain fatty acids contain proportionately less oxidizable hydrocarbon.

Even-carbon-numbered unsaturated fatty acids are metabolized in the same general way as even-numbered saturated fatty acids. Polyunsaturated fatty acids (PUFA) pose some metabolic problems because of the multiple unsaturated double bonds and their location. Nevertheless, these problems are surmounted by enzymes present in the mitochondrial matrix, and polyunsaturated fatty acids also follow the same general pathway of β-oxidation. Monounsaturated and polyunsaturated fatty acids have a slightly lower caloric value than do saturated fatty acids of similar carbon number, as unsaturation results in the reduction of the amount of reduced coenzymes formed and hydrogen traversing the ETC for ATP synthesis. Odd-carbon-numbered fatty acids (C:15, 17, 19, etc.) are oxidized in the usual β-oxidation pathway until the 3-carbon unit propionyl-CoA (instead of butryl-CoA) is reached. Propionyl-CoA is then carboxylated (involves biotin and vitamin B_{12}) and enters the TCA cycle as succinyl-CoA or succinate.

Catabolic Pathways of Proteins

Protein metabolism is continuous and constant in the normal and adequately nourished adult and can be biochemically assessed by measurement of nitrogen balance (nitrogen consumed minus nitrogen excreted). In the absence of food (calories) for an extended period, carbohydrates stored as glycogen in the muscle, heart, and liver are rapidly depleted. This loss of carbohydrate is followed by the hydrolysis of triglycerides, the mobilization of body depot fat, and the oxidation of fatty acids by β-oxidation. In the advent of extended starvation and catexia, massive amounts of the body's protein stores (e.g., muscle tissue) are mobilized for the body's energy requirements. Such events are serious when they occur and may result in extreme negative nitrogen balance.

Metabolically, proteins are enzymatically converted intracellularly to amino acids. Each of the 21 commonly found amino acids in protein follows catabolic routes after either transamination or deamination. Transamination from one amino acid leads to the synthesis of another amino acid, with the concurrent generation of a new α-keto acid. Vitamin B_6 functions in transamination and deamination of amino acids. In transamination reactions, nitrogen is not lost, only transferred from one amino acid in the synthesis of another amino acid. In deamination reactions, however, the loss of the amino moiety results in the production of ammonia (NH_3) as ammonium ions (NH_4^+), and as in transamination reactions, the synthesis of an α-keto acid. A deamination reaction requiring vitamin B_6 is the initial metabolic reaction common to the elimination of nitrogen from amino acids. Deamination is shown in Equation 12.14 for phenylalanine. The amino acids may be oxidized via amino acid oxidases, requiring the flavoprotein coenzymes FAD or FMN, specific for each amino acid.

EQUATION 12.14
Deamination of Phenylalanine.

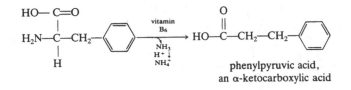

phenylpyruvic acid,
an α-ketocarboxylic acid

Reprinted with permission from CRC Press. Spallholz, J. E., Boylan, L. M., and Driskell, J. A., *Nutrition: Chemistry and Biology,* © 1999 by CRC Press, Boca Raton, FL.

The metabolism of the hydrocarbon portion of each of the deaminated amino acids is different and for many amino acids quite complex. Their ultimate oxidation, however, follows the established final common pathways of the TCA cycle and the ETC. The hydrocarbon portion of all 21 amino acids commonly found in protein enters catabolic pathways as either pyruvate, acetyl-CoA, α-ketoglutarate, succinyl-CoA, fumarate, or oxaloacetate. With the exception of pyruvate, these metabolites are all associated with the TCA cycle. The hydrocarbon portions of all deaminated amino acids, therefore, enter common catabolic pathways as either pyruvate or intermediates of the TCA cycle. Points of entry of the hydrocarbon portions of the amino acids into the TCA cycle are shown in Figure 12.10.

It may be apparent from Figure 12.10 that the caloric value and yield of ATP from each amino acid can be somewhat different depending on the point of entry of its hydrocarbon skeleton into the TCA cycle. Alanine, glycine, lysine, and so on, whose hydrocarbon skeletons become pyruvate, will yield more ATP than will the hydrocarbons of other amino acids, whose entry to the TCA cycle occurs later. The size of the hydrocarbon portion of the amino acid also has a bearing on caloric yield. For example, phenylalanine and tyrosine, larger-molecular-weight amino acids, are divided and enter the TCA cycle as two hydrocarbon fragments, acetyl-CoA and fumarate. Such variations in amino acid metabolism contribute to the average caloric value of 4 kcal/g for proteins.

Elimination of Ammonia: The Urea Cycle

Ammonia produced from the deamination of amino acids and other amines is strongly basic and very toxic. Cells of the liver and to a lesser degree, the kidney and brain, detoxify

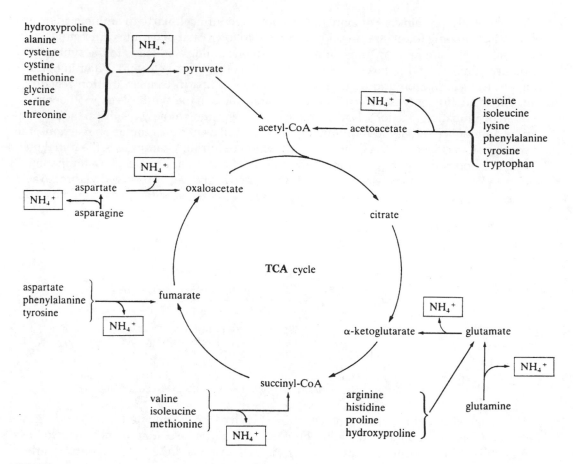

FIGURE 12.10
Deamination of amino acids and hydrocarbon entry into the TCA cycle. Reprinted with permission from CRC Press. Spallholz, J. E., Boylan, L. M., and Driskell, J. A., *Nutrition: Chemistry and Biology,* © 1999 by CRC Press, Boca Raton, FL.

ammonia by its conversion to the less toxic and water-soluble compound, ***urea***. The conversion of ammonia to urea from amino acids proceeds in the liver, kidney, and brain, predominantly through a single common pathway of a glutamic acid transamination-deamination and the urea cycle. Ammonia arising from deamination reactions in tissues other than the liver, kidney, or brain is coupled to the amino acid glutamate and is carried in the blood plasma to the liver or kidney as the basic amino acid glutamine (Equation 12.15).

EQUATION 12.15
Conversion of Ammonia to Glutamine.

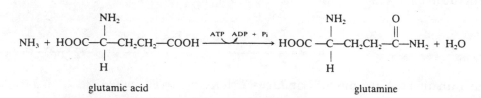

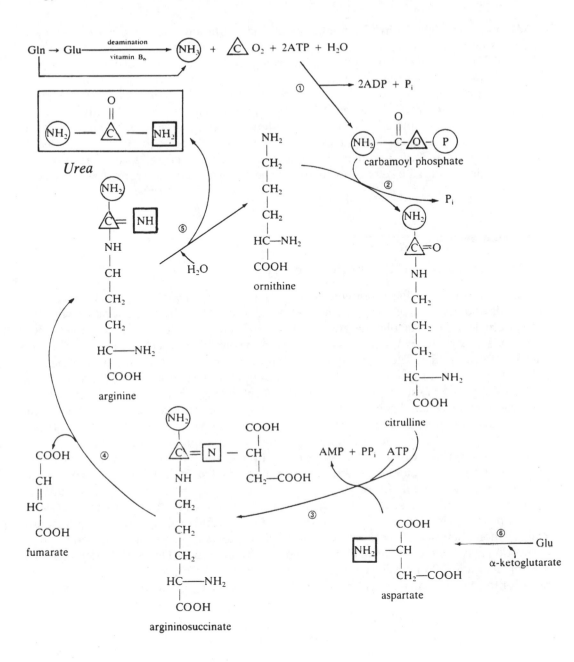

FIGURE 12.11
Urea cycle. 1. Carbamoyl phosphate synthetase. 2. Ornithine-carbamoyl transferase. 3. Argininosuccinate synthetase. 4. Argininosuccinate lyase. 5. Arginase. 6. Aminotransferase. Reprinted with permission from CRC Press. Spallholz, J. E., Boylan, L. M., and Driskell, J. A., *Nutrition: Chemistry and Biology*, © 1999 by CRC Press, Boca Raton, FL.

The formation of glutamine in Equation 12.15 requires ATP and results from the ammonia being coupled to glutamate. Glutamine, via a deamination reaction (involves vitamin B$_6$) in liver or kidney, yields ammonia, which is converted into carbamoyl phosphate, the first reaction of the urea cycle (Figure12.11). This reaction requires two molecules of ATP and carboxybiocytin. The remaining amine of glutamic acid enters the urea cycle either through carbamoyl phosphate or via a transamination from glutamic acid to aspartic acid, which then enters the urea cycle via coupling to citrulline in the formation of arginosuccinic acid. The latter reaction also requires an energy expenditure of one molecule of ATP for completion. The urea cycle, beginning with the synthesis of carbamoyl phosphate and ending with urea and the regeneration of ornithine, requires the expenditure of three molecules of ATP per molecule of urea generated. The derived ammonia (amino groups from glutamine, glutamate, and aspartate) in urea is contributed equally from a molecule of carbamoyl phosphate and aspartic acid. Manganese functions as a cofactor of the enzyme arginase with the ketone moiety of urea being derived from carbon dioxide (C) and water (O).

Energy, ATP, and the Catabolic Pathways

We have examined how the caloric energy of food (starch $\rightarrow$ glucose; lipids (or fats and oils) $\rightarrow$ fatty acids and glycerol; proteins $\rightarrow$ amino acids) is converted in the catabolic pathways to a more useful form of metabolic energy, ATP. The unanswered question throughout this discussion of energy transfer is: Where was the energy in the organic nutrients that was transferred and conserved as ATP? The energy transferred from the organic nutrients to ATP in the catabolic pathways was originally stored by plants during photosynthesis and was retained in the covalent bonds of the starch, lipids, proteins, and other organic molecules. Table 12.4 lists some representative bond energies that are present in organic nutrients. Examination of this table reveals that the organic nutrients of foods, which contain predominantly C–C, C–H, C–S, C–N, and C–O bonds, contain a great deal of stored energy expressed as kcal/mol.

The *caloric value* of food — carbohydrates, lipids, and proteins — is the amount of potential energy stored in the molecule's covalent bonds. During catabolic metabolism, the potential energy available for release and transfer to ATP is related to the total amount of hydrocarbon within molecules. The hydrocarbon content ($-CH_2-$) of the organic nutrients determines the caloric value of foods. The lipids, i.e., fats and oils, contain 9 cal/g (actually kcal/g), more than twice the caloric value of carbohydrates and protein (4 cal/g) because they proportionately contain about twice the amount of hydrocarbon. Figure 12.12 demonstrates the approximate 2.25:1:1 caloric ratios for lipids, carbohydrates, and protein, respectively, represented by the fatty acids hexonic and palmitic acids, glucose, and the dipeptide

TABLE 12.4

Representative Bond Energies That Are Present in Nutrients and Important Molecules

Bond	kcal/mol	Bond	kcal/mol
H–C	81	HC–H	108
C–C	144	HO–H	119
C–S	175	OC≠O	128
C–N	174	O–O	119
C–O	257	O–P	144
H_2N–H	103	S–S	102
HOH_2C–H	92	N≡N	226

Reprinted with permission from CRC Press. Spallholz, J. E., Boylan, L. M., and Driskell, J. A., *Nutrition: Chemistry and Biology.* © 1999 by CRC Press, Boca Raton, FL.

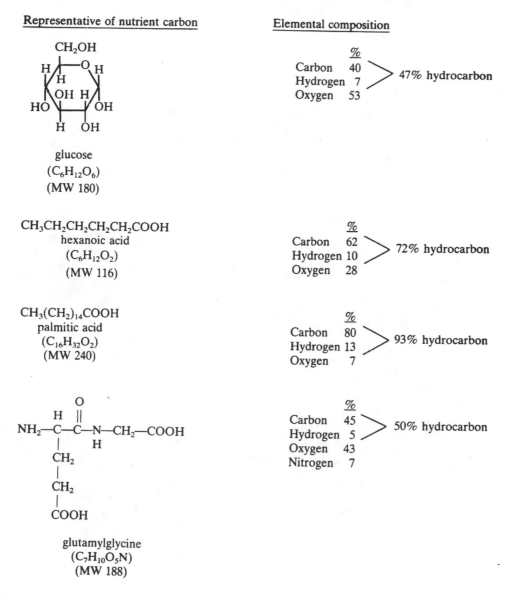

FIGURE 12.12

Hydrocarbon content of organic nutrients. Reprinted with permission from CRC Press. Spallholz, J. E., Boylan, L. M., and Driskell, J. A., *Nutrition: Chemistry and Biology,* © 1999 by CRC Press, Boca Raton, FL.

glutamylglycine. These small molecules approximate the elemental composition of the energy nutrients, the dietary fats, starch, and protein. Figure 12.12 shows the hydrocarbon ratios of palmitic acid, glucose, and glutamylglycine to be 1.98:1:1.2, which approaches the average caloric ratio of 2.25:1:1 for lipids, carbohydrates, and protein. When hexonic acid, with the same number of carbons (six) as glucose, and glutamylglycine are used in such calculations, the energy ratios go down because of a higher percentage of oxygen in hexanoic acid (27.6 percent) than palmitic acid (13.3 percent), which does not contribute to caloric value, yet hexanoic acid (MW 116) still has nearly 72 percent hydrocarbon. As Figure 12.12 indicates, as the molecular weight of fatty acids increases, the percentage of hydrocarbon, and hence calories, also increases. Herein lies the partial reason for the reduced caloric content of triglycerides like Solatrim®.

13

Weight Control

Most people talk about *weight control* with their friends, family, and health professionals. Weight control is a major concern of individuals of all ages. Frequently, people think that they are overweight, but they are not. Figure 13.1 summarizes the percentage of overweight people 20+ years of age who believe that they are overweight and are overweight according to NHANES III (a national survey) data of 1988-91, while Figure 13.2 summarizes the percentage of people 20+ years of age in the same survey who mistakingly believe they are overweight. Before individuals decide to attempt to lose weight, they should seek information as to their optimal body weight.

Healthy Body Weight

A couple of decades ago, the ideal body weight was thought to be within 10 or 20 percent of ideal weight values listed in one of two or three tables. Today, the definition is not so well-defined.

Several different tables have been utilized in estimating appropriate body weights. Those applicable to adults will be discussed in this chapter; however, tables do exist for infants, children, and adolescents.

The *1995 Dietary Guidelines for Americans* uses the term *healthy weight ranges*. Increased health risks are associated with being overweight and underweight. Figure 13.3 gives the healthy weight range as well as ranges for moderate and severe overweight. The higher weights in the ranges are intended for people who have more muscle and bone. In estimating healthy weight using this figure, height is taken without shoes and weight without or with light clothes.

The *Metropolitan Life Insurance Table* (Table 13.1) is another standard utilized for estimating healthy weights for adults. Values for this table were obtained by obtaining height and weight measurements of individuals 25 to 59 years having the lowest mortality. The data were derived using height and weight values of purchasers of life insurance. The height measurement is taken with 1 inch heels. The weight measurement includes 3 pounds of clothing for women and 5 pounds for men. *Frame size* categories were derived from elbow breadth measurements such that 50 percent of the population had medium; 25 percent, small; and 25 percent large, frames. Table 13.2 lists the elbow breadth measurements associated with each of the frame sizes.

The preferred method for evaluation of body weight is the *body mass index* (BMI). Theoretically, the BMI mathematically accounts for differences in body composition with respect to adiposity. The BMI is useful in identifying obese individuals, but is less useful in evaluating adiposity in nonobese individuals, such as many types of athletes, particularly

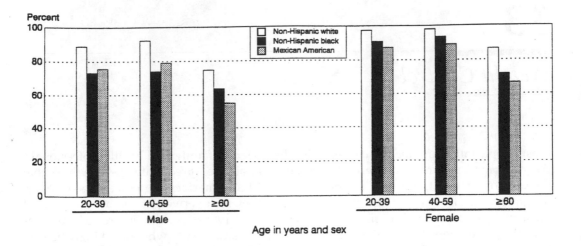

FIGURE 13.1
Self-perceived overweight: percentage of overweight people 20 years of age and older who think they are overweight by age, sex, and race/ethnicity, 1989-91. From Department of Health and Human Services, NHANES III, 1988-91. Reprinted with permission from Life Sciences Research Office. Federation of American Societies for Experimental Biology, *Third Report on Nutrition Monitoring in the United States,* © 1995. U.S. Government Printing Office, Washington, DC.

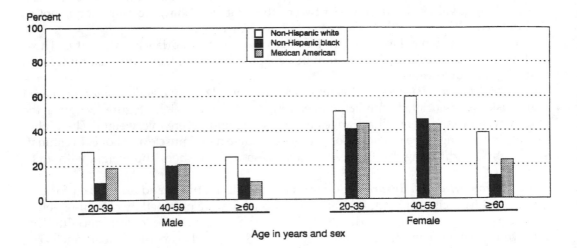

FIGURE 13.2
Self-perceived overweight: percentage of people 20 years of age and older who think they are overweight, but are not overweight, by age, sex, and race/ethnicity, 1988-91. From Department of Health and Human Services, NHANES III, 1988-91. Reprinted with permission from Life Sciences Research Office. Federation of American Societies for Experimental Biology, *Third Report on Nutrition Monitoring in the United States,* © 1995. U.S. Government Printing Office, Washington, DC.

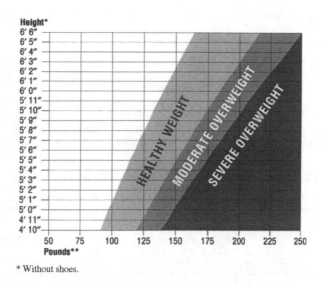

* Without shoes.

** Without clothes. The higher weights apply to people with more muscle and bone, such as many men.

FIGURE 13.3

Ranges for healthy weight, moderate overweight, and severe overweight. Taken from U.S. Department of Agriculture and of Health and Human Services, *Nutrition and Your Health: Dietary Guidelines for Americans*, 1995.

TABLE 13.1

1983 Metropolitan Height and Weight Tables

| MEN | | | | | WOMEN | | | | |
| Height | | Small Frame | Medium Frame | Large Frame | Height | | Small Frame | Medium Frame | Large Frame |
Feet	Inches				Feet	Inches			
5	2	128-134	131-141	138-150	4	10	102-111	109-121	118-131
5	3	130-136	133-143	140-153	4	11	103-113	111-123	120-134
5	4	132-138	135-145	142-156	5	0	104-115	113-126	122-137
5	5	134-140	137-148	144-160	5	1	106-118	115-129	125-140
5	6	136-142	139-151	146-164	5	2	108-121	118-132	128-143
5	7	138-145	142-154	149-168	5	3	111-124	121-135	131-147
5	8	140-148	145-157	152-172	5	4	114-127	124-138	134-151
5	9	142-151	148-160	155-176	5	5	117-130	127-141	137-155
5	10	144-154	151-163	158-180	5	6	120-133	130-144	140-159
5	11	146-157	154-166	161-184	5	7	123-136	133-147	143-163
6	0	149-160	157-170	164-188	5	8	126-139	136-150	146-167
6	1	152-164	160-174	168-192	5	9	129-142	139-153	149-170
6	2	155-168	164-178	172-197	5	10	132-145	142-156	152-173
6	3	158-172	167-182	176-202	5	11	135-148	145-159	155-176
6	4	162-176	171-187	181-207	6	0	138-151	148-162	158-179

[a] Weights for adults 25 to 59 years based on lowest mortality. See Table 13.2 for determination of frame size.

The data are from the *1979 Build Study* of the Society of Actuaries and Association of Life Insurance Medical Directors of America and is Courtesy of the Metropolitan Life Insurance Company, *Statistical Bulletin*, © 1983.

TABLE 13.2

Determination of Frame Size

The patient's right arm is extended forward perpendicular to the body, with the arm bent so the angle at the elbow forms a 90° angle with the fingers pointing up and the palm turned away from the body. The greatest breadth across the elbow joint is measured with a sliding caliper along the axis of the upper arm, on the two prominent bones on either side of the elbow. The tables given below give the elbow breadth measurements for medium-framed men and women of various heights. Measurements lower than those listed indicate a small frame size; higher measurements indicate a large frame size.

Men		Women	
Height in 1 inch heels	Elbow Breadth	Height in 1 inch heels	Elbow Breadth
5′2″–5′3″	2½″–2⅞″	4′10″–4′11″	2¼″–2½″
5′4″–5′7″	2⅝″–2⅞″	5′0″–5′3″	2¼″–2½″
5′8″–5′11″	2¾″–3″	5′4″–5′7″	2⅜″–2⅝″
6′0″–6′3″	2¾″–3⅛″	5′8″–5′11″	2⅜″–2⅝″
6′4″	2⅞″–3¼″	6′0″	2½″–2¾″

The data are from the *1979 Build Study* of the Society of Actuaries and Association of Life Insurance Medical Directors of America and is Courtesy of the Metropolitan Life Insurance Company, *Statistical Bulletin,* © 1983.

those who have "built up" their bodies. However, BMI values are well correlated with health risk. The formula for calculating BMI is given below.

$$\text{BMI} = \frac{\text{weight in kg}}{(\text{height in meters})^2} \quad \text{or} \quad \text{BMI} = \frac{\text{weight in pounds}}{(\text{height in inches})^2} \times 705$$

An individual's height should be measured in stocking feet, with feet together and heels and back against the wall or a board (Figure 13.4). A bar on the top of a *statiometer* should be lowered to rest flat on the top of the head. The individual, wearing light clothing, should have body weight measured using a *beam balance scale*. In 1998 The National Heart, Lung, and Blood Institute in cooperation with the National Institute of Diabetes and Digestive and Heart Disease, both part of the National Institutes of Health, released the first federal guidelines on identification, evaluation, and treatment of overweight and obesity in adults. These guidelines identified *desirable body weights* (also known as desirable BMIs) as being a BMI between 20 and 24.9, *overweight* as a BMI of 25 to 29.9, and *obesity* as being a BMI of 30 and above. Individuals with BMIs below 20 are considered to be *underweight*. Individuals should not be concerned if their BMIs are slightly lower than 20 or slightly higher than 25. Once again, BMIs are not appropriate for use with muscular individuals.

These two institutes also indicated that assessment of overweight involves evaluation of BMI, waist circumference, and a patient's risk factors for diseases/conditions associated with obesity. *Waist circumferences* (see Figure 13.5) above 40 inches in men and 35 inches in women is indicative of increased risk in adults having BMIs above 25.

Better methods exist for evaluating body composition, but are rarely used in estimating optimal body weight. These methods involve the use of equipment frequently not available in a nonresearch setting or a trained individual is needed to perform these measurements. Other methods for evaluating body composition are discussed in Chapter 14.

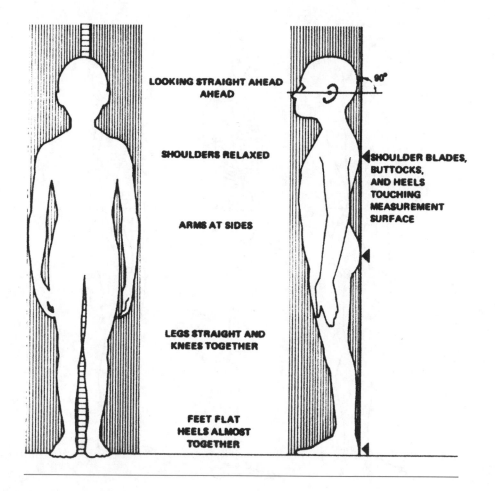

FIGURE 13.4

Positioning of subject for height measurement. Reprinted with permission of J. A. Gilbride. Simko, M. D., Cowell, C., and Gilbride, J. A., *Nutrition Assessment: A Comprehensive Guide for Planning Intervention*, © 1984. Aspen Publishers, Gaithersburg, MD.

Energy Balance

Energy balance is when energy (cal) intake is equal to energy (cal) output or expenditure. Maintaining energy balance is critical with regard to maintaining body weight. One of the 1995 *Dietary Guidelines for Americans* is to "balance the food you eat with physical activity — maintain or improve your weight." Health problems have been associated with being overweight or underweight. Obesity and underweight will be discussed in detail in Chapters 14 and 15, respectively.

Regular *aerobic exercise* results in more desirable body weight and body composition. *Resistance training* results in better maintenance of lean body mass. Exercise can also alter body composition, such that there is decreased adipose tissue and even a small increase in lean body mass. Frequency, intensity, and duration of specific exercises are important considerations in weight control. There is no one best exercise. One should begin slowly and

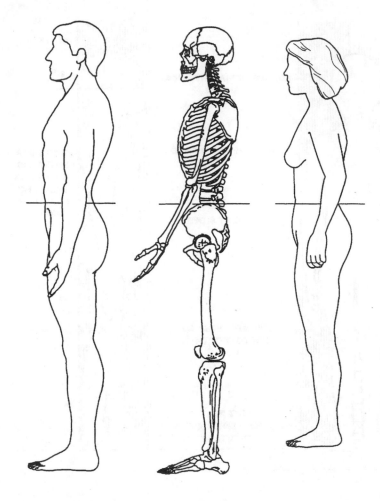

FIGURE 13.5
Measuring tape position for waist circumference. Taken from National Heart, Lung, and Blood Institute's *Clinical Guidelines Report*, 1998.

progress steadily. Each exercise bout should expend or burn *at least 300 cal*. The calorie-expending effects of exercise are additive. Exercise needs to be part of the daily routine.

Caloric Intake and Body Weight Changes

Theoretically, 1 pound of body weight is lost when energy expenditure exceeds caloric intake by *3,500 cal*, and 1 pound of body weight is gained when caloric intake exceeds energy expenditure by 3,500 cal. However, great individual variation exists as to how efficient one's body is in converting food energy (or energy intake) to energy expenditure (or energy output).

Weight Loss

When less food energy is consumed than the body expends, the body utilizes its stored energy sources. It is advantageous to eat periodically, store energy, and then use up all that energy between meals. The body uses up its readily available liver glycogen every four to six hours while one is awake. If one consumes about 500 cal less than one expends, but consumes an otherwise adequate diet, the body will use adipose stores for energy production and gradual weight loss will occur. One can also increase their normal energy expenditure by about 500 cal. It is best to lose weight gradually. The recommended weight loss for adults is 1 to 2 pounds weekly. If one loses body weight fast, the loss is in primarily water and perhaps electrolytes. Also, if one uses primarily fat for energy production, ketosis occurs. Fasting is not the best way to lose weight, as lean body mass is decreased. Diets low in carbohydrates are not advised as there are losses of water and lean body mass as well as physiological problems such as hypoglycemia and mineral imbalances. Liquid protein diets are not advised unless adequate amounts of other essential nutrients are included. Adults should consume a *minimum of 1,000 to 1,200 cal* unless they are under the direct care of a physician. Adults consuming less than 1,000 to 1,200 should take a multivitamin/multimineral supplement daily. Many pharmaceutical products are available that are proposed to help one lose weight; most of these are ineffective and some are dangerous. Sometimes, surgeons may perform gastric bypasses and gastroplasties on individuals who are morbidly obese and who have been unsuccessful in losing weight.

There are three basic principles that should be followed in losing weight. These are as follows:

- Decrease caloric intake
- Increase energy expenditure
- Behavior modification

Frequently, individuals need to modify their usual eating and exercise habits so they can lose weight and maintain a desirable body weight. With regard to successful *weight loss plans*, the following are recommended:

- Persons should make their own decisions that they want to lose weight.
- Persons should have positive attitudes about weight loss and believe that they can lose the weight.
- Persons should develop weight loss programs for themselves that favor success.
- Persons should set reasonable goals for weight loss for themselves.
- Persons should combine decreased caloric intake and increased physical activity, taking a gradual, but sustained approach.
- Persons should improve their eating and exercise habits.
- Persons should develop appropriate ways for themselves to gradually shift to more desirable eating and exercise habits.

The composition of the diet influences how efficiently the body converts excessive energy from caloric intake to adipose tissue. About a quarter of the energy from ingested carbohydrates is needed to convert it to adipose tissue, while only 3 percent of the energy of ingested fats is needed for this conversion. It is best to consume a diet high in complex carbohydrate, high in fiber, moderately low in fat, and moderate in protein that contains sufficient quantities of all of the essential micronutrients. No food plan is magical; food plans must be individualized.

Many Americans have difficulty curbing their appetites and increasing physical activity. When one is deciding to change their eating and exercise behaviors, they need to plan behaviors that they can follow the rest of their lives.

Weight cycling or *"yo-yo" dieting* is when there are repeated rounds of weight loss and weight regain. This is not good for one's health, and it tends to make the body more efficient at manufacturing and storing fat.

A person has to take personal ownership and responsibility for their weight loss plan or the program will not be successful. Individuals are responsible for controlling their own body weights.

Weight Gain

Weight gain, similar to weight loss, plans follow three basic principles; these are as follows:

- Increasing caloric intake
- Decreasing physical activity
- Behavior modification

First, a person needs to decide whether weight gain is warranted. Then they need to decide if they want to gain total body weight or primarily lean tissue weight (muscular tissues). Individuals trying to gain weight should eat foods that are less nutrient-dense than those eaten by people wanting to lose weight. Individuals wanting to gain weight should eat more frequently and have higher-calorie snacks than individuals not wanting to gain weight. An altered exercise regimen may also be part of the weight gain plan if one wants to increase their lean tissues. Resistance training can result in increases, usually small, in lean body mass.

Behavior Modification

Behavior modification is an essential component of both weight loss and weight gain plans. Behavior modification is very important with regard to weight control. Individuals need to modify their eating and exercise habits such that they can practice them for life, and even prefer their newly modified habits to their old habits. After all, eating and exercise should be pleasurable activities.

Today, Americans exercise less than they did one or two decades ago. Watching television and using the computer are popular activities for individuals of all ages. Research shows that individuals of all ages who maintain a physically active lifestyle maintain a desirable body weight.

Body Composition

Body Composition

The composition of the body may be evaluated by methods other than those based upon body weight and height (discussed in Chapter 13) of an individual. These methods are more appropriate for use with individuals who have built up their bodies. These methods involve determinations or estimations of the fat and/or the lean components of the body by either *direct or indirect assessment*. Generally, indirect assessment methods are utilized in evaluating body composition. The "gold standard" for evaluation of body composition is *hydrostatic weighing*, also known as underwater weighing. Body composition is frequently estimated by a trained technician performing one to five site-specific *skinfold measurements*, also known as fatfold measurements. *Girth measurements*, also known as circumference measurements, are also sometimes taken of specific areas of the body in evaluating body composition, frequently in combination with skinfold measurements. Other direct methods occasionally used in assessing body composition are ultrasound, bio-electrical impedance, and computer tomography and magnetic resonance imaging scanning. All of the above listed methods for assessing body composition are thought to be better than methods based on height and weight measurements, particularly for the athletic population. However, measurements other than height and weight are more expensive, time consuming, and must be done by individuals with specific training.

Overweight and *obesity* are prevalent in many age:gender groups, particularly in Western countries. A quarter to a half of the adults in the United States are overweight. *Underweight* and *eating disorders* are often observed in adolescents and young adults, particularly those who are athletes. Health problems have been associated with being overweight and underweight. Nutrition and exercise is of importance in weight loss and weight gain programs. Nutrition and exercise therapists frequently treat individuals who are overweight and underweight. In the case of eating disorders and severe obesity, psychoanalysis is an essential part of the treatment. Nutrition and exercise therapists are essential members of the health care team in the treatment of individuals who are overweight and underweight.

Conditioning influences body composition. Individuals who are conditioned are able to much more easily perform physical and perhaps even mental tasks than unconditioned individuals. Physical conditioning is important in obtaining and maintaining fitness and a desirable quality of life.

14

Assessment of Body Composition

The use of height-weight measurements and calculations for evaluating body composition were discussed in Chapter 13. Other methods for evaluation of body composition are available and are superior, particularly for the athletic population.

The body contains two chemically distinct compartments: *fat mass* and *fat-free mass*. Fat-free mass (FFM) consists of skeletal and nonskeletal muscles and soft lean tissues as well as the skeleton. Methods exist to directly and indirectly assess fat mass and fat-free mass.

Direct Assessment of Body Composition

Direct assessment of body composition is often utilized with animals, but rarely with humans. Direct assessment involves chemical analysis of carcasses, which is time-consuming and requires specialized equipment. Ethical and legal problems exist with regard to utilizing human cadavers in body composition studies.

Indirect Assessment of Body Composition

Most methods utilized to evaluate body composition of humans are indirect. Values obtained utilizing these *indirect assessment* methods are estimates of body composition. However, generally several of these indirect assessment methods are utilized so that more accurate estimates of body composition are obtained. These indirect assessment methods will be discussed in this chapter.

Hydrostatic Weighing

Hydrostatic weighing, also known as underwater weighing, is the "gold standard" for the assessment of body composition. Archimedes Principle is applied in estimating body composition by hydrostatic weighing. In hydrostatic weighing, the body weight of a person is compared with their body volume as estimated by the amount of water that the body displaces (see Figure 14.1); hence, *whole body density* may be estimated. In hydrostatic weighing, basically the subject is first weighed, and then is submerged either totally (the best) or up to just below the nose (often used) in water in a large tank, and water displacement is measured. The subject should expel as much air as possible before immersion, thus removing residual air. This measurement is usually repeated three times and a mean value utilized. Warm water is generally used and correction factors are utilized to correct to cold

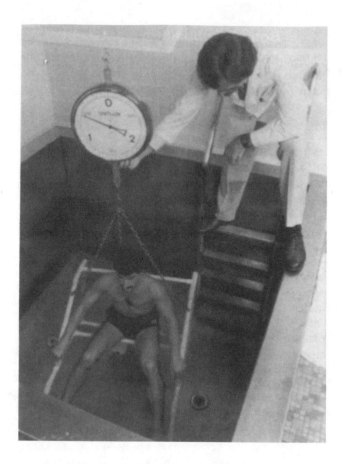

FIGURE 14.1
Equipment for hydrostatic weighing. Reprinted with permission from Mayfield Publishing Company. Nieman, D. C., *Fitness and Sports Medicine: An Introduction,* © 1990. Bull Publishing Company, Palo Alto, CA.

water densities. The values are also corrected for intestinal gas (from the subjects). Various equations have been developed for calculating *percent body fat* and *lean body mass* from these measurements. The densities of fat and fat-free tissues theoretically remain constant with fat tissue = 0.90 g/ml and fat-free tissue = 1.10 g/ml. The most commonly used equation is that developed by W. Siri, which is: percent body fat = 495 ÷ body density − 450. Lean body mass (LBM) is equal to body mass (or body weight) minus fat mass (fat weight). The density values of 0.90 and 1.10 g/ml were obtained in studies using young to middle-aged White adults. Racial differences are thought to exist with regard to densities of fat and fat-free mass, and equations have been proposed for use with the Black population. It may also be that these density values are different for the elite athlete. Underwater weighing is not appropriate for use by some population groups including young children, obese individuals, the elderly, and the unhealthy. Hydrostatic weighing methods yield reproducible results, within about 5 percent, provided that the technicians performing the measurement and the subjects are trained with regard to appropriate procedures.

Other Methods for Evaluating Body Density

Body density may be evaluated by hydrostatic weighing as discussed previously. Body density may also be evaluated by plasma dilution, ^{40}K counting, urinary creatinine excretion,

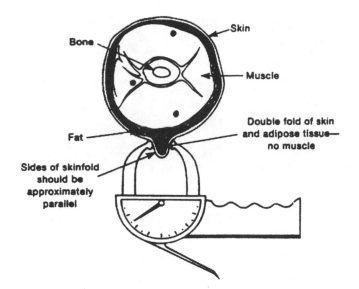

FIGURE 14.2

Skinfold measurements. Reprinted with permission from McGraw-Hill Companies. Lee, R. D., and Nieman, D. C., *Nutritional Assessment*, © 1993. William C. Brown Communications, Dubuque, IA.

total body electrical conductivity, bioelectrical impedence, dual-energy x-ray absorptiometry (DEXA), computerized axial tomography (CAT), and nuclear magnetic resonance (MRI). These methods for evaluating body density are not often utilized because of the expense of the equipment and/or the required personnel expertise. Also, norms for comparison, particularly for nonwhite populations, are not as readily available for data obtained by these methods.

Skinfold Thickness Measurements

Approximately one-third of the total body fat in the reference man and women is present as subcutaneous fat. Hence, *skinfold thickness* (also called fatfold thickness) measurements provide estimates of both subcutaneous and total body fat (Figure 14.2). Expensive equipment is not required for these measurements, but the individuals performing these measurements need to be trained. Skinfold thicknesses are best made utilizing precision calibrated skinfold calipers (Figure14.3), most commonly the Lange calipers. The trained technician grasps a fold of skin plus the underlying fat at specific sites, pulling it away from the underlying muscle tissues, and then the jaws of the calipers are applied at right angles exactly at the midpoint site (Figure 14.4). The measurement is usually taken repeatedly until the same value is obtained twice.

Skinfold thickness measurements are most often obtained for the triceps; however, often three to five or even more sites are utilized. Skinfold measurements are most often taken on the right side of the body, but may be taken on the left or on both sides. The sites commonly used in measuring skinfolds are detailed along with instructions for obtaining these measurements:

- Triceps skinfold measurement — obtained utilizing a vertical fold at the midpoint of the upper arm (see Figures 14.5 and 14.6).
- Subscapular skinfold measurement — obtained utilizing an oblique fold just below and lateral to the angle of the shoulder blade with the arm and shoulder relaxed (Figures 14.7).

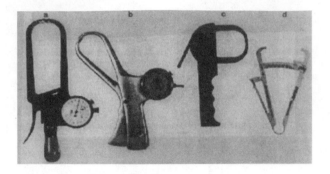

FIGURE 14.3
Skinfold calipers. (a) Harpenden, (b) Holtain, (c) Lange, and (d) McGaw skinfold calipers. Reprinted with permission from R. S. Gibson. Gibson, R. S., *Principles of Nutritional Assessment*, © 1990. Oxford Press, New York, NY.

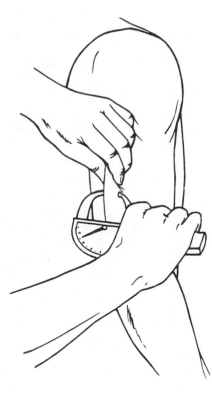

Grasp a double fold of skin and subcutaneous adipose tissue with the thumb and index finger of the left hand.

Place the caliper tips on the site where the sides of the skinfold are approximately parallel and 1 cm distal to where the skinfold is grasped.

Position the caliper dial so that it can be read easily. Obtain the measurement about 4 sec after placing the caliper tips on the skinfold.

FIGURE 14.4
Measurement of skinfold thickness using caliper. Reprinted with permission from McGraw-Hill Companies. Lee, R. D., and Nieman, D. C., *Nutritional Assessment*, © 1993. William C. Brown Communications, Dubuque, IA.

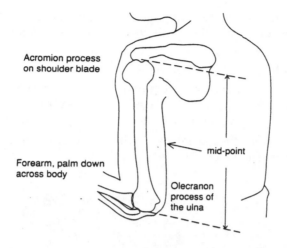

FIGURE 14.5

Location of the midpoint of upper arm. Reprinted with permission of J. A. Gilbride. Simko, M. D., Cowell, C., and Gilbride, J. A., *Nutrition Assessment: A Comprehensive Guide for Planning Intervention,* © 1984. Aspen Publishers, Gaithersburg, MD.

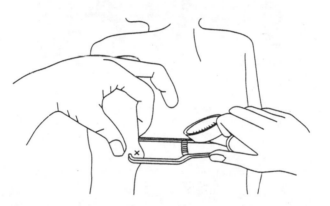

FIGURE 14.6

Measurement of the triceps skinfold. Reprinted with permission of J. A. Gilbride. Simko, M. D., Cowell, C., and Gilbride, J. A., *Nutrition Assessment: A Comprehensive Guide for Planning Intervention,* © 1984. Aspen Publishers, Gaithersburg, MD.

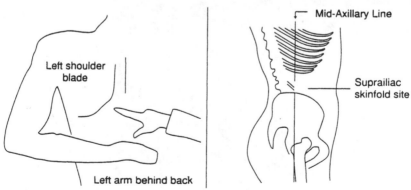

FIGURE 14.7

Location of subscapular and suprailiac skinfold sites. Reprinted with permission from R. S. Gibson. Gibson, R. S., *Principles of Nutritional Assessment,* © 1990. Oxford Press, New York, NY.

- Suprailiac skinfold measurement — obtained utilizing a slightly oblique fold in the midaxillary line immediately above the iliac crest (Figures 14.7).

- Abdominal skinfold measurement — obtained using a horizontal fold one inch to the right of the umbilicus (Figure 14.8).

- Thigh skinfold measurement — obtained using a vertical fold at the thigh mid-line (Figure 14.9). • Biceps skinfold measurement — obtained using a vertical fold on the front of the upper arm, at the same level as the triceps skinfold.

- Midaxillary skinfold measurement —obtained using a horizontal fold on the midaxillary line at the xiphoid process.

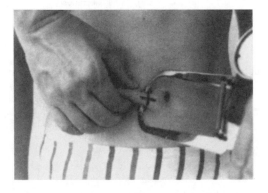

FIGURE 14.8
Measurement of abdominal skinfold. Reprinted with permission from Human Kinetics. Harrison, G. G. et al. Skinfold thicknesses and measurement technique, In: Lohman, T. et al., Eds., *Anthropometric Standardization Reference Manual*, © 1988. Human Kinetics Books, Champaign, IL.

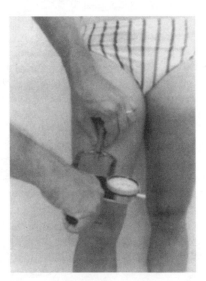

FIGURE 14.9
Measurement of thigh skinfold. Reprinted with permission from Human Kinetics. Harrison, G. G. et al. Skinfold thicknesses and measurement technique, In: Lohman, T. et al., Eds., *Anthropometric Standardization Reference Manual*, © 1988. Human Kinetics Books, Champaign, IL.

TABLE 14.1

Triceps Skinfolds (mm) for Males 18 to 74 Years of Age, By Race and Age: United States, 1976–80

Race and age	Number of examined persons	Mean	Standard deviation	Percentile								
				5th	10th	15th	25th	50th	75th	85th	90th	95th
All races[a]												
18-74 years	5,916	12.9	6.7	5.0	6.0	6.5	8.0	12.0	16.0	19.5	22.0	25.5
18-24 years	988	11.6	6.5	4.5	5.0	6.0	6.5	10.0	15.0	17.5	20.0	24.5
25-34 years	1,067	12.9	7.0	4.5	5.5	6.5	7.5	11.5	16.5	20.0	23.0	26.0
35-44 years	745	13.8	7.1	5.0	6.0	7.0	9.0	12.5	17.0	20.0	23.0	27.0
45-54 years	690	13.5	6.7	5.5	6.5	7.0	9.0	12.0	16.5	20.0	22.0	25.5
55-64 years	1,227	13.2	6.3	5.0	6.0	7.5	9.0	12.0	16.0	19.5	21.5	25.5
65-74 years	1,199	12.7	6.1	5.0	6.0	7.0	8.0	11.5	16.0	18.5	21.0	25.0
White												
18-74 years	5,148	13.0	6.6	5.0	6.0	7.0	8.0	12.0	16.0	19.5	22.0	25.5
18-24 years	846	11.9	6.5	4.5	5.0	6.0	7.0	10.0	15.0	18.0	20.0	25.0
25-34 years	901	13.1	6.9	5.0	6.0	7.0	8.0	12.0	16.5	20.0	22.5	26.0
35-44 years	653	13.9	7.0	5.5	6.5	7.0	9.0	12.5	17.0	21.0	23.0	27.0
45-54 years	617	13.4	6.5	5.5	6.5	7.5	9.0	12.0	16.5	20.0	21.0	25.0
55-64 years	1,086	13.1	5.9	5.5	6.5	7.5	9.0	12.0	16.0	19.0	21.0	24.5
65-74 years	1,045	12.9	6.0	5.0	6.5	7.0	8.0	12.0	16.0	19.0	21.0	25.0
Black												
18-74 years	649	12.1	7.8	4.0	4.5	5.0	6.5	10.0	16.0	19.0	23.0	27.0
18-24 years	121	9.7	6.4	4.0	4.0	4.5	5.0	7.5	13.0	15.0	18.5	21.5
25-34 years	139	11.5	7.5	3.5	4.0	5.0	6.0	10.0	15.5	19.0	23.0	24.5
35-44 years	70	13.0	8.1	*	5.0	6.5	9.0	11.0	16.0	18.5	20.0	*
45-54 years	62	15.0	8.7	*	5.5	6.0	9.0	13.0	18.0	25.5	27.5	*
55-64 years	129	12.9	7.8	3.5	4.5	5.5	7.0	10.5	17.5	22.0	25.0	29.0
65-74 years	128	11.6	6.7	4.0	4.5	5.5	7.0	10.0	14.5	16.0	19.5	27.5

[a] Includes all other races not shown as separate categories.

Taken from U.S. Department of Health and Human Services, *Anthropometric Reference Data and Prevalence of Overweight: United States, 1976–80*, 1987. Sample size was 25–44 and does not meet the reliability standard.

Skinfold measurements of an individual or group of individuals may be compared to published tables to determine whether values are within the normal ranges. The tables most often used for these comparisons are those from the NHANES II national survey of 1976-80, and the normal range is generally interpreted as being between the 15th and 85th percentiles. NHANES II tables for triceps and subscapular skinfold measurements for adults are given in Tables14.1 to 14.4. Similar tables are available for children and adolescents.

Sum of skinfolds (fatfolds) are often utilized in evaluating body composition. Skinfold measurements from three or more sites are summed (added) together. A combination of skinfold measurements may also provide information on body fat distribution. Multiple skinfold measurements are advised for the evaluation of individuals undergoing body weight changes and physical training programs, with selected skinfold measurements being taken before and at intervals during the training program.

TABLE 14.2

Triceps Skinfolds (mm) for Females 18 to 74 Years of Age, By Race and Age: United States, 1976–80

Race and age	Number of examined persons	Mean	Standard deviation	Percentile								
				5th	10th	15th	25th	50th	75th	85th	90th	95th
All races[a]												
18-74 years	6,588	24.9	9.8	11.0	13.0	15.0	17.5	24.0	31.0	35.1	38.0	43.0
18-24 years	1,066	20.7	8.6	10.0	11.5	12.5	15.0	19.0	25.0	29.5	32.0	37.0
25-34 years	1,170	23.6	9.9	10.0	13.0	14.0	16.5	22.0	29.0	33.5	36.6	43.5
35-44 years	844	26.3	9.8	12.0	14.5	16.5	19.5	25.0	32.6	37.0	40.5	44.5
45-54 years	763	27.5	9.7	12.5	15.0	17.0	20.5	27.0	34.0	38.0	40.5	45.0
55-64 years	1,329	27.2	9.5	12.0	15.0	17.5	21.0	26.5	33.0	37.0	40.0	43.6
65-74 years	1,416	25.7	9.0	12.0	14.5	16.5	19.0	25.0	31.0	35.0	37.6	42.0
White												
18-74 years	5,686	24.7	9.5	11.5	13.5	15.0	17.5	23.5	30.5	35.0	37.5	42.5
18-24 years	892	20.8	8.5	10.5	11.5	13.0	15.0	19.0	25.0	29.0	32.0	37.1
25-34 years	1,000	23.3	9.4	10.5	13.0	14.0	16.5	22.0	28.5	33.0	36.0	42.1
35-44 years	726	26.1	9.6	12.0	14.5	16.0	19.0	24.5	32.0	36.5	40.0	44.0
45-54 years	647	27.2	9.4	13.0	15.0	16.5	20.5	27.0	33.0	37.0	40.0	43.1
55-64 years	1,176	27.0	9.4	12.5	15.0	17.5	21.0	26.0	32.6	36.5	39.1	43.1
65-74 years	1,245	25.5	8.8	12.0	14.5	16.5	19.0	25.0	30.5	34.0	37.0	41.1
Black												
18-74 years	782	26.6	11.6	10.0	12.0	14.0	17.5	25.5	35.0	39.0	42.5	48.0
18-24 years	147	20.6	8.8	8.0	10.0	11.0	14.0	19.0	27.0	31.0	35.0	37.0
25-34 years	145	25.5	12.2	8.0	11.0	13.0	16.0	24.0	32.0	37.0	47.0	49.5
35-44 years	103	28.7	11.4	9.0	14.0	15.5	20.5	29.5	36.6	40.5	45.0	48.0
45-54 years	100	31.6	11.8	10.5	16.0	20.0	23.5	31.5	40.0	43.5	48.5	53.1
55-64 years	135	29.5	10.8	12.0	14.0	18.0	22.0	28.5	38.5	42.0	43.0	46.0
65-74 years	152	29.0	10.5	11.5	14.5	17.0	21.5	29.0	37.0	38.6	44.0	47.5

[a] Includes all other races not shown as separate categories.

Taken from U.S. Department of Health and Human Services, *Anthropometric Reference Data and Prevalence of Overweight: United States, 1976–80,* 1987.

TABLE 14.3

Subscapular Skinfolds (mm) for Males 18 to 74 Years of Age, By Race and Age: United States, 1976–80

Race and age	Number of examined persons	Mean	Standard deviation	Percentile								
				5th	10th	15th	25th	50th	75th	85th	90th	95th
All races[a]												
18-74 years	5,916	17.4	8.8	7.0	8.0	9.0	10.5	15.0	22.5	26.0	30.0	34.6
18-24 years	988	13.7	7.5	6.5	7.0	7.5	8.5	11.5	16.0	20.0	23.0	30.0
25-34 years	1,067	16.9	8.6	7.0	8.0	9.0	10.0	15.0	22.0	25.5	29.0	34.0
35-44 years	745	18.7	9.2	7.0	8.5	10.0	12.0	17.0	24.0	28.0	30.5	37.0
45-54 years	690	19.4	8.9	7.5	9.0	10.0	12.5	18.0	25.0	29.0	31.0	36.0
55-64 years	1,227	18.9	8.4	7.5	9.0	10.0	12.5	18.0	24.0	27.0	30.0	34.5
65-74 years	1,199	17.9	8.7	7.0	8.0	9.5	11.0	16.0	23.0	27.5	30.5	35.1
White												
18-74 years	5,148	17.3	8.5	7.0	8.0	9.0	11.0	15.5	22.0	26.0	29.5	34.0
18-24 years	846	13.8	7.5	6.5	7.0	7.5	8.5	11.5	16.5	20.5	24.0	30.0
25-34 years	901	16.9	8.3	7.0	8.0	9.0	10.5	15.0	22.0	25.5	29.0	32.5
35-44 years	653	18.5	8.7	7.0	9.0	10.0	12.0	17.0	23.5	27.0	30.0	35.0
45-54 years	617	19.1	8.6	8.0	9.0	10.0	12.5	17.5	24.0	28.5	30.5	35.1
55-64 years	1,086	18.9	8.3	7.5	9.5	10.5	12.5	18.0	24.0	27.0	29.5	34.0
65-74 years	1,045	18.0	8.5	7.0	8.0	9.5	11.5	16.0	23.0	27.5	30.0	35.0
Black												
18-74 years	649	17.8	10.5	6.5	7.5	8.5	10.0	14.0	24.0	30.0	32.1	38.1
18-24 years	121	12.6	6.6	6.5	7.5	8.0	9.0	10.5	14.5	16.5	19.5	25.0
25-34 years	139	17.2	10.1	7.0	8.0	8.5	9.0	13.0	23.0	27.0	34.0	38.0
35-44 years	70	20.3	12.2	*	8.5	9.5	11.0	17.0	26.0	35.0	40.0	*
45-54 years	62	22.8	11.1	*	8.0	10.0	13.0	21.5	30.0	37.0	37.0	*
55-64 years	129	18.7	9.9	6.0	7.0	8.0	9.5	18.0	26.0	30.0	32.1	37.0
65-74 years	128	18.4	10.4	5.5	7.0	8.0	10.0	15.0	26.5	30.5	33.0	37.0

[a]Includes all other races not shown as separate categories.
*Sample size was 25–44 and does not meet the reliability standard.
Taken from U.S. Department of Health and Human Services, *Anthropometric Reference Data and Prevalence of Overweight: United States, 1976–80*, 1987.

TABLE 14.4

Subscapular Skinfolds (mm) for Females 18 to 74 Years of Age, By Race and Age: United States, 1976–80

Race and age	Number of examined persons	Mean	Standard deviation	Percentile								
				5th	10th	15th	25th	50th	75th	85th	90th	95th
All races[a]												
18-74 years	6,588	21.2	12.0	7.0	8.0	9.5	11.5	18.0	29.0	35.0	38.5	45.0
18-24 years	1,066	16.6	9.9	7.0	7.5	8.0	10.0	13.0	20.5	26.0	31.0	38.0
25-34 years	1,170	20.0	12.2	7.0	8.0	8.5	10.5	16.0	27.0	33.5	38.0	45.0
35-44 years	844	22.3	12.4	7.0	8.5	10.0	12.0	19.0	31.0	36.6	40.1	46.5
45-54 years	763	24.1	12.2	7.0	10.0	11.0	14.5	22.0	32.5	37.5	40.5	47.6
55-64 years	1,329	23.7	12.3	7.5	9.0	11.0	13.5	22.0	32.0	37.0	41.0	47.0
65-74 years	1,416	22.3	11.1	7.0	8.5	10.0	13.0	21.0	30.0	35.0	37.1	43.0
White												
18-74 years	5,686	20.5	11.7	7.0	8.0	9.0	11.0	17.0	27.5	34.0	37.5	43.5
18-24 years	892	16.1	9.6	7.0	7.5	8.0	10.0	13.0	19.0	25.0	29.5	37.5
25-34 years	1,000	19.1	11.7	7.0	7.5	8.5	10.5	15.0	25.0	32.0	36.0	43.0
35-44 years	726	21.4	12.1	7.0	8.0	9.5	11.5	17.5	30.0	36.0	39.5	46.0
45-54 years	647	23.1	11.8	7.0	9.5	11.0	14.0	20.5	31.0	36.6	40.0	45.0
55-64 years	1,176	23.0	12.0	7.0	9.0	11.0	13.0	21.5	31.0	36.0	39.5	45.6
65-74 years	1,245	21.8	10.9	6.5	8.5	10.0	13.0	20.5	29.5	34.0	36.1	41.1
Black												
18-74 years	782	26.1	13.3	8.0	9.5	11.0	14.0	25.0	35.5	40.6	45.0	50.0
18-24 years	147	19.1	10.6	7.0	8.0	9.0	11.0	15.0	26.0	31.0	34.0	37.0
25-34 years	145	25.4	13.3	8.5	9.5	11.0	14.0	22.5	35.5	40.6	44.5	48.1
35-44 years	103	27.9	13.0	7.0	10.5	12.0	17.0	28.0	36.5	42.5	46.5	52.0
45-54 years	100	32.0	13.1	11.0	15.0	17.0	22.5	30.5	39.5	45.6	50.5	56.0
55-64 years	135	30.0	13.5	8.0	12.5	13.0	19.5	31.0	40.6	45.0	47.5	50.5
65-74 years	152	27.1	12.1	7.5	9.5	12.0	18.0	27.0	35.5	41.0	44.5	47.0

[a] Includes all other races not shown as separate categories.

Taken from U.S. Department of Health and Human Services, *Anthropometric Reference Data and Prevalence of Overweight: United States, 1976–80*, 1987.

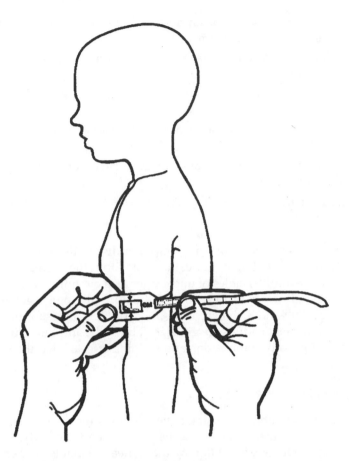

FIGURE 14.10

Measurement of mid-upper arm circumference. Reprinted with permission of J. A. Gilbride. Simko, M. D., Cowell, C., and Gilbride, J. A., *Nutrition Assessment: A Comprehensive Guide for Planning Intervention*, © 1984. Aspen Publishers, Gaithersburg, MD.

Girth Measurements

Girth measurements (also called circumference measurements) are also utilized in evaluating body composition. Girth measurements estimate body fat on a limb or larger area of the body than skinfold measurements, which are site-specific. Sometimes girth measurements are used in combination with skinfold measurements in the evaluation of body composition.

Girth measurements are taken using a flexible, but nonstretchable measuring tape. The measuring tape is pulled tight enough to compress the body hair, but not squeeze the skin. The subject should be standing, but relaxed for most girth measurements. Girth measurements of specific areas of the body should be taken by a trained technician, with measurements generally being repeated until the same value is obtained twice.

The body areas commonly utilized for girth measurements (often on the right side of the body) are detailed along with instructions for obtaining these measurements:

- Mid-upper arm circumference (MAC) — taken at the midpoint of the arm (where biceps skinfold was taken) (Figure 14.10).
- Chest circumference — taken at the level of the fourth costosternal (rib) joint.

- Abdominal circumference — taken midway between the inferior margin of the last rib and the crest of the ileum.
- Buttock or hip circumference — taken at maximum protrusion of hips with arms at sides and feet together.
- Calf circumference — taken at widest girth of calf (subjects sits on a table for this measurement).
- Thigh circumference — taken at upper thigh just below buttocks (largest girth of thigh).
- Forearm circumference — taken at maximum girth of forearm with arm extended in front of body open palm.
- Head circumference — taken just above eyebrows going posteriorly to give greatest circumference.

Girth measurements of an individual or group of individuals may be compared to published tables to determine whether or not values are within the normal ranges. As with triceps and subscapular skinfolds, tables of mid-upper arm circumference are available from the NHANES II national survey of 1976-80, and the normal range is generally interpreted as being between the 15th and 85th percentiles. NHANES II tables for mid-upper arm circumference measurements for adults are given in Tables 14.5 and 14.6. Girth measurements are useful in evaluating body composition and training effects in adults.

Breadth Measurements

Breadth measurements are obtained using a flexible nonstretchable measuring tape. Generally, breadth measurements are taken on the right side of the body. Common breadth measurements and instructions for obtaining these measurements are detailed:

- Bitrochanteric breadth — taken at the greater femoral trochanters.
- Elbow breadth — taken at the greatest breadth across the elbow joint with subject extending arm forward at a 90° angle.

Breadth measurements are generally utilized in evaluating growth of children and adolescents and in determining frame size. Breadth values between the 15th and 85th percentiles from the NHANES II study are generally used as norms in evaluating bitrochanteric and elbow breadth measurements.

TABLE 14.5

Mid-upper Arm Circumference (cm) for Males 18 to 74 Years of Age, By Race and Age: United States, 1976–80

Race and age	Number of examined persons	Mean	Standard deviation	Percentile								
				5th	10th	15th	25th	50th	75th	85th	90th	95th
All races[a]												
18-74 years	5,916	32.4	3.4	27.0	28.2	29.0	30.1	32.3	34.5	35.7	36.7	38.1
18-24 years	988	31.1	3.4	26.2	27.3	27.9	28.9	30.9	33.1	34.4	35.4	36.6
25-34 years	1,067	32.7	3.4	27.5	28.6	29.3	30.4	32.5	34.8	35.9	37.1	38.4
35-44 years	745	33.2	3.3	27.7	29.2	30.0	31.1	33.2	35.3	36.5	37.3	38.8
45-54 years	690	33.1	3.3	28.0	29.0	29.9	31.0	32.9	35.2	36.4	37.2	38.5
55-64 years	1,227	32.5	3.2	27.4	28.7	29.4	30.4	32.3	34.3	35.5	36.3	37.9
65-74 years	1,199	31.3	3.4	25.4	26.8	28.0	29.2	31.5	33.5	34.8	35.6	37.0
White												
18-74 years	5,148	32.4	3.3	27.1	28.3	29.1	30.2	32.3	34.5	35.7	36.6	38.0
18-24 years	846	31.2	3.3	26.3	27.3	28.0	29.0	31.0	33.2	34.6	35.6	36.6
25-34 years	901	32.7	3.3	27.7	28.8	29.3	30.5	32.6	34.7	35.9	37.0	38.2
35-44 years	653	33.3	3.1	28.3	29.5	30.1	31.3	33.1	35.1	36.4	37.1	38.4
45-54 years	617	33.0	3.2	28.1	29.2	29.9	31.0	32.8	35.1	36.1	37.1	38.2
55-64 years	1,086	32.5	3.1	27.5	28.9	29.5	30.5	32.3	34.3	35.4	36.2	37.6
65-74 years	1,045	31.4	3.4	25.5	27.0	28.1	29.3	31.6	33.6	34.8	35.6	36.8
Black												
18-74 years	649	32.7	4.2	26.5	27.7	28.7	30.0	32.6	35.3	37.0	38.2	39.5
18-24 years	121	30.7	3.5	26.1	26.9	27.6	28.7	30.7	32.6	33.3	34.4	35.9
25-34 years	139	33.1	4.2	27.5	28.3	29.0	30.2	32.6	35.3	36.6	38.1	39.8
35-44 years	70	34.4	3.9	*	30.0	30.2	31.6	33.9	37.5	38.2	39.3	*
45-54 years	62	34.3	3.9	*	28.8	30.5	31.9	34.6	36.4	38.5	39.5	*
55-64 years	129	32.8	3.8	27.2	28.4	29.2	30.1	32.6	34.4	37.1	37.9	39.6
65-74 years	128	31.1	4.1	24.6	26.1	27.4	28.4	30.6	33.6	35.6	36.9	38.2

[a] Includes all other races not shown as separate categories.

* Sample size was 25–44 and does not meet the reliability standard.

Taken from U.S. Department of Health and Human Services, *Anthropometric Reference Data and Prevalence of Overweight: United States, 1976–80*, 1987.

TABLE 14.6

Mid-upper Arm Circumference (cm) for Females 18 to 74 Years of Age, By Race and Age: United States, 1976–80

Race and age	Number of examined persons	Mean	Standard deviation	Percentile								
				5th	10th	15th	25th	50th	75th	85th	90th	95th
All races[a]												
18-74 years	6,588	30.1	4.7	23.9	24.9	25.6	26.7	29.3	32.6	34.8	36.4	38.7
18-24 years	1,066	27.7	3.8	23.0	23.8	24.4	25.3	27.1	29.2	31.2	32.4	34.8
25-34 years	1,170	29.2	4.4	23.6	24.5	25.2	26.2	28.3	31.3	33.4	35.6	37.9
35-44 years	844	30.7	4.9	24.4	25.5	26.2	27.2	29.6	33.3	35.8	37.5	39.6
45-54 years	763	31.3	4.8	24.9	25.8	26.5	28.2	30.6	34.1	36.1	37.5	39.7
55-64 years	1,329	31.5	4.7	25.1	26.3	27.1	28.3	30.9	34.1	36.3	37.6	39.7
65-74 years	1,416	31.1	4.4	24.4	26.0	27.0	28.3	30.8	33.6	35.4	36.8	38.8
White												
18-74 years	5,686	29.9	4.5	23.9	24.9	25.6	26.6	29.2	32.3	34.5	36.2	38.4
18-24 years	892	27.7	3.7	23.0	23.9	24.5	25.4	27.1	29.2	30.8	32.2	34.7
25-34 years	1,000	29.0	4.3	23.5	24.5	25.1	26.2	28.1	31.1	33.1	35.1	37.3
35-44 years	726	30.4	4.7	24.3	25.5	26.1	27.1	29.4	32.7	35.4	37.3	39.1
45-54 years	647	31.1	4.6	24.8	25.7	26.3	28.0	30.3	33.8	35.8	37.2	39.3
55-64 years	1,176	31.3	4.5	25.1	26.2	27.0	28.1	30.8	34.0	35.7	37.3	39.4
65-74 years	1,245	31.0	4.4	24.3	26.0	26.8	28.2	30.5	33.3	35.2	36.4	38.8
Black												
18-74 years	782	31.7	5.5	24.1	25.0	25.9	27.6	31.2	34.9	37.1	38.5	41.9
18-24 years	147	28.2	4.2	23.0	23.9	24.3	25.2	27.1	30.5	32.2	34.3	36.4
25-34 years	145	30.8	5.2	24.1	25.1	25.9	27.4	29.7	33.9	36.2	37.8	40.4
35-44 years	103	33.0	5.7	24.5	25.1	27.0	29.2	32.1	36.4	37.6	40.6	44.4
45-54 years	100	34.4	5.4	27.0	28.4	28.5	31.1	34.0	36.4	38.5	40.4	45.8
55-64 years	135	33.9	5.5	25.5	28.2	28.9	30.2	33.5	36.9	38.6	41.8	45.1
65-74 years	152	33.1	4.1	26.1	27.5	28.8	30.4	32.7	36.3	37.1	37.4	39.1

[a] Includes all other races not shown as separate categories.

Taken from U.S. Department of Health and Human Services, *Anthropometric Reference Data and Prevalence of Overweight: United States, 1976–80,* 1987.

15

Overweight and Obesity

More American adults, adolescents, and children are overweight now than ever before. The Interagency Board for Nutrition Monitoring and Related Research defined *overweight* as being above the 85th percentile of BMI values from NHANES II, a national survey conducted in 1976-80. This definition is also being used for evaluating the Healthy People 2000 Objective relating to overweight. Men are considered to be overweight when their BMIs are ≥27.8 and women, when their BMIs are ≥27.3. Figure 15.1 gives the age-adjusted percentage of people 20 to 74 years of age who are overweight by sex and race in the national surveys conducted in 1960-62 up to 1988-91. In 1998, new federal guidelines were released, as discussed in Chapter 13, identifying overweight in adults as having a BMI of 25 to 29.9 and obesity as a BMI above 30. According to the National Heart, Lung, and Blood Institute 55 percent of the adult population in the United States is overweight or obese as evaluated using these guidelines. Similar data are given for children and adolescents 2 to 19 years of age in Figure 15.2. Other methods for defining overweight include being more than 10 percent above standard body weight with the standard being defined by various methods.

Overweight is caused by *energy imbalance*, with caloric intake exceeding energy expenditure. Research has shown that individuals frequently under-report their caloric intakes. The prevalence of physical activity among people 20+ years of age and the percentage of these meeting the Healthy People 2000 Objective for vigorous physical activity in 1992 is given in Figure 15.3. The frequency of participation in vigorous activity over the past 14 days among high school students by sex and race is given in Figure 15.4. The vast majority of adults and high school students do not participate in sufficient vigorous physical activity. This lack of sufficient physical activity is thought to be the major cause of overweight.

Obesity is a state of adiposity. *Obesity* is frequently defined as being 20 percent above desirable body weight. Sometimes, obesity is referred to as severe overweight. The Interagency Board for Nutrition Monitoring and Related Research defined *severe overweight* as BMI values from NHANES II, the national survey conducted in 1976-80, equal to or greater than the 95th percentile. Men are considered to be severely overweight when their BMIs are ≥31.1 and women when their BMIs are ≥32.3. About 8 percent of men and 11 percent of women in the NHANES II study were found to be severely overweight, with the percentages being higher for Blacks than Whites.

Obesity can also be defined in terms of percent body fat. Five percent is added to the average percent body fat for an age group in estimating lower limits for obesity. Thus, the lower limits for obesity would be about 20 percent body fat for young men, 30 percent for older men and young women, and 37 percent for older women. However, the current thinking is that these limits should not be adjusted for age, making the lower limits for obesity 20 percent body fat for men and 30 percent for women.

Overweight (and obesity) is a current public health concern. A goal of a Healthy People 2000 Objective is "to reduce the prevalence of overweight in adults to no more than 20 percent and in adolescents to no more than 15 percent." Goals for Healthy People 2000 Objectives also exist with regard to physical activity. These are "to increase to at least

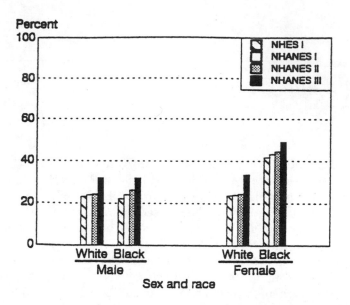

FIGURE 15.1

Age-adjusted percentage of people 20 to 74 years of age who are overweight (high BMI), by sex and race, 1960-72, 1971-74, 1976-80, and 1988-91. Source: HHS, NHES I, 1960-62; NHANES I, 1971-74; NHANES II, 1976-80; NHANES III, 1988-91. Reprinted with permission from Life Sciences Research Office. Federation of American Societies for Experimental Biology, *Third Report on Nutrition Monitoring in the United States*, © 1995. U.S. Government Printing Office, Washington, DC.

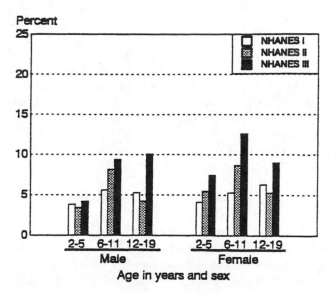

FIGURE 15.2

Percentage of children and adolescents, 2 to 19 years of age who have high weight for height (2 to 5 years of age) or are overweight (6 to 19 years of age), by age and sex, 1971-1974, 1976-80, and 1988-91. Source: HHS, NHANES I, 1971-74; NHANES II, 1976-80; NHANES III, 1988-91. Reprinted with permission from Life Sciences Research Office. Federation of American Societies for Experimental Biology, *Third Report on Nutrition Monitoring in the United States*, © 1995. U.S. Government Printing Office, Washington, DC.

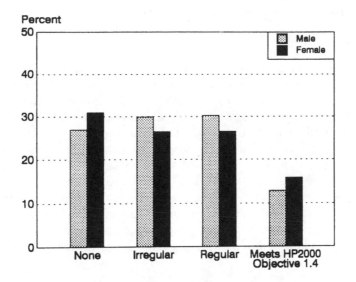

FIGURE 15.3
Prevalence of physical activity among people 20 years of age and older and percentage meeting the Healthy People 2000 (HP2000) objective for vigorous physical activity, by sex, 1992. Source: HHS, BRFSS, 1992. Reprinted with permission from Life Sciences Research Office. Federation of American Societies for Experimental Biology, *Third Report on Nutrition Monitoring in the United States,* © 1995. U.S. Government Printing Office, Washington, DC.

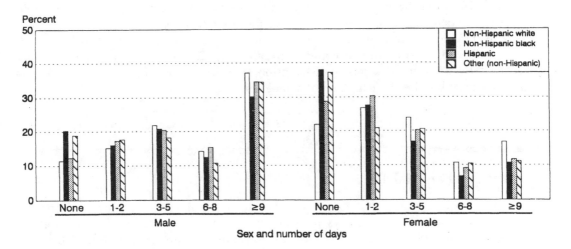

FIGURE 15.4
Frequency of participation in vigorous physical activity over the past 14 days among high school students, by sex, and race/ethnicity, 1990. Source: HHS, YRBS, 1990. Reprinted with permission from Life Sciences Research Office. Federation of American Societies for Experimental Biology, *Third Report on Nutrition Monitoring in the United States,* © 1995. U.S. Government Printing Office, Washington, DC.

20 percent the proportion of people 18 years and older, and to at least 75 percent the proportion of children and adolescents aged 6-17 years who participate in vigorous activity." Another objective is "to reduce to no more than 15 percent the proportion of people 6 years of age and older who engage in no leisure-time physical activity." Increased percentages of overweight individuals result in increased health care costs.

Body Fat Distribution

Where fat is stored on the body relates to adiposity and possible health risk. Individuals can measure the circumferences of their waists and hips and then calculate *waist-to-hip ratios*. Health risks are increased when the ratio exceeds 0.80 for women and 0.95 for men. In *central obesity* (also called abdominal, android, and upper-body obesity), the excess fat is located in the abdominal areas. In *peripheral obesity* (also called gluteal, gynoid-type, and lower-body obesity or "pear-shaped"), excess fat is located in the hips and thighs. Obese men are more likely to have central obesity, while obese women are more likely to have peripheral obesity. The health risks of central obesity are greater than those of peripheral obesity. High blood levels of the hormone testosterone enhances central obesity. After menopause, blood estrogen levels decrease, enhancing central obesity. To some extent an individual's pattern of fat distribution is genetic and likely is controlled by the regional activity of *lipoprotein lipase*, the rate-limiting enzyme for triglyceride uptake by the adipocyte.

Health Concerns of Overweight Individuals

The health risks are increased in overweight individuals and are even higher in those who are severely overweight or obese. Health risks are reported to be very low in individuals with BMIs <25 (normal weight), low with BMIs of 25 to 30, moderate with BMIs of 30 to 35, high with BMIs of 35 to 40, and very high with BMIs >40. Figure 15.5 summarizes the relationships between health risk and fat distribution. Health complications that have been frequently observed in the obese are given in Table 15.1.

Obesity as a Familial Trait

Obesity is a familial trait. Family members generally share dietary and other environmental exposures as well as having somewhat similar genetic makeup. A strong interaction has often been reported between genetic predisposition and environmental stimuli with regard to obesity. Specific body types are thought to be inherited. These specific body types are ectomorphs (tall, slender), mesomorphs (medium muscular build), and endomorphs (short, stocky build). Some individuals utilize their energy intakes more efficiently than others. Lower resting metabolic rates are found in members of some families than in other families, indicating a probable genetic component. Identical twins have more similar body weights and fat distributions than fraternal twins, which in turn are more similar with regard to body weights and fat distributions than unrelated individuals. Husbands and wives, having different genetic backgrounds, frequently have similar specific body shapes. Family members often have similar eating habits.

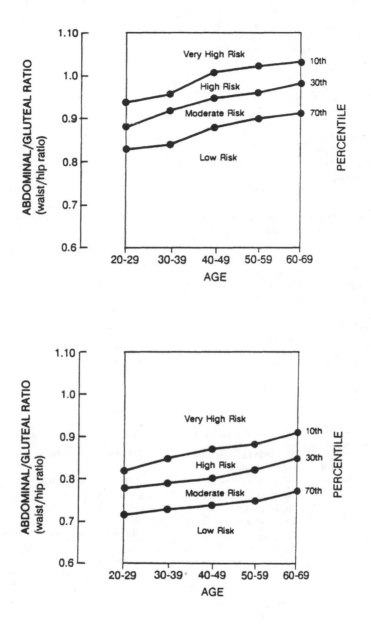

FIGURE 15.5

Percentiles of fat distribution. The percentiles of the ratio of abdominal-to-gluteal circumference (waist-to-hip ratio) are depicted for men and women by age groups along with relative risk. Reprinted with permission from The Western Journal of Medicine, San Francisco, CA. Bray, G. A. and Gray, D. S., *Western Journal of Medicine* 149, 429, © 1988.

Determinants of Obesity

Many factors influence an individual's likelihood of being obese. Determinants known to influence obesity are given in Table 15.2. Some of these are more controlled by genetic or

TABLE 15.1

Health Complications Frequently Observed in Obese Individuals

Hypertension
Stroke
Cardiovascular diseases
Kidney disease
Gallbladder disease
Diabetes mellitus
Respiratory diseases
Pulmonary function
Osteoarthritis
Bone, joint, and skin disorders
Gout
Cancers   In women: gallbladder, biliary duct, endometrium, ovary, cervix, and breast
               In men: prostate and colon
Abnormal immune response
Impaired temperature regulation and heat loss
Complications of pregnancy
Menstrual irregularities
Ovarian abnormalities
Sleep apnea
Psychological trauma
Organ compression by adipose tissues
Early death

TABLE 15.2

Determinants and Correlates of Excess Body Weight or Fat

Age	More prevalent in adults and middle-aged individuals.
Gender	Females have more fat.
Positive energy balance	An absolute requirement over a relatively long period.
Amount of energy intake	Overfeeding leads to gain in weight and fat mass.
Composition of intake	High-fat intake may be a contributing factor.
Physical activity level	Low or decreasing level of activity.
Resting metabolic rate	A low value with respect to body mass and fat-free mass is correlated with weight gain.
Thermic effect of food	Low for energy intake in some obesity cases.
Lipid oxidation	A high respiratory quotient is correlated with body fat and weight gain.
Ratio of fat to lean tissue	A high fat mass-to-fat free mass ratio is correlated with excess weight or weight gain.
Adipose tissue lipoprotein lipase activity	High in obese individuals and remains high (perhaps even increases) with weight loss.
Variety of social and behavioral factors	Obesity is associated with socioeconomic status, familial conditions, network of friends, pattern of leisure activities, television time, smoking habits, alcohol intake, etc.
Undetermined genetic characteristics	These affect energy balance particularly via the energy expenditure, the deposition of the energy surplus as fat or as lean tissue, and the relative proportion of lipids and carbohydrates oxidized.

Reprinted with permission from the International Life Sciences Institute, Washington, DC. Bouchard, C., *Nutrition Reviews* 53, 1562S, © 1991.

nongenetic factors than others. It is difficult to separate genetics and environment when searching for the causes of obesity.

Obesity as a Lifestyle

Obesity frequently begins when one is a child. As indicated earlier, around 10 percent of children and adolescents are overweight. If one is obese as a child, the chance of being obese as an adult is increased threefold. We develop our dietary and exercise habits as children and often continue these same habits into adulthood. It is important that children learn and participate in desirable dietary and exercise habits. As adults age, they frequently become less physically active. Creeping obesity happens in many adults, even though they may not have been obese as a child. Increases in body fat in adults are thought to be more a function of physical activity level than of age.

Treatment of Obesity

Treatment of obesity requires lifestyle changes. A person needs to set personal short-term and long-term goals with regard to weight loss. As indicated in Chapter 13, it is best to lose weight slowly but steadily. Desirable weight loss of 1 to 2 pounds weekly can be obtained by reducing caloric intake by 500 cal daily or increasing energy expenditure by 500 cal daily or both. Some people can lose weight more easily if they are part of a group of people trying to lose weight. Psychological support from others is important in helping one lose weight.

Weight loss diets should be nutritionally adequate. The diet should be high (>20 g daily) in fiber. In addition, over 50 percent of the caloric intake should come from complex carbohydrates, and less than 30 percent of the caloric intake should come from fats. If the dietary intake is less than 1,000 to 1,200 cal daily, a multivitamin/multimineral supplement is recommended. Perhaps most important, individuals trying to lose weight should increase their physical activity level. The physical activities should be fun-type experiences and be enjoyable. Obese individuals need to permanently modify their eating and exercise behavior. The principles of weight control were discussed in more detail in Chapter 13. One needs to adopt desirable eating and exercise plans for life.

16

Underweight and Eating Disorders

Underweight is generally defined as being 15 percent or more below expected body weight. Sometimes, underweight is defined as having a BMI of less than 20. Underweight is frequently caused by an insufficient energy intake and/or excessive physical activity. Underweight may also be caused by inadequate absorption and utilization of food, wasting diseases, and emotional stress. The cause(s) of the underweight must be determined before treatment is initiated. Medical tests should be performed in assessing the etiology of one's being underweight. Frequently, the underweight individual also needs psychiatric treatment.

Health Concerns

A BMI of less than 19 or 20 has been associated with greater disease and mortality risks; these risks increase as the BMI decreases. Health complications frequently observed in underweight individuals are given in Table 16.1.

Anorexia Nervosa

Anorexia nervosa is an eating disorder that is characterized by the person having a body weight that is >10 or >15 percent lower than normal, having distorted attitudes toward food, having a distorted body image, and denying the illness. Anorexics believe that all foods are bad and cause weight gain. Anorexics believe that they are fat when they are not. Anorexics frequently exercise excessively. Anorexic women frequently miss menstrual periods. The underweight person frequently wears baggy clothes to disguise their thinness.

The following health complications have been reported in anorexics: amenorrhea, lanugo (downy body hair), dizziness or fainting upon standing, insomnia, tachycardia (rapid heart beat), edema particularly in arms and legs (from lack of protein), anemia, peripheral cold intolerance, dull brittle hair, impaired immune response, digestive problems, decreased thyroxine synthesis, and decreased bone density. One female in 400 to 500 in the United States has anorexia nervosa, and 1 in 4 dies. About 1 in 100 adolescent girls have anorexia nervosa. About 5 to 10 percent of the cases of anorexia nervosa have been reported in men.

TABLE 16.1

Health Complications Frequently
Observed in Underweight Individuals

Respiratory disease
Digestive diseases
Some cancers
Reproductive complications
Impaired immune function
Tuberculosis
AIDS (Acquired immune deficiency syndrome)
If person has surgery, infections are more likely

Bulimia

Bulimia, also called binge eating or binge-purge syndrome, is an eating disorder in which individuals eat excessively and then induce vomiting, use laxatives, or exercise excessively. This behavior happens repeatedly, a minimum of twice weekly for at least three months. The behavior is secretive. Bulimics feel a lack of control during binging. The bulimic often ends the binge-purge by sleeping. Bulimia is addictive. Bulimics have persistent overconcerns with their body shape and weight. Bulimics usually undergo large weight fluctuations. Bulimics may be thin, normal weight, or obese.

A variety of health problems are observed in bulimics, including fainting, obesity, hypoglycemia, parotid gland enlargement, internal bleeding, and gastric rupturing. If the bulimic vomits, they may experience heartburn, esophageal rupture, tooth decay, metabolic alkalosis, constipation, and heart arrhythmias. If the bulimic uses excessive laxatives, they may experience dehydration, constipation, mineral imbalances, and cathartic colon. About 20 percent of college women and about 5 percent of college men have reportedly had at least one binge/purge syndrome.

About half of the females with anorexia nervosa also develop symptoms of bulimia. Bulimia exists concomitantly with anorexia nervosa and as a separate disorder.

Exercise Dependency

Some people, particularly young women and sometimes young men, exercise too much. Their eating is disordered. Individuals with the disorder have amenorrhea and lower than normal bone densities. These individuals may also be anorexic or bulimic.

Nutritional and Exercise Therapy

Nutrition and exercise therapeutists need to know the symptoms of anorexia nervosa, bulimia, and exercise dependency; they may refer individuals with these conditions to their physicians. The diagnosis of eating disorders should be done by a psychiatrist.

Nutrition and exercise therapies are appropriate and effective along with or after treatment of the underlying physical or psychological disorder(s). High calorie, yet nutritionally balanced diets should be consumed as part of this therapy. The meals should be well planned and served on a schedule in an environment that is nonthreating and as tension-free as possible. Appropriate snacks are desirable. Sometimes, liquid supplements are consumed as part of a meal or a snack. The underweight person needs to be relaxed and under little to no stress, especially at eating times. Underweight persons frequently need to be encouraged to eat whether or not they are hungry. The underweight person should strive to gain 1 to 2 pounds weekly by increasing their caloric intake by 500 cal or decreasing their energy expenditure by 500 cal or both. The nutritional and exercise therapist should work with a physician or psychiatrist with regard to the treatment program. Sometimes, a psychologist is also part of the team. The underweight person needs to modify their behavior by identifying the problem(s), controlling the problem(s), and modifying the undesirable behavior(s). Weight gain is not the only goal of the treatment, but rather having an overall increase in the quality of life.

After having some psychiatric treatment, individuals with eating disorders may gain by learning more about caloric intake and expenditures as well as normal body weights and body images. The person may gain a better attitude toward foods and a better understanding of their functions in the body. These individuals may also gain a better appreciation of moderate exercise.

17

Conditioning

Individuals need to exercise aerobically to maintain fitness of their bodies. Fitness is a state of physical well-being such that one can perform various types of physical activity. Physical fitness entails having adequate muscular strength and endurance, sufficient joint flexibility, efficient cardiovascular and respiratory systems, and a desirable body composition and weight. Strength, muscle endurance, joint flexibility, and cardiovascular endurance are the four components of fitness.

- *Strength* is the ability of the muscles to work against resistance.
- *Muscle endurance* is the ability of the muscles to contract repeatedly without becoming exhausted during a given time period.
- *Joint flexibility* is the capacity that the joints have to move through a full range of motion and recover without injury.
- *Cardiovascular endurance* is the ability of the cardiovascular and respiratory systems to sustain effort over a given time period.

A physically fit person needs to have sufficiency of these components plus a little extra to spare. Exercise training enhances physical fitness and performance in sports. *Training* is the routine practice of any physical activity leading to physiological adaptations of the body, thus improving the various components of fitness.

Fitness and Health

Exercise is an integral component of health and a healthy lifestyle. The American College of Sports Medicine has recommended exercise as a way to enhance physical fitness and health as have the American Heart Association, Public Health Service, and National Institutes of Health. The President's Council on Physical Fitness and Sports and the Centers for Disease Control collaboratively developed a report on the relationships between physical activity and health. This report, known as the *Surgeon General's Report Addressing Physical Activity and Health*, was released in 1996. The report indicates "that people of all ages can improve the quality of their lives through a lifelong practice of moderate physical activity."

Muscle Contraction

The body contains smooth muscles (often called viscereal muscles), skeletal muscles, and cardiac muscles. Smooth muscles are under involuntary control as are cardiac muscles. Skeletal muscles are voluntary in that one does have conscious control over these muscles.

Skeletal muscle cells are extremely long and are often referred to as *muscle fibers*. Each muscle fiber is packed with *myofibrils*, which are arrangements of *myofilaments* ("myo" meaning muscle). Embedded in the intracellular fluid of the muscle fiber cells is ATP, creatine phosphate, glycogen, and the enzymes of glycolysis. The thin myofilaments are made up of the protein *actin*, while the thick myofilaments are made up of the larger protein *myosin*. The whole muscle unit, containing both actin and myosin is called the *sarcomere* ("sarco" meaning flesh), which is the contractile unit of the muscle. Neural impulses result in stimulation of the flexion of the muscle, causing contraction and relaxation, which is continuous, and at rest "muscle tone" is maintained.

The contraction of skeletal muscles is initiated by a neural impulse. Acetylcholine passes across the neuromuscular junction from the nerve to the muscle initiating the process that causes muscle to contract. Muscle contraction occurs when the actin and the myosin within the sacromere slide across each other, with neither actin or myosin changing in length but resulting in a shortening of the muscle fiber or contraction. Actually actin and myosin interact via crossbridges forming *actomyosin*. Calcium plays a central role in the regulation of muscle contraction. The joining of ATP to actomyosin results in the separation of actin and myosin. Relaxation occurs when the calcium concentration drops and also ATPase converts *ATP* to adenosine diphosphate (ADP) and inorganic phosphate.

Skeletal muscle contains Type I and Type II fibers. Type I fibers are *slow twitch*, also called red fibers. Slow twitch fibers have a higher myoglobin concentration and higher oxidative capacity than *fast twitch* (Type II) fibers. Type II fibers, also called white fibers, exist as Type IIA and IIB, with IIB having the higher glycolytic capacity. The contraction speed of slow-twitch fibers is about half that of fast-twitch fibers, but slow-twitch fibers have the greater capacity to generate ATP aerobically. Slow-twitch fibers are utilized more in endurance and fast-twitch more in short-term sprint activities.

Principles of Conditioning

An effective training program is based on the *overload principle*. By exercising a body system at a level above that at which it normally operates, the system physiologically adapts and functions more efficiently. It is best if it is a *progressive overload*. Muscle cells respond to the overload by undergoing *hypertrophy*, or increasing in size. If training is stopped, the muscles will *atrophy* or decrease in size. The best overall fitness is achieved by performing a variety of physical activities. Different muscle groups should be worked from day to day. In general, weight or resistance training and calisthenics develop muscular strength and endurance, stretching enhances flexibility, and aerobic exercises enhance cardiovascular endurance.

Conditioning for Muscular Strength

In conditioning for muscular strength, muscle overload is applied by increasing the *resistance*, increasing the *repetitions* of an exercise, increasing the *muscle contraction speed*, or most likely, a combination of these factors. Muscle strength may be developed using resistance, isometric, and isokinetic resistance training. *Resistance training*, also known as weight training, is a dynamic exercise, whereas isometric training is static. Barbells, weight plates, or exercise machines are used in resistance training, with the resistance being progressive. In *isometric training* there is little body movement and strength increases in the exact position at which the training took place. It is best if isometric force is applied at several different angles through the range of the motion. *Isokinetic resistance training* allows the muscle to mobilize its maximum force-generating capacity at all points in the range of motion. Isokinetics is frequently used in rehabilitation, more so than by the athlete.

Several factors are known to influence muscle strength. Genetics sets the limits, while other factors influence one's potential to reach the limits. Other factors include nutrition and muscular training as well as environmental, hormonal, and psychological influences. Women usually have about 70 percent of the muscular strength of men. "Psyching" one's self up is important with regard to muscle strength and overall physical performance.

Resistance Training Programs

Individuals should seek professional advice from persons trained in exercise sciences or at least read some "how to" type books on the subject before initiating a physical training program of any type. Obese, elderly, and unhealthy individuals should seek advice from their physicians prior to participating in a physical training program.

Appropriate loose-fitting clothing and comfortable shoes should be worn when exercising. *Warm-up* exercises such as slow stretching and slow jogging for 5 to 10 minutes help reduce the possibility of injury and improves the cardiovascular response to more rigorous physical activity. Proper weights should be utilized, with lighter weights being used when starting the program. The power of the legs should be used in lifting heavy objects so as to decrease lower back injuries. Appropriate equipment should be used with the exerciser being familiar with its operation and proper utilization. An *exercise circuit* in which different muscles are worked is desirable. A progressive overload should be maintained. The workout should end with a *cool-down* period with exercises being done similar to those of the warm-up.

Conditioning for Muscle Endurance

Energy needs to be continuously, and frequently rapidly, generated to maintain the various forms of physical activity. Energy production may be *aerobic*, requiring oxygen, or *anaerobic*, not requiring oxygen. The reader is referred to Chapter 12 for information on energy production in the body. ATP is the "energy currency" of the cell; however, very little ATP is present in the body. ATP can be generated by any or all of the three energy systems of the body — ATP-creatine phosphate cycle or system, anaerobic glycolysis system (also known as lactic acid system), and aerobic systems. The relative contributions of each of these systems depends on the duration and intensity of the physical activity. ATP and creatine phosphate are primarily utilized during short bursts of physical effort lasting only a few seconds. The ATP produced from anaerobic glycolysis provides a rapid source of energy for muscular activity that is particularly useful in short-duration, high-intensity activities lasting one to four minutes. Lactic acid is produced in anaerobic glycolysis. After about four minutes of physical activity, the body becomes more dependent on aerobic pathways of energy production. The physical activity in which a person wants to participate should be evaluated in terms of the energy system needed for that activity before a training program for that specific activity is initiated. Many activities operate on an anaerobic-to-aerobic continuum, first being anaerobic and then becoming aerobic without first stopping anaerobic energy production.

Training activities to improve energy production by the *ATP-creatine phosphate cycle* or system of a muscle(s) involve working that muscle(s) in movement patterns desired for improved power. This facilitates needed neuromuscular adaptations appropriate for the specific muscle movement pattern and enables one to have bursts of energy that are important in some sports.

Training to improve *anaerobic glycolysis* involves performing up to a minute or so of intense cycling, running, swimming, or such activity, then stopping the activity 30 to 40 seconds prior to exhaustion, resting about 3 to 5 minutes, and then repeating the activity, stopping, resting, and repeating again several times. This causes lactic acid to accumulate (often called *lactate stacking*) and the muscle adapts to and tolerates higher than usual concentrations of lactic acid. Thus, the muscle does not experience *fatigue* at as low a lactic acid level as before. As with training for maximal efficiency of the ATP-creatine phosphate cycle, it is important that appropriate muscle(s) be utilized in training for maximal efficiency of anaerobic glycolysis. Sometimes this process is called anaerobic conditioning.

Aerobic training improves the ability of the body to produce ATP from pyruvate and breakdown products of fat and protein metabolism via the tricarboxylic acid cycle (TCA) (also called Krebs cycle, carboxylic acid cycle, and citric acid cycle) and the electron transport chain (ETC) (also called electron transport system). Oxygen is required for these two energy pathways. It is important that a training regimen include at least some aerobic training because muscle fatigue occurs if lactic acid accumulates. Aerobic training of the large muscle groups entails training for cardiovascular endurance. More oxygen and nutrients, supplied by the cardiovascular or circulatory system, are needed by exercising muscles including those in the large muscle groups; also the increased quantities of end-products including water, carbon dioxide, and waste products produced by the exercising muscles must be removed by the circulatory system.

Joint flexibility is enhanced by stretching. Stretches should be held for 10 to 20 seconds. Stretches should not be choppy, bouncy, or painful; they also should not twist or put pressure on body joints.

Cardiovascular Endurance Training

As mentioned earlier, aerobic conditioning improves the endurance of the cardiovascular system as well as the active large muscle groups. Cardiovascular endurance relates to the heart, lungs, and the systems that serve them. Sometimes, cardiovascular endurance is referred to as cardiorespiratory endurance. Cardiovascular endurance training enables the following:

- Heart muscle to become stronger so that it can empty its chambers more completely and pump more blood per beat, thus making fewer beats necessary and decreasing *resting pulse rate*.
- Muscles that inflate and deflate the lungs to become stronger, thus making respiration or breathing more efficient.
- Blood to circulate more easily through the blood vessels because the heart contracts more powerfully, thus normalizing *blood pressure*.

Increased blood HDL cholesterol levels are often a result of cardiovascular training; HDL cholesterol is the so-called "good" cholesterol.

Training for cardiovascular endurance requires sustained activity that elevates the heart rate for at least 30 minutes and uses most of the body's large muscle (legs, buttocks, abdomen) groups. Effective activities include fast walking, jogging, cross-country skiing, swimming, fast bicycling, and a wide variety of physically active sports. The American College of Sports Medicine indicates that each training session should include continuous exercise of sufficient intensity to expend around 300 kcal. Cardiovascular endurance training should be done a minimum of three times weekly. Some athletes may train for athletic endurance two to three hours daily five or more times weekly. Improvements are not immediate, but start to be evident in about six to eight weeks. These improvements are actually physiological adaptations and they start to plateau as individuals reach their genetically determined maximum. These improvements are also reversible if cardiovascular training is discontinued.

Intensity of training is important with regard to cardiovascular endurance. Healthy individuals in their early 20s should increase their heart rate to at least 130 beats per minute, which is generally equivalent to about 50 percent of VO_2 max (maximal oxygen uptake) or 70 percent of *maximum heart rate*, and is representative of *moderate exercise*. Maximum heart rate is generally estimated by subtracting an individual's age from 220 beats per minute. This is the *threshold for aerobic improvement*. Training levels which induce an exercise heart rate of 70 percent maximum are sometimes called *conversational exercise* and do lead to improved cardiovascular fitness. More rigorous exercise is more effective. Exercising at intensities less than this threshold level can also increase fitness. Lower exercise intensity appears to be usually offset by longer exercise duration. The guidelines for aerobic conditioning programs are similar to those for resistance training. It is important that a gradual cool-down period be included to avoid the pooling of blood in the large veins of previously exercised muscles.

Aerobic training programs may also be continuous or intermittent. Continuous aerobic conditioning, also called long-slow distance, involves performing sustained moderate or high-intensity exercise activities. Intermittent or interval aerobic training involves appropriate spacing of exercise and rest periods, much like that previously described for resistance training as "lactate-stacking" also occurs. Most of the time aerobic conditioning is continuous; however, both methods can be used interchangeably as both are effective.

Training Programs

Training programs should be planned with the individual in mind. Factors which should be taken into account include their initial fitness level, overall health status, age, gender, and muscle groups to be "built up."

Training improves the utilization of glycogen by the body. Training through repeated aerobic activity encourages the muscles of the body to develop more fat-burning enzymes, and thus, to utilize more fat for energy formation. The use of fat for energy formation during physical activity makes glycogen reserves last longer. The moderating effect of training on glucose metabolism is helpful to diabetics. Anaerobic training also helps an individual be less fatigued. Training, both anaerobic and aerobic, is important in obtaining and maintaining fitness. Resistance training at moderate levels can help prevent osteoporosis. Importantly, training decreases obesity and the diseases associated with obesity.

Diet and Exercise Recommendations

Diet and Exercise Recommendations

Several professional organizations have recommended guidelines for diet and for exercise. The most recent recommendations are discussed in this section. Some of these recommendations are "in process" in various expert committees in these organizations and are forthcoming.

Nutrition and exercise are environmental factors that influence health and disease. Other environmental and genetic factors also influence health and disease. These factors interact with each other.

Early in life, individuals should develop good nutrition and exercise habits. Physical fitness is a characteristic that has to be obtained and maintained throughout one's life span. The food that individuals eat should be balanced with physical activity, so they can maintain or improve their body weights. One of the hardest things to accomplish is to modify poor eating and exercise habits so that they become beneficial to the improvement and maintenance of good health. Although athletes generally are physically fit, they still need to continuously practice good nutrition and exercise habits. Needs of athletes with regard to specific nutrients were discussed in earlier chapters.

Health care costs are reduced when individuals practice good nutrition and exercise habits. Good nutrition and exercise habits enhance one's chances of having life-long good health and having a good quality of life.

18

Nutritional Status of Athletes

Few studies have been conducted on the nutrient intakes and nutritional status of athletes. The studies that have been done generally indicate that the nutrient intakes and nutritional status of athletes are similar to that of the population as a whole.

Median Daily Nutrient Intakes of Adults

Table 18.1 gives the median daily intakes of energy-yielding nutrients, U.S. population, of individuals 20 to 59 years of age included in the national survey (NHANES III) of 1988-91 as well as the recommended intakes (discussed in Chapters 4 to 6). Median daily intakes of both men and women were lower than recommended for carbohydrates and higher than recommended for total fats and saturated fats. The median daily protein intakes of both groups were within the recommended range. The median daily dietary fiber intakes of men and women (Table 18.2) were lower than the recommended level of intake, with intake values for women being lower than those of men.

The median daily intakes of vitamins and minerals, U.S. population, of individuals 20 to 59 years of age for the national survey (NHANES III) of 1988-91 are given in Table 18.2. This table also lists the recommended intakes of these nutrients; detailed discussions of vitamin and mineral needs were included in Chapters 7 and 8. The median daily intakes of men for vitamin A, vitamin E, folate, calcium, and zinc were lower than recommended, but sodium intakes were higher than recommended. The median daily intakes of women for vitamin A, vitamin E, folate, calcium, magnesium, iron, zinc, and copper were lower than recommended, but sodium intakes were higher than recommended. The median daily intakes of women were lower than those of men for these vitamins and minerals.

Use of Vitamin/Mineral Supplements by Athletes

About three-quarters of athletes surveyed by Grandjean et al. believed that they needed more vitamins and minerals than nonathletes. Information presented in Chapters 7 and 8 indicates that athletes may need more than recommended intake levels of some vitamins and minerals than nonathletes.

Surveys indicate that one-third to one-half of adults in the United States use vitamin/mineral supplements. Sobal and Marquart, using a meta-analysis design, combined data obtained in 51 studies that included 10,274 male and female athletes. These studies included subjects from 15 different sports at the high school, college, and Olympic levels. The mean

TABLE 18.1

Median Daily Intakes of Energy-Yielding Nutrients,
U.S. Population, 20-59 Years of Age, 1988-91

	Men	Women	Recommended intakes[a] (Percentage of kcal)
Carbohydrates	46.8	49.5	55-65
Total fats	35.2	34.5	<30
Saturated fats	11.8	11.7	<10
Proteins	14.7	14.6	1-2 × RDA

[a] Recommendations are discussed in Chapters 4-6.
Taken from NHANES III data provided by the U.S. Department of Agriculture's Food Survey Research Group as given by Federation of American Societies for Experimental Biology, 1995.

TABLE 18.2

Median Daily Intakes of Dietary Fiber, Vitamins, and Minerals,
U.S. Population, 20-59 Years of Age, 1988-91

	Males	Females	Recommended intakes[a,b]
Dietary fiber (g)	16.49	11.86	20-35
Vitamin A (μg RE)	739	581	1000/800[c]
Carotene (μg RE)	235	172	—[d]
Vitamin E (mg α-TE)	8.63	6.26	10/8
Vitamin C (mg)	85	67	60
Thiamin (mg)	1.77	1.23	1.2/1.1
Riboflavin (mg)	2.11	1.49	1.3/1.1
Niacin (mg NE)	26.20	17.47	16/14
Vitamin B_6 (mg)	1.97	1.31	1.3
Folate (μg)	280	189	400
Vitamin B_{12} (μg)	4.83	3.03	2.4
Calcium (mg)	847	617	1000
Phosphorus (mg)	1466	1026	700
Magnesium (mg)	326	230	400(420)/310(320)[e]
Iron (mg)	15.83	10.93	10/15
Zinc (mg)	12.68	8.32	15/12
Copper (mg)	1.45	1.02	1.5-2.5
Potassium (mg)	3060	2230	2000 (minimum)
Sodium (mg)	3813	2641	>500 <2400

[a] Recommendations are discussed in Chapters 4, 7, 8, and 19.
[b] Recommended intakes for vitamins and minerals are for individuals 19 to 50 years of age.
[c] Recommendations for males/females.
[d] Recommendations have not been made.
[e] For those 19 to 30 years and those for 31 to 50 years in ().
Taken from NHANES III data provided by the U.S. Department of Agriculture's Food Survey Research Group as given by Federation of American Societies for Experimental Biology, 1995.

prevalence of vitamin and/or mineral supplement use among these male subjects was 47 percent while that for females was 57 percent. Prevalence figures varied among the different sports from 30 percent for basketball players to 69 percent for body builders. The most commonly used supplements were (in descending order) multivitamins, vitamin C, iron, B-complex vitamins, vitamin E, calcium, and vitamin A. Schulz reported that the most commonly cited reasons by a group of college athletes for taking vitamin-mineral supplements were (in descending order) nutritional insurance, avoiding illness, increasing energy/vitality/strength, and compensating for stress. Sobal and Marquart reported that their meta-analysis study indicated that coaches, other athletes, parents, physicians, and other athletic personnel such as trainers were the most frequent sources of supplement information for the surveyed athletes.

We recently completed a study of vitamin/mineral supplement usage by athletes at the University of Nebraska. Athletes in all 11 female and 11 male varsity teams served as subjects. Approximately 59 percent of the female athletes and 55 percent of the males indicated that they were taking a vitamin and/or mineral supplement. The most frequently given reasons for taking supplements were because of a recommendation from friend or family member and to improve athletic performance. The most frequently given reasons for not taking supplements were that vitamin and mineral content of the diet was adequate and personal or religious beliefs. Multivitamins with minerals was the most commonly taken supplement, followed by vitamin C, multivitamins (no minerals), and B-complex vitamins. The athletes reported that they got their information on nutrition from (in descending order) nutritionist/dietitian, family or friend, coach or trainer, and physician or pharmacist. The Athletic Department of the University of Nebraska has performance nutritionists, coaches/trainers, and physicians on their staff. Hence, advice on nutrition, including supplement use, is easily available to their athletes. I am only aware of two other NCAA institution that has one or more full-time nutritionist/dietitian on their athletic staff. Athletes need advice from appropriate professionals with regard to their nutritional needs.

Nutritional Status of Athletes

Although most studies examined only dietary intakes of athletes, a few reports have been published on the nutritional status of athletes. Biochemical and dietary levels of nutrients and anthropometric data and sometimes clinical data are evaluated in nutritional status studies (also called nutritional assessment or evaluation). *Iron deficiency* is fairly prevalent in athletes and nonathletes alike, particularly in females. *Calcium deficiency* is frequently observed in both athletic and nonathletic females. Iron and calcium needs during exercise as well as that of other minerals and the vitamins were discussed in Chapters 7 and 8.

Eating disorders are frequently observed in the athletic population (see Chapter 16). Beals and Manore observed that a group of female athletes with subclinical eating disorders had dietary intakes of energy, protein, carbohydrates, calcium, zinc, iron, and magnesium below recommendations. The nutritional status of these women with respect to these minerals was relatively unaffected as indicated by serum levels of the nutrients, as many of the subjects took mineral supplements. Vitamin/mineral supplementation appears to be quite prevalent in athletes and this supplementation may be of importance in helping athletes to have adequate intakes of these essential micronutrients.

19

Nutrition and Exercise Recommendations

Nutrition and exercise guidelines have existed for many years. The most recent guidelines are discussed in this chapter. During the last decade, the organizations and governmental groups that have made recommendations on a topic have generally made their recommendations similar to those of other reputable groups making recommendations on the same topic. Frequently, the groups have collaborated. Sometimes, the groups have adopted the recommendations of other reputable groups. This has enabled the public to get the same message rather than conflicting messages, even though the conflict may be minute.

Dietary Recommendations

Humans get the vast majority of their nutrients from *foods*. Many individuals may get some of their nutrients from various types of *dietary supplements*.

Dietary recommendations and guidelines for the consumption of a diet that meets an individual's requirements for nutrients as well as promotes health and reduces the risks of chronic disease are available. Information regarding dietary recommendations and guidelines developed by the committees/subcommittees of the National Academy of Sciences, U.S. Department of Agriculture, and U.S. Department of Health and Human Services will be briefly described in this chapter. The reader is referred to the original publications if additional information is desired. Other organizations and individuals also have issued dietary recommendations and guidelines.

Recommended Dietary Allowances

The nutrient standards used in the United States are developed by a committee/subcommittee of the Food and Nutrition Board of the National Academy of Sciences. The *Recommended Dietary Allowances*, tenth edition, published in 1989, is currently being updated. According to the 1989 edition, the Recommended Dietary Allowances (RDAs) are "the levels of intake of essential nutrients that, on the basis of scientific knowledge, are judged by the Food and Nutrition Board to be adequate to meet the known nutrient needs of practically all healthy persons." The 1989 *Recommended Dietary Allowances* dealt with the minimal amounts, plus safety margins, of nutrients needed to protect against possible nutrient deficiency. Currently, the Recommended Dietary Allowances are being updated and expanded. According to V. Young, the recommended intakes will be levels believed to help people "achieve measurable physical indicators of good health." To date, revised dietary recommendations are available for calcium and related nutrients as well as B-vitamins and choline. Until revised dietary recommendations are released, the 1989 *Recommended Dietary Allowances* will remain in use.

The *1989 Recommended Dietary Allowances* presently being used are listed in Table 19.1. The 1989 RDA revision also included the category *Estimated Safe and Adequate*

TABLE 19.1

Recommended Dietary Allowances,[a] Revised 1989. Designed for the maintenance of good nutrition of practically all healthy people in the United States

Category	Age (years) or Condition	Weight[b] (kg)	Weight[b] (lb)	Height[b] (cm)	Height[b] (in)	Protein (g)	Fat-Soluble Vitamins Vitamin A (µg RE)[c]	Fat-Soluble Vitamins Vitamin E (mg α-TE)[d]	Fat-Soluble Vitamins Vitamin K (µg)	Minerals Iron (mg)	Minerals Zinc (mg)	Minerals Iodine (µg)	Minerals Selenium (µg)	Vitamin C (mg)
Infants	0.0-0.5	6	13	60	24	13	375	3	5	6	5	40	10	30
	0.5-1.0	9	20	71	28	14	375	4	10	10	5	50	15	35
Children	1-3	13	29	90	35	16	400	6	15	10	10	70	20	40
	4-6	20	44	112	44	24	500	7	20	10	10	90	20	45
	7-10	28	62	132	52	28	700	7	30	10	10	120	30	45
Males	11-14	45	99	157	62	45	1,000	10	45	12	15	150	40	50
	15-18	66	145	176	69	59	1,000	10	65	12	15	150	50	60
	19-24	72	160	177	70	58	1,000	10	70	10	15	150	70	60
	25-50	79	174	176	70	63	1,000	10	80	10	15	150	70	60
	51+	77	170	173	68	63	1,000	10	80	10	15	150	70	60
Females	11-14	46	101	157	62	46	800	8	45	15	12	150	45	50
	15-18	55	120	163	64	44	800	8	55	15	12	150	50	60
	19-24	58	128	164	65	46	800	8	60	15	12	150	55	60
	25-50	63	138	163	64	50	800	8	65	15	12	150	55	60
	51+	65	143	160	63	50	800	8	65	10	12	150	55	60
Pregnant						60	800	10	65	30	15	175	65	70
Lactating	1st 6 mo					65	1,300	12	65	15	19	200	75	95
	2nd 6 mo					62	1,200	11	65	15	16	200	75	90

[a] The allowances, expressed as average daily intakes over time, are intended to provide for individual variations among most normal persons as they live in the United States under usual environmental stresses. Diets should be based on a variety of common foods in order to provide other nutrients for which human requirements have been less well-defined.

[b] Weights and heights of Reference Adults are actual medians for the U.S. population of the designated age, as reported by NHANES II. The median weights and heights of those under 19 years of age were taken from Hamill et al. (1979). The use of these figures does not imply that the height-to-weight ratios are ideal.

[c] Retinol equivalents. 1 retinol equivalent = 1 µg retinol or 6 µg β-carotene.

[d] α-Tocopherol equivalents. 1 mg d-α-tocopherol = 1 α-TE.

Adapted from National Research Council, *Recommended Dietary Allowances*, 10th ed., © 1989 by the National Academy of Sciences. Courtesy of the National Academy Press, Washington, DC.

The 1989 Recommended Dietary Allowances for vitamin D, calcium, phosphorus, and magnesium were replaced by Dietary Reference Intakes in 1997.
The 1989 Recommended Dietary Allowances for thiamin, riboflavin, niacin, vitamin B₆, folate, vitamin B₁₂, pantothenic acid, biotin, and choline were replaced by Dietary Reference Intake in 1998.

Daily Dietary Intakes (ESADDIs). Estimated Safe and Adequate Daily Dietary Intakes for essential nutrients are used when data were deemed to be sufficient for estimating a range of requirements but not a Recommended Dietary Allowance. The 1989 Estimated Safe and Adequate Daily Dietary Intakes are listed in Table 19.2. The 1989 revision also included *Estimated Minimum Requirements* for three electrolytes. These Estimated Minimum Requirements are given in Table 19.3.

In the 1989 RDAs, the *recommended energy allowances* are reflective of the mean requirement of each category:age group. These allowances are for reference adults with light to moderate physical activity. These recommended energy intakes were discussed in Chapter 11. Safety margins were not added to these allowances as was done with those for the nutrients. This is because doing so could lead to obesity in most individuals.

Dietary Reference Intakes

The new recommended intakes are known as *Dietary Reference Intakes* (DRIs). There are four types of Dietary Reference Intakes — *Estimated Average Requirements* (EARs), *Recommended Dietary Allowances* (RDAs), *Adequate Intakes* (AIs), and *Tolerable Upper Intake Levels* (ULs). Together these four categories constitute a complete set of reference values. Definitions and intended uses of these Dietary Reference Intake values are given in Table 19.4. *The Recommended Dietary Allowance (RDA) and the Adequate Intake (AI) are the values intended for use in "guiding individuals to achieve adequate nutrient intake."*

TABLE 19.2

Estimated Safe and Adequate Dietary Intakes of Selected Nutrients[a,b,c]

Category	Age (y)	Trace Elements[d]			
		Copper (mg)	Manganese (mg)	Chromium (µg)	Molybdenum (µg)
Infants	0-0.5	0.4-0.6	0.3-0.6	10-40	15-30
	0.5-1	0.6-0.7	0.6-1.0	20-60	20-40
Children and	1-3	0.7-1.0	1.0-1.5	20-80	25-50
Adolescents	4-6	1.0-1.5	1.5-2.0	30-120	30-75
	7-10	1.0-2.0	2.0-3.0	50-200	50-150
	11+	1.5-2.5	2.0-5.0	50-200	75-250
Adults		1.5-3.0	2.0-5.0	50-200	75-250

a Because there is less information on which to base allowances, these figures are not given in the main table of the RDA and are provided here in the form of ranges of recommended intakes.

b The Estimated Safe and Adequate Daily Dietary Intakes of fluoride were replaced by Dietary Reference Intakes in 1997.

c The Estimated Safe and Adequate Daily Dietary Intakes of biotin and pantothenic acid were replaced by Dietary Reference Intakes in 1998.

d Since the toxic levels for many trace elements may be only several times usual intakes, the upper levels for the trace elements given in this table should not be habitually exceeded.

Adapted from National Research Council, *Recommended Dietary Allowances*, 10th ed., © 1989 by the National Academy of Sciences. Courtesy of the National Academy Press, Washington, DC.

TABLE 19.3

Estimated Sodium, Chloride, and Potassium
Minimum Requirements of Healthy Persons[a]

Age	Weight (kg)[a]	Sodium (mg)[a,b]	Chloride (mg)[a,b]	Potassium (mg)[c]
Months				
0-5	4.5	120	180	500
6-11	8.9	200	300	700
Years				
1	11.0	225	350	1000
2-5	16.0	300	500	1400
6-9	25.0	400	600	1600
10-18	50.0	500	750	2000
>18[d]	70.0	500	750	2000

[a] No allowance has been included for large, prolonged losses from the skin through sweat.

[b] There is no evidence that higher intakes confer any health benefit.

[c] Desirable intakes of potassium may considerably exceed these values (~3,500 mg for adults).

[d] No allowance included for growth.

Reprinted with permission from National Research Council, *Recommended Dietary Allowances*, 10th ed., © 1989 by the National Academy of Sciences. Courtesy of the National Academy Press, Washington, DC.

TABLE 19.4

Dietary Reference Intakes and Their Intended Usage[a]

Estimated Average Requirements (EAR) — the intake that meets the estimated nutrient need of 50 percent of the individuals in a specific life-stage group. This reference value is to be used as the basis for developing the Recommended Dietary Allowances and is to be used by policy-makers in the evaluation of the adequacy of nutrient intakes of the group and for planning how much the group should consume.

Recommended Dietary Allowance (RDA) — the intake that meets the nutrient need of almost all (97 to 98 percent) individuals in a specific life-stage group. This reference value should be used in guiding individuals to achieve nutrient intake aimed at decreasing the risk of chronic disease. It is based on estimating an average requirement plus an increase to account for the variation within a particular group.

Adequate Intake (AI) — average observed or experimentally derived intake by a defined population or subgroup that appears to sustain a defined nutritional state, such as normal circulating nutrient values, growth, or other functional indicators of health. Adequate Intakes have been set when sufficient scientific evidence is not available to estimate an average requirement. Individuals should use the Adequate Intake as a goal for intake where no Recommended Dietary Allowances exist.

Tolerable Upper Intake Level (UL) — the maximum intake by an individual that is unlikely to pose risks of adverse health effects in almost all (97 to 98 percent) individuals in a specified life-stage group. This figure is not intended to be a recommended level of intake, and there is no established benefit for individuals to consume nutrients at levels above the Recommended Dietary Allowances or Adequate Intakes. For most nutrients, this figure refers to total intakes from food, fortified food, and nutrient supplements.

[a] Refers to daily intakes averaged over time.

Reprinted with permission from Institute of Medicine, *Uses of Dietary Reference Intakes* and *New Report Recasts Dietary Requirements for Calcium and Related Nutrients*. © 1997 by the National Academy of Sciences. Courtesy of the National Academy Press, Washington, DC.

An RDA for a given nutrient is set when scientific evidence is convincing enough to set an Estimated Average Requirement (EAR) from which the RDA is derived. Individuals should use AIs as goals for intakes when RDAs are not available. Having a set of Dietary Reference Intakes should permit health professionals to utilize the appropriate reference value designed for the intended usage

The Dietary Reference Intakes for calcium and related nutrients were released in 1997. The recommended levels for individual intakes of calcium, phosphorus, magnesium, vitamin D, and fluoride are given in Table 19.5.

TABLE 19.5

Recommended Levels for Individual Intakes of Calcium, Phosphorus, Magnesium, Vitamin D, and Fluoride

Life-Stage Group	Calcium (mg/d)	Phosphorus (mg/d)	Magnesium (mg/d)	Vitamin D (μg/d)[a,b]	Fluoride (mg/d)
Infants					
0-5 mo	210*	100*	30*	5*	0.01*
6-11 mo	270*	275*	75*	5*	0.5*
Children					
1-3 y	500*	**460**	**80**	5*	0.7*
4-8 y	800*	**500**	**130**	5*	1.0*
Males					
9-13 y	1,300*	**1,250**	**240**	5*	2*
14-18 y	1,300*	**1,250**	**410**	5*	3*
19-30 y	1,000*	**700**	**400**	5*	4*
31-50 y	1,000*	**700**	**420**	5*	4*
51-70 y	1,200*	**700**	**420**	10*	4*
>70 y	1,200*	**700**	**420**	15*	4*
Females					
9-13 y	1,300*	**1,250**	**240**	5*	2*
14-18 y	1,300*	**1,250**	**360**	5*	3*
19-30 y	1,000*	**700**	**310**	5*	3*
31-50 y	1,000*	**700**	**320**	5*	3*
51-70 y	1,200*	**700**	**320**	10*	3*
>70 y	1,200*	**700**	**320**	15*	3*
Pregnancy					
≤18 y	1,300*	**1,250**	**400**	5*	3*
19-30 y	1,000*	**700**	**350**	5*	3*
31-50 y	1,000*	**700**	**360**	5*	3*
Lactation					
≤18 y	1,300*	**1,250**	**360**	5*	3*
19-50 y	1,000*	**700**	**310**	5*	3*
31-50 y	1,000*	**700**	**320**	5*	3*

Note: This table presents Recommended Dietary Allowances (RDAs) in bold type and Adequate Intakes (AIs) in ordinary type followed by an asterisk (*). RDAs and AIs may both be used as goals for individual intake. RDAs are set to meet the needs of almost all (97 to 98 percent) individuals in a group. For healthy breastfed infants, the AI is the mean intake. The AI for other life-stage groups is believed to cover their needs, but lack of data or uncertainty in the data prevent clear specification of this coverage.

a As cholecalciferol, 1 μg cholecalciferol = 40 IU vitamin D.

b In the absence of adequate exposure to sunlight.

Adapted from Institute of Medicine, *Dietary Reference Intakes: Calcium, Phosphorus, Magnesium, Vitamin D, and Fluoride.* © 1997 by the National Academy of Sciences. Courtesy of the National Academy Press, Washington, DC.

Dietary Reference Intakes for B-vitamins and choline were released in 1998. The recommended levels for individual intakes of B-vitamins a nd choline are given in Table 19.6.

TABLE 19.6

Recommended Levels for Individual Intakes of the B-Vitamins and Choline

Life-Stage Group	Thiamin (mg/d)	Riboflavin (mg/d)	Niacin (mg/d)[a]	Vitamin B_6 (mg/d)	Folate (μg/d)[b]	Vitamin B_{12} (μg/d)	Pantothenic Acid (mg/d)	Biotin (μg/d)	Choline[c] (mg/d)
Infants									
0-5 mo	0.2*	0.3*	2*	0.1*	65*	0.4*	1.7*	5*	125*
6-11 mo	0.3*	0.4*	3*	0.3*	80*	0.5*	1.8*	6*	150*
Children									
1-3 y	0.5	0.5	6	0.5	150	0.9	2*	8*	200*
4-8 y	0.6	0.6	8	0.6	200	1.2	3*	12*	250*
Males									
9-13 y	0.9	0.9	12	1.0	300	1.8	4*	20*	375*
14-18 y	1.2	1.3	16	1.3	400	2.4	5*	25*	550*
19-30 y	1.2	1.3	16	1.3	400	2.4	5*	30*	550*
31-50 y	1.2	1.3	16	1.3	400	2.4	5*	30*	550*
51-70 y	1.2	1.3	16	1.7	400	2.4[d]	5*	30*	550*
>70 y	1.2	1.3	16	1.7	400	2.4[d]	5*	30*	550*
Females									
9-13 y	0.9	0.9	12	1.0	300	1.8	4*	20*	375*
14-18 y	1.0	1.0	14	1.2	400[e]	2.4	5*	25*	400*
19-30 y	1.1	1.1	14	1.3	400[e]	2.4	5*	30*	425*
31-50 y	1.1	1.1	14	1.3	400[e]	2.4	5*	30*	425*
51-70 y	1.1	1.1	14	1.5	400[e]	2.4[d]	5*	30*	425*
>70 y	1.1	1.1	14	1.5	400	2.4[d]	5*	30*	425*
Pregnancy (all ages)	1.4	1.4	18	1.9	600[f]	2.6	6*	30*	450*
Lactation (all ages)	1.5	1.6	17	2.0	500	2.8	7*	35*	550*

Note: This table presents Recommended Dietary Allowances (RDAs) in bold type and Adequate Intakes (AIs) in ordinary type followed by an asterisk (*). RDAs and AIs may both be used as goals for individual intake. RDAs are set to meet the needs of almost all (97 to 98 percent) individuals in a group. For healthy breastfed infants, the AI is the mean intake. The AI for other life-stage groups is believed to cover their needs, but lack of data or uncertainty in the data prevent clear specification of this coverage.

[a] As niacin equivalents. 1 mg of niacin = 60 mg of tryptophan.

[b] As dietary folate equivalents (DFE). 1 DFE = 1 μg food folate = 0.6 μg of folic acid (from fortified food or supplement) consumed with food = 0.5 μg of synthetic (supplemental) folic acid taken on an empty stomach.

[c] Although AIs have been set for choline, there are few data to assess whether a dietary supply of choline is needed at all stages of the life cycle, and it may be that the choline requirement can be met by endogenous synthesis at some of these stages.

[d] Since 10 to 30 percent of older people may malabsorb food-bound Vitamin B_{12}, it is advisable for those older than 50 years to meet their RDA mainly by taking foods fortified with Vitamin B_{12} or a Vitamin B_{12}-containing supplement.

[e] In view of evidence linking folate intake with neural tube defects in the fetus, it is recommended that all women capable of becoming pregnant consume 400 μg of synthetic folic acid from fortified foods and/or supplements in addition to intake of food folate from a varied diet.

[f] It is assumed that women will continue taking 400 μg of folic acid until their pregnancy is confirmed and they enter prenatal care, which ordinarily occurs after the end of the periconceptional period — the critical time for formation of the neural tube.

Reprinted with permission from Institute of Medicine, *Dietary Reference Intakes for Thiamin, Riboflavin, Niacin, Vitamin B_6, Folate, Vitamin B_{12}, Pantothenic Acid, Biotin, and Choline.* © 1998 by the National Academy of Sciences. Courtesy of the National Academy Press, Washington, DC.

Tolerable Upper Intake Levels for calcium, phosphorus, magnesium, vitamin D, and fluoride are given in Table 19.7, and those for niacin, vitamin B$_6$, synthetic folic acid, and choline are given in Table 19.8. Dietary Reference Intakes will be released in the next couple of years or so for the following nutrient groups: energy and macronutrients (tentative); antioxidants, carotenoids, vitamin E, vitamin C, and selenium; trace elements; electrolytes; and other food components (tentative).

TABLE 19.7

Tolerable Upper Intake Levels for Calcium, Phosphorus, Magnesium, Vitamin D, and Fluoride

Life-Stage Group (y)	Calcium (g/d)	Phosphorus (g/d)	Magnesium[a] (mg/d)	Vitamin D (µg/d)[b]	Fluoride (mg/d)
0-0.5	ND[c]	ND	ND	25	0.7
0.5-1	ND	ND	ND	25	0.9
1-3	2.5	3.0	65	50	1.3
4-8	2.5	3.0	110	50	2.2
9-18	2.5	4.0	350	50	10.0
19-70	2.5	4.0	350	50	10.0
>70	2.5	3.0	350	50	10.0
Pregnant	2.5	3.5	350	50	10.0
Lactating	2.5	4.0	350	50	10.0

[a] The Tolerable Upper Intake Level for magnesium represents intake from a pharmacological agent.
[b] As cholecalciferol, 1 µg cholecalciferol = 40 IU vitamin D.
[c] ND = not determinable due to lack of data of adverse effects in this age group and concern with regard to lack of ability to handle excess amounts. Source of intake should be from food only in order to prevent high levels of intake.

Adapted from Institute of Medicine, *Dietary Reference Intakes for Calcium, Phosphorus, Magnesium, Vitamin D, and Fluoride.* © 1997 by the National Academy of Sciences. Courtesy of the National Academy Press, Washington, DC.

TABLE 19.8

Tolerable Upper Intake Levels for Niacin, Vitamin B$_6$, Synthetic Folic Acid, and Choline

Life-Stage Group (y)	Niacin (mg/d)	Vitamin B$_6$ (mg/d)	Synthetic Folic Acid (µg/d)	Choline (g/d)
1-3	10	30	300	1.0
4-8	15	40	400	1.0
9-13	20	60	600	2.0
14-18	30	80	800	3.0
≥19	35	100	1,000	3.5
Pregnant	35	100	1,000	3.5
Lactating	35	100	1,000	3.5

Reprinted with permission from Institute of Medicine, *Dietary Reference Intakes for Thiamin, Riboflavin, Niacin, Vitamin B$_{12}$, Folate, Vitamin B$_{12}$, Panthothenic Acid, Biotin, and Choline.* © 1998 by the National Academy of Sciences. Courtesy of the National Academy Press, Washington, DC.

Dietary Guidelines for Americans

These guidelines are designed to be used in advising healthy Americans, two years of age and older, about "food choices that promote health and prevent disease." The ***Dietary Guidelines for Americans***, in its fourth edition in 1995, was prepared jointly by the U.S. Departments of Agriculture and of Health and Human Services. The 1995 Dietary Guidelines for Americans are given in Figure 19.1. A committee of health professionals is now working on the 2000 Dietary Guidelines for Americans. The Dietary Guidelines for Americans are meant to apply to diets eaten over several days not just a 24-hour period.

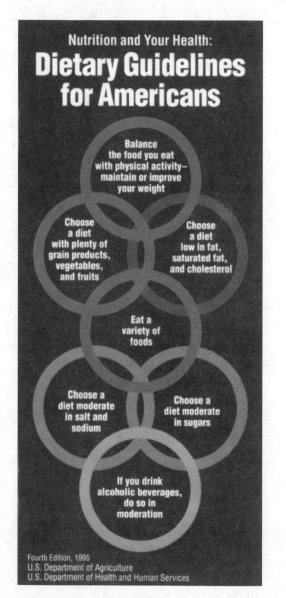

FIGURE 19.1
Taken from Dietary Guidelines for Americans, 1995.

Food Guide Pyramid

The Food Guide Pyramid is a food guidance system developed by the U.S. Department of Agriculture and supported by the U.S. Department of Health and Human Services. It was published in 1992. The Food Guide Pyramid provides information for putting the Dietary Guidelines for Americans into action. The Food Guide Pyramid recommends "what and how much to eat from each food group to get the nutrients you need and not too many calories, or too much fat, saturated fat, cholesterol, sugar, sodium, or alcohol." The Food Guide Pyramid helps individuals design a healthful diet that is appropriate for them. The Food Guide Pyramid focuses on fat in that most individuals in the United States consume diets high in fat. The consumption of diets low in fat has been associated with decreased incidence of chronic diseases. The Food Guide Pyramid is given in Figure 19.2.

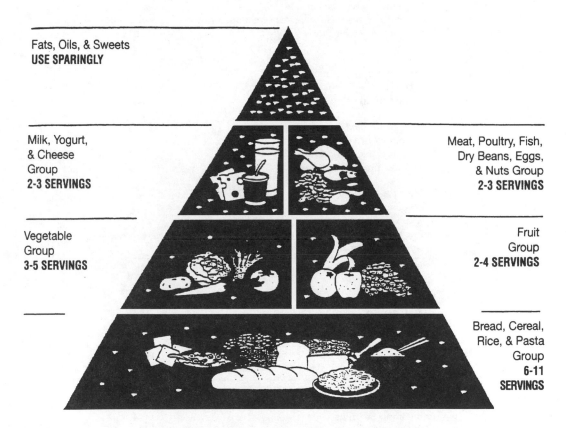

A Guide to Daily Food Choices

FIGURE 19.2
Food Guide Pyramid. Taken from *The Food Guide Pyramid*, 1992.

In using the Food Guide Pyramid in dietary planning, one needs to know what counts as a *serving* (see Table 19.9). These serving sizes are general guidelines. If you consumed a sandwich, you would be consuming foods from several of the food groups. A typical sandwich might contain 2 servings of the bread group, half a serving of the meat group, half a serving of the milk group, and perhaps a partial serving of the vegetable group. Table 19.10 lists daily sample diets at three different calorie levels. The amount of fat in the daily diet can be estimated using information given in Table 19.11. The total fat consumed can be compared to the number of calories listed in Table 19.9 for your caloric intake or you may calculate how many *grams of fat* represents <30 percent of your caloric intake.

TABLE 19.9

What Counts as a Serving of Each of the Food Groups

Bread, Cereal, Rice, and Pasta
1 slice bread
1 ounce ready-to-eat cereal
½ cup cooked cereal rice, or pasta

Vegetable
1 cup raw leafy vegetables
½ cup other vegetables, cooked or chopped raw
¾ cup of vegetable juice

Fruit
1 medium apple, banana, orange
½ cup chopped, cooked, or canned fruit
¾ cup fruit juice

Milk, Yogurt, and Cheese
1 cup milk or yogurt
1½ ounces natural cheese
2 ounces processed cheese

Meat, Poultry, Fish, Dry Beans, Eggs, and Nuts
2-3 ounces cooked lean meat, poultry, or fish
½ cup cooked dry beans
1 egg
4-6 Tablespoons peanut butter

Taken from USDA's *The Food Guide Pyramid*, 1992.

TABLE 19.10

Sample Diets for a Day at Three Calorie Levels

	Lower ~1,600	Moderate ~2,200	Higher ~2,800
Bread Group Servings	6	9	11
Vegetable Group Servings	3	4	5
Fruit Group Servings	2	3	4
Milk Group Servings	2-3[a]	2-3[a]	2-3[a]
Meat Group[b] (ounces)	5	6	7
Total Fat (grams)	53	73	93
Total Added Sugars (teaspoons)	6	12	18

[a] Women who are pregnant or breastfeeding, teenagers, and young adults to age 24 need 3 servings.
[b] See Table 19.8 as to what constitutes a serving.
Taken from USDA's *The Food Guide Pyramid*, 1992.

TABLE 19.11

Counting Grams of Fat

	Servings	Grams Fat
Bread, Cereal, Rice, and Pasta Group		
Bread, 1 slice	1	1
Hamburger roll, bagel, English muffin	2	2
Tortilla, 1	1	3
Rice or pasta, cooked, ½ cup	1	trace
Plain crackers, small, 3-4	1	3
Breakfast cereal, 1 oz.	1	*
Pancakes, 4″ diameter, 2	2	3
Croissant, 1 large, 2 oz.	2	12
Doughnut, 1 medium, 2 oz.	2	11
Danish, 1 medium, 2 oz.	2	13
Cake, frosted, ⅟₁₆ average	1	13
Cookies, 2 medium	1	4
Pie, fruit, 2-crust, ⅙ 8″ pie	2	19
*Check product label		
Vegetable Group		
Vegetables, cooked, ½ cup	1	trace
Vegetables, leafy, raw, 1 cup	1	trace
Vegetables, nonleafy, raw, chopped, ½ cup	1	trace
Potatoes, scalloped, ½ cup	1	4
Potato salad, ½ cup	1	8
French fries, 10	1	8
Fruit Group		
Whole fruit: medium apple, orange, banana	1	trace
Fruit, raw or canned, ½ cup	1	trace
Fruit juice, unsweetened, ¾ cup	1	trace
Avocado, ¼ whole	1	9
Milk, Yogurt, and Cheese Group		
Skim milk, 1 cup	1	trace
Nonfat yogurt, plain, 8 oz.	1	trace
Lowfat milk, 2%, 1 cup	1	5
Whole milk, 1 cup	1	8
Chocolate milk, 2%, 1 cup	1	5
Lowfat yogurt, plain, 8 oz.	1	4
Lowfat yogurt, fruit, 8 oz.	1	3
Natural cheddar cheese, 1½ oz.	1	14
Processed cheese, 2 oz.	1	18
Mozzarella, part skim, 1½ oz.	1	14
Ricotta, part skim, ½ cup	1	10
Cottage cheese, 4% fat, ½ cup	¼	5
Ice cream, ½ cup	⅓	7
Ice milk, ½ cup	⅓	3
Frozen yogurt, ½ cup	½	2
Meat, Poultry, Fish, Dry Beans, Eggs, and Nuts Group		
Lean meat, poultry, fish, cooked	3 oz.*	6
Ground beef, lean, cooked	3 oz.*	16
Chicken, with skin, fried	3 oz.*	13
Bologna, 2 slices	1 oz.*	16
Egg, 1	1 oz.*	5
Dry beans and peas, cooked, ½ cup	1 oz.*	trace
Peanut butter, 2 Tbsp.	1 oz.*	16
Nuts, ⅓ cup	1 oz.*	22
*Ounces of lean meat these items count as		
Fat, Oils, and Sweets		
Butter, margarine, 1 Tsp.	—	4
Mayonnaise, 1 Tbsp.	—	11
Salad dressing, 1 Tbsp.	—	7
Reduced calorie salad dressing, 1 Tbsp.	—	*
Sour cream, 2 Tbsp.	—	6
Cream cheese, 1 oz.	—	10
Sugar, jam, jelly, 1 Tsp.	—	0
Cola, 12 fl. oz.	—	0
Fruit drink, ade, 12 fl. oz.	—	0
Chocolate bar, 1 oz.	—	9
Sherbet, ½ cup	—	2
Fruit sorbet, ½ cup	—	0
Gelatin dessert, ½ cup	—	0
*Check product label		

Taken from USDA's *The Food Guide Pyramid*, 1992.

Nutritional Labeling

The Nutrition Labeling and Education Act of 1990 indicated that all processed foods must have food labels. The U.S. Department of Agriculture is responsible for the regulation of meat and poultry products and eggs, while the U.S. Food and Drug Administration regulates all other foods, nutrient supplements, and drugs.

Information provided on food products as *Nutrition Facts* may be used by the consumer in planning and consuming healthful diets. An example of a Nutrition Facts label is shown in Figure 19.3. The label provides information as to the serving size of the product and the calories and percentage of the *Daily Value* (DV) of selected nutrients per serving. Daily Values for selected nutrients were derived from the 1973 *U.S. Recommended Daily Allowances* (U.S. RDA). The 1973 U.S. RDAs are based on the 1968 RDAs and what was available at the time as to 1974 RDAs. U.S. RDAs are given for four life cycle groupings: infants, children, adults and children 4+ years of age, and pregnant or lactating women. The Nutrition Facts label utilizes the life cycle category for which the food is intended, which is primarily adults and children 4+ years of age. The U.S. RDAs, which also function as Daily Values, are given in Table 19.12. These Daily Values are meant to be used as a rough guide to ensure that daily nutrient needs are met. The U.S. Food and Drug Administration has regulations in which serving sizes are defined.

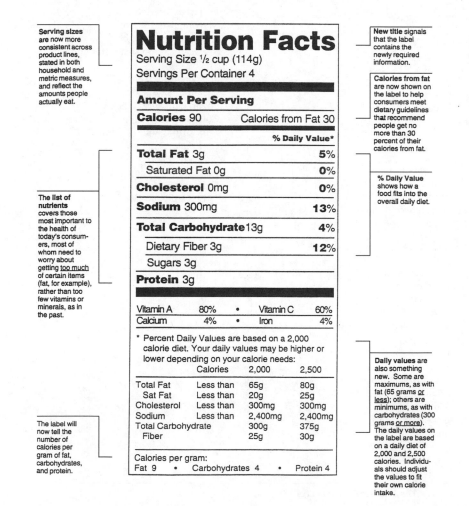

FIGURE 19.3
An example of the Nutrition Panel. Figure is courtesy of the Food and Drug Administration.

TABLE 19.12

U.S. Recommended Daily Allowances[a]

	Age in Years	Vitamin A (IU)	Vitamin D (IU)	Vitamin E Activity (IU)	Ascorbic Acid (mg)	Folacin (µg)	Niacin (mg)	Riboflavin (mg)	Thiamin (mg)	Vitamin B$_6$ (mg)
Infants	0.0-1.0	1,500	400	5	35	100	8	0.6	0.5	0.4
Children	1-3	2,500	400	10	40	200	9	0.8	0.7	0.7
Adults and Children 4+ years of age	—	5,000	400	30	60	400	20	1.7	1.5	2.0
Pregnant or Lactating Women	—	8,000	400	30	60	800	20	2.0	1.7	2.5

	Vitamin B$_{12}$ (µg)	Biotin (mg)	Pantothenic Acid (mg)	Calcium (mg)	Phosphorus (mg)	Iodine (µg)	Iron (mg)	Magnesium (mg)	Copper (mg)	Zinc (mg)
Infants	2.0	0.15	3	600	500	45	15	70	0.6	5
Children	3.0	0.15	5	800	800	70	10	200	1.0	8
Adults and Children 4+ years of age	6.0	0.30	10	1,000	1,000	150	18	400	2.0	15
Pregnant or Lactating Women	8.0	0.30	10	1,300	1,300	150	18	450	2.0	15

[a] U.S. Recommended Daily Allowances are used as Daily Values.

From Food and Drug Administration, Food labeling, *Federal Register*, 38, 2161, 1973.

Standardized *descriptors for nutrient content* to be used on food labels were set by the Food and Drug Administration as a result of the Nutrition Labeling and Education Act of 1990. These terms are given in Table 240

19.13. The food industry also is allowed only to make appropriate health claims. These *approved health claims* are listed in Table 19.14.

The dietary recommendations and guidelines are useful in advising individuals regarding the consumption of nutritionally adequate diets. By appropriate planning, healthy individuals can obtain all the nutrients needed by the body from foods. Everyday individuals

TABLE 19.13

Nutrient Content Descriptors that May be Used on Food Labels

Descriptor	Definition
Free	A serving contains no or a physiologically inconsequential amount: <5 calories; <5 mg sodium; <5 g fat; <0.5 g saturated fat; <2 mg cholesterol; or <0.5 g sugar.
Low	A serving (and 50 g food if the serving size is small) contains no more than 40 calories; 140 mg sodium; 3 g fat; 1 g saturated fat and 15% of calories from saturated fat; or 20 mg cholesterol; not defined for sugar; for "very low sodium," no more than 35 mg sodium.
Lean	A serving (and 100 g) of meat, poultry, seafood, and game meats contains <10 g fat, <4 g saturated fat, and <95 mg cholesterol.
Extra lean	A serving (and 100 g) of meat, poultry, seafood, and game meats contains <5 g fat, <2 g saturated fat, and <95 mg cholesterol.
High	A serving contains 20% or more of the Daily Value (DV) for a particular nutrient. Also referred to as "major source of" and "rich in."
Good source	A serving contains 10-19% of the DV for the nutrient. Also referred to as "source of" and "important source of."
Reduced	A nutritionally altered product contains 25% less of a nutrient or 25% fewer calories than a reference food; cannot be used if the reference food already meets the requirement for a "low" claim.
Less	A food contains 25% or less of a nutrient or 25% fewer calories than a reference food.
Light	An altered product contains ⅓ fewer calories or 50% of the fat in a reference food; if 50% or more of the calories come from fat, the reduction must be 50% of the fat;
	or
	The sodium content of a low-calorie, low-fat food has been reduced by 50% (the claim "light in sodium" may be used)
	or
	The term describes such properties as texture and color, as long as the label explains the intent (examples — "light brown sugar" and "light and fluffy").
More	A serving contains at least 10% of the Daily Value (DV) of a nutrient more than a reference food. Also applied to fortified, enriched, and added claims for altered foods.
% Fat-Free	A product must be low-fat or fat-free, and the percentage must accurately reflect the amount of fat in 100 g of food. Thus, 2.5 g of fat in 50 g of food results in a "95% fat-free" claim.
Fresh	A food is raw, has never been frozen or heated, and contains no preservatives (irradiation at low levels is allowed)
	or
	The term accurately describes the product (examples — "fresh milk" and "freshly baked bread").
Fresh frozen	The food has been quickly frozen while still fresh; blanching is allowed before freezing to prevent nutrient breakdown.

Adapted from Mermelstein, N. H., *Food Technology* 47(2), 81-92, © 1993. With permission from the Institute of Food Technologists, Chicago, IL.

TABLE 19.14

Approved Health Claims

Claims for the following relationships between diet and disease are allowed on appropriate food products:

- Calcium and osteoporosis

- Fat and cancer

- Saturated fat and cholesterol and coronary heart disease

- Fruits, vegetables, and grain products and cancer

- Fruits, vegetables, and grain products and coronary heart disease

- Fruits and vegetables and cancer

- Sodium and hypertension

- Folic acid during pregnancy and neural tube defects

- Dietary sugar alcohol and dental caries

- Dietary soluble fiber (whole oats and psyllium seed husks) and coronary heart disease

The claim must use "may" or "might" in describing the relationship and must add that other factors play a role in that disease.

make food choices that affect their health for better or worse. The making of beneficial choices may decrease the risk of chronic diseases. Good nutrition is important to good health.

Dietary Supplements

The Dietary Supplement Health and Education Act of 1994 called for the labeling of *dietary supplements*. These labeling regulations are effective March 23, 1999. Figure 19.4 summarizes the composition of these dietary supplement labels. All dietary supplements will be labeled with *Supplement Facts*. The Supplement Facts will include serving size, a listing of nutrients and forms of the nutrients in the supplement, and other ingredients in the supplement. A sample Supplement Facts for a multivitamin/multimineral product is given in Figure 19.5.

When appropriate, supplement manufacturers may use three types of claims: nutrient-content, disease, and nutrient support, which includes structure-function. The quantity of a nutrient in a dietary supplement may be described in a nutrient-content claim; for example, a supplement containing at least 200 mg calcium could have the claim "high in calcium" on its label. Supplements may carry disease claims that show a link between: 1) folic acid and decreased risk of neural tube defect-affected pregnancy if the supplement contains sufficient quantities of folic acid; 2) calcium and a lower risk of osteoporosis if the supplement contains sufficient quantities of calcium; and, 3) psyllium seed husk and coronary heart disease if the supplement contains sufficient quantities of psyllium seed husk. The label may include structure-function claims. These claims should avoid suggesting that a disease or health-related condition exists or can be prevented. The claim should be written in a manner that presumes the body is healthy or functioning normally. For example, "helps improve cardiovascular performance" would be permissible, but "helps improve blood circulation" implies a drug claim rather than a structure-function claim. Structure-function claims must be accompanied by the following disclaimer: "This statement has not been evaluated by the Food and Drug Administration. This product is not intended to diagnose, treat, cure, or prevent any disease." Supplement product labels contain information that is useful to the consumer.

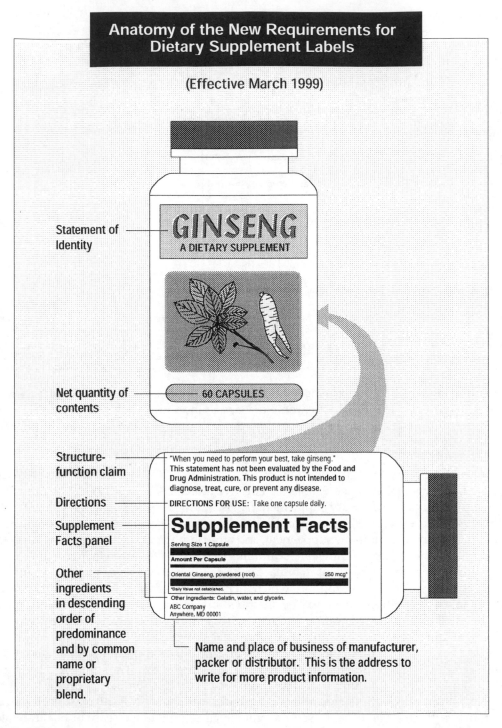

FIGURE 19.4
Anatomy of the new requirements for dietary supplement labels. Food and Drug Administration, *Federal Register*, 62, 49856, 1997.

Supplement Facts

Serving Size 1 Packet

Amount Per Packet		% Daily Value
Vitamin A (from cod liver oil)	5,000 IU	100%
Vitamin C (as ascorbic acid)	250 mg	417%
Vitamin D (as ergocalciferol)	400 IU	100%
Vitamin E (as d-alpha tocopherol)	150 IU	500%
Thiamin (as thiamin mononitrate)	75 mg	5000%
Riboflavin	75 mg	4412%
Niacin (as niacinamide)	75 mg	375%
Vitamin B$_6$ (as pyridoxine hydrochloride)	75 mg	3750%
Folic Acid	400 mcg	100%
Vitamin B$_{12}$ (as cyanocobalamin)	100 mcg	1667%
Biotin	100 mcg	33%
Pantothenic Acid (as calcium pantothenate)	75 mg	750%
Calcium (from oystershell)	100 mg	10%
Iron (as ferrous fumarate)	10 mg	56%
Iodine (from kelp)	150 mcg	100%
Magnesium (as magnesium oxide)	60 mg	15%

Amount Per Packet		% Daily Value
Zinc (as zinc oxide)	15 mg	100%
Selenium (as sodium selenate)	25 mcg	36%
Copper (as cupric oxide)	1 mg	50%
Manganese (as manganese sulfate)	5 mg	250%
Chromium (as chromium chloride)	50 mcg	42%
Molybdenum (as sodium molybdate)	50 mcg	67%
Potassium (as potassium chloride)	10 mg	< 1%
Choline (as choline chloride)	100 mg	*
Betaine (as betaine hydrochloride)	25 mg	*
Glutamic Acid (as L-glutamic acid)	25 mg	*
Inositol (as inositol monophosphate)	75 mg	*
para-Aminobenzoic acid	30 mg	*
Deoxyribonucleic acid	50 mg	*
Boron	500 mcg	*

* Daily Value not established

Other Ingredients: Cellulose, stearic acid and silica.

FIGURE 19.5
Supplement Facts (serving size 1 packet). Food and Drug Administration, *Federal Register*, 62, 49857, 1997.

Exercise Recommendations

Individuals do not have to exercise vigorously to reap the health rewards of exercise. Generally, individuals who *exercise moderately* live longer than those who are sedentary. Exercising excessively, sometimes known as *exercise-dependency*, can also have adverse health effects.

Evolution of Physical Activity Guidelines

The evolution of physical activity recommendations, as given in the *1996 Surgeon General's Report on Physical Activity and Health*, is summarized in Table 19.15. The report's summary of the physiologic responses and long-term adaptations to exercise is given i n Table 19.16.

TABLE 19.15

Evolution of Physical Activity Recommendations

- Physical activity for better health and well-being has been an important theme throughout much of Western history.
- Public health recommendations have evolved from emphasizing vigorous activity for cardiorespiratory fitness to include the option of moderate levels of activity for numerous health benefits.
- Recommendations from experts agree that for better health, physical activity should be performed regularly. The most recent recommendations advise people of all ages to include a minimum of 30 minutes of physical activity of moderate intensity (such as brisk walking) on most, if not all, days of the week. It is also acknowledged that for most people, greater health benefits can be obtained by engaging in physical activity of more vigorous activity or of longer duration.
- Experts advise previously sedentary people embarking on a physical activity program to start with short durations of moderate-intensity activity and gradually increase the duration or intensity until the goal is reached.
- Experts advise consulting with a physician before beginning a new physical activity program for people with chronic disease, such as cardiovascular disease and diabetes mellitus, or for those who are at high risk for these diseases. Experts also advise men over age 40 and women over age 50 to consult a physician before they begin a vigorous activity program.
- Recent recommendations from experts also suggest that cardiorespiratory activity should be supplemented with strength-developing exercises at least twice per week for adults in order to improve musculoskeletal health, maintain independence in performing the activities of daily life, and reduce the risk of falling.

Reprinted with permission from the International Life Sciences Institute, Washington, DC. All rights reserved. Summary of the Surgeon General's report addressing physical activity and health, *Nutrition Reviews* 54, 280-284, © 1996.

TABLE 19.16

Physiologic Responses and Long-term Adaptations to Exercise

- Physical activity has numerous beneficial physiologic effects. Most widely appreciated are its effects on the cardiovascular and musculoskeletal systems, but beneficial effects on the metabolic, endocrine, and immune systems are also considerable.
- Many of the beneficial effects of exercise training — from both endurance and resistance activities — diminish within two weeks if physical activity is substantially reduced, and effects disappear within two to eight months if physical activity is not resumed.
- People of all ages, both male and female, undergo beneficial physiologic adaptations to physical activity.

Reprinted with permission from the International Life Sciences Institute, Washington, DC. All rights reserved. Summary of the Surgeon General's report addressing physical activity and health, *Nutrition Reviews* 54, 280-284, © 1996.

Physical Activity Guidelines

The 1995 *Dietary Guidelines for Americans* indicates that Americans should perform 30 minutes or more of physical activity on most, preferably all, days of the week. Examples of moderate physical activities for healthy adults are given in Table 19.17.

The American College of Sports Medicine recommends that most people follow an ***aerobic training program***. This training program should be conducted at least three days weekly 30 to 60 minutes daily and be of sufficient intensity to expend about ***300 kcal***. Generally, the individual exercises at about 70 percent of their maximum heart rate. Table 19.18 lists the number of minutes required in performing different physical activities to expend 300 kcal for three different body weights. In 1998, the American College of Sports Medicine updated their recommendations for the quantity and quality of exercise for developing and maintaining cardiorespiratory and muscular fitness and flexibility in adults (see Table 19.19). The American College of Sports Medicine and the Centers for Disease Control recommend that adults in the United States accumulate 20 to 30 minutes or more of moderate-intensity physical activity on most, preferably all, days of the week.

Resistance or weight training enables one to develop and maintain strength and endurance. Both strength and endurance training utilize anaerobic energy. Resistance or weight training were discussed in Chapter 17. The lifting of weights builds up the muscles that are worked.

TABLE 19.17

Examples of Moderate Physical Activities for Healthy U.S. Adults

Walking briskly (3-4 miles per hour)

Cycling for pleasure or transportation (≤10 miles per hour)

Swimming, moderate effort

Conditioning exercise, general calisthenics

Racket sports such as table tennis

Golf, pulling cart or carrying clubs

Fishing, standing/casting

Canoeing, leisurely (2.0-3.9 miles per hour)

Home care, general cleaning

Mowing lawn, power mower

Home repair, painting

From Pate, R. R. et al., *Physical activity and public health: A recommendation from the Centers for Disease Control and Prevention and the American College of Sports Medicine*, 1995.

TABLE 19.18

Minutes Required of Different Activities to Expend 300 kcal for Three Different Body Weights

	Minutes for 300 kcal				Minutes for 300 kcal		
	59 kg	68 kg	77 kg		59 kg	68 kg	77 kg
Aerobic dancing				7.0 min/mile	22	19	17
medium intensity	49	43	38	6.0 min/mile	20	17	15
high intensity	38	33	29	5.0 min/mile	18	15	13
Cycling				Nordic skiing, hard snow			
leisure, 5.5 mph	79	69	61	level, moderate speed	43	37	33
leisure, 9.4 mph	51	44	39	level, walking speed	36	31	27
racing	30	26	23	level, maximum speed	19	16	14
In-line skating	32	27	24	Swimming, freestyle			
Jumping rope				20 yd/min	73	63	55
70/min	31	27	24	25 yd/min	58	50	44
125/min	29	25	22	35 yd/min	47	41	36
145/min	26	22	20	50 yd/min	33	28	25
Rowing	55	47	42	treading, fast	30	26	23
Running, horizontal				treading, normal	82	71	63
11.5 min/mile	38	33	29	Walking, normal pace			
9.0 min/mile	26	23	20	asphalt road	63	55	49
8.0 min/mile	24	21	19	fields and hills	62	54	47

Reprinted with permission from CRC Press, Jackson, C., Ed., *Nutrition for the Recreational Athlete*, © 1994. CRC Press, Boca Raton, FL.

TABLE 19.19

Recommendations for the Quantity and Quality of Exercise for Developing and Maintaining Cardiorespiratory and Muscular Fitness and Flexibility in Healthy Adults

Cardiorespiratory Fitness and Body Composition
- Frequency of Training: 3 to 5 days weekly
- Intensity of Training: 55 to 90% of maximum heart rate or 40 to 85% of maximum oxygen uptake reserve.
- Duration of Training: 20 to 60 minutes total of activity (can be 10 minute intermittent bouts accumulating to 20 to 60 minutes a day). Lower-intensity activity should be for 30+ minutes and higher-intensity activity, 20+ minutes.
- Mode of Activity: any activity that uses large muscle groups, which can be maintained continuously, and is aerobic and rhythmical in nature.

Muscle Strength and Endurance, Body Composition, and Flexibility
- Resistance Training: of all major muscle groups 2 to 3 days weekly.
- Flexibility Training: exercises should stretch the major muscle groups maintaining range of motion and should be performed a minimum of 2 to 3 days weekly.

Adapted from American College of Sports Medicine, *Medical Science Sports Exercise* 30, 275, 1998.

20

Recommendations for Individuals in the Various Stages of Their Life Cycles

Dietary and exercise recommendations exist for individuals at various stages of their life cycles, sometimes referred to as *life stages*. As noted in Chapter 19, the ***Dietary Guidelines for Americans*** are intended for use in advising Americans 2+ years of age. The Food Guide Pyramid is a food guidance system for individuals 2+ years of age. Recommended intakes for the various essential nutrients for individuals in different stages of their life spans were also included in the tables presented in Chapter 19. Good nutrition and exercise habits are important throughout one's life span.

Pregnancy

The pregnant woman consumes foods both for herself and her future offspring. Adequate nutrition is vital for the pregnant woman. Poor dietary habits during this time can cause a birth defects and influence the growth and development of the child. Women need to consume 300 cal more daily than they expend during the second and third trimesters of pregnancy. The woman of normal weight should gain 25 to 35 pounds during pregnancy.

The woman's need for protein, vitamins, and essential minerals increases during ***pregnancy***. Many women need to take iron, calcium, and folate supplements during pregnancy. Frequently, physicians prescribe prenatal multivitamin/multimineral supplements.

Women who are physically fit can continue to exercise moderately during pregnancy. If one is not physically fit, pregnancy is not the time to initiate an exercise program. Pregnancy even slightly increases aerobic capacity. Vigorous exercise by the pregnant woman may potentially harm a fetus that has umbilical circulatory problems. It is important that ***exercising pregnant women*** consume adequate fluids.

Lactation

The American Academy of Pediatrics recommends that women ***breastfeed*** their babies during their first year of life. Only a few women are unable physiologically or psychologically to breastfeed. Mothers' milk provides immune factors that are beneficial to infants throughout their lives. Also, breast milk is manufactured to meet the nutritional needs of human infants. Breast milk from a healthy mother contains adequate quantities of essential fatty acids, proteins, vitamins, and essential minerals.

Lactating women need to consume 500 cal more than their prepregnancy recommendation. Lactating women need to consume adequate quantities of all of the vitamins and essential minerals.

Lactating women who were physically fit prior to and during pregnancy can safely participate in moderate exercise programs. These women should talk with their physicians about their exercise programs. Exercising lactating women should be sure that they consume plenty of fluids and they should not exercise when fatigued.

Infancy

An infant is zero to one years of age. Body weight in infants doubles birth weight by four to six months of age and triples within a year. The general development of infants is generally followed by measuring heights and weights and comparing these values to appropriate tables.

Table 20.1 gives the *Dietary Guidelines for Infants* by the American Academy of Pediatrics. During the first four months or so of life the infant consumes only breast milk or formula. Commercial infant formulas meet American Academy of Pediatrics recommendations for nutrient composition. Infant formulas are designed to resemble human breast milk. Special formulas are available for allergic infants and those with certain medical problems. Infants need to get adequate amounts of all essential nutrients, particularly vitamin D, calcium, iron, zinc, and fluoride.

At four to six months of age, infants start eating *solid foods* in addition to breast milk or formula. It is essential that the infant consume sufficient water. The body of the infant contains more water by percent than that of adults; hence, infants are easily dehydrated. New foods should be added to an infant's diet one at a time so that *allergies* or other sensitivities can be detected. Iron-fortified cereals are usually the first foods given to infants. Strained fruits and vegetables and their juices are usually given to 5- to 7-month-old infants. Soft or strained meats, egg yolks, and dairy products are usually given to 6- to 8-month-old infants, with finely chopped meats, toasts/crackers, and soft table foods being added at 8 to 10 months. One-year-old infants can consume most table foods. All infants are individuals and do not develop control of their jaw muscles, tongue, and manual dexterity at the same time. One should be sure that infants do not choke on the foods.

Older infants (7 to 12 months of age) will start physically moving on their own. Parents and caregivers should not discourage the physical efforts of infants. Parents and caregivers can include their infants in some of their exercise programs.

TABLE 20.1

Dietary Guidelines for Infants

- Build to a variety of foods
- Pay attention to your infant's appetite to avoid overfeeding or underfeeding
- Infants need fat
- Choose fruits, vegetables, and grains, but don't overdo high-fiber foods
- Infants need sugar in moderation
- Infants need sodium in moderation
- Choose foods containing iron, zinc, and calcium

Reprinted with permission from International Life Sciences Institute, Washington, DC. From Glinsmann, W. H. et al., *Nutrition Reviews*, 54, 50 © 1996.

Childhood

Nutrient recommendations are issued by the National Research Council for children in the following age groups: 1 to 3, 4 to 6, and 7 to 10 years of age (see Chapter 19). The average weight gain during childhood is about 3.5 to 6.5 pounds yearly and the average height gain is 3 to 4 inches yearly. However, all children do not grow at the same rates. Growth charts are available for evaluating heights, weights, and other anthropometric measurements of children.

Parents and caregivers should help children to choose nutritious foods. Children need to develop good food habits. Children often learn by example. Nutritious snacks should be readily available for children to eat. Meals should be happy sociable occasions. A food plan appropriate for children based on the Food Guide Pyramid has been developed by the U.S. Department of Agriculture and is given in Table 20.2. The two most common nutritional problems of children are obesity and iron-deficiency anemia.

Good exercise habits should be developed during childhood. Young children may exercise with other members of their families and/or with their peers. Children should think of exercise as being fun.

Adolescence

Rapid growth spurts are observed in girls between the ages of 10 and 13 years and in boys between the ages of 12 and 15 years. Girls reach menarche (start menstruating) during this growth spurt. Girls tend to accumulate lean and fat tissues during this growth spurt while boys accumulate primarily lean tissues.

As teenagers grow, they eat more. It is important that teenagers eat nutritious foods. Food habits of teenagers are influenced by their peers and adult role models that they select. Teenagers frequently snack and eat out with their friends. They need to know how to make good food choices at fast-food establishments and restaurants.

Teenagers are very interested in their body images. Sometimes teenagers develop anorexia nervosa and bulimia.

The Food Guide Pyramid should be used in planning diets for teenagers utilizing adult serving sizes. Female teenagers frequently do not consume enough calcium and iron. Teenagers frequently consume too many calories. Poor dietary habits formed during the teen years frequently continue into adulthood.

Teenagers need to exercise at least at moderate levels. Teenagers primarily exercise with their peers as opposed to their families. Poor exercise habits tend to continue into adulthood.

Young and Middle Adulthood

Adulthood is generally categorized into young, middle, and older (or elderly) classifications. The nutrition and exercise needs of adults have been discussed throughout this book. Median daily nutrient intakes of adults in the United States who are 20 to 59 years of age

TABLE 20.2

Meal Pattern for Children

	1 to 2 years	3 to 5 years	6 to 12 years
Breakfast			
Milk, fluid	½ cup	¾ cup	1 cup
Juice, fruit or vegetable	¼ cup	½ cup	½ cup
Grains/Breads			
Bread: whole-grain, bran, germ or enriched	½ slice	½ slice	1 slice
Cereal: cold, dry	¼ cup[a]	⅓ cup[b]	¾ cup[c]
or hot, cooked	¼ cup	¼ cup	½ cup
Supplement (snack) (select 2 components)			
Milk, fluid	½ cup	½ cup	1 cup
Meat or meat alternate[d]	½ ounce	½ ounce	1 ounce
Juice, fruit or vegetable	½ cup	½ cup	¾ cup
Grains/Breads			
Bread: whole-grain, bran, germ or enriched	½ slice	½ slice	1 slice
Cereal: cold, dry	¼ cup[a]	⅓ cup[b]	¾ cup[c]
or hot, cooked	¼ cup	¼ cup	½ cup
Lunch or Supper			
Milk, fluid	½ cup	¾ cup	1 cup
Meat or meat alternate			
Meat, poultry or fish, cooked (lean without bone)	1 ounce	1½ ounces	2 ounces
Cheese	1 ounce	1½ ounces	2 ounces
Egg	1	1	1
Cooked dry beans/peas	¼ cup	⅜ cup	½ cup
Peanut butter or other nut or seed butters	2 Tbsp	3 Tbsp	4 Tbsp
Nuts and/or seeds	½ ounce[e]	¾ ounce[e]	1 ounce[e]
Vegetable and/or fruit (2 or more)	¼ cup total	½ cup total	¾ cup total
Grains/Breads:			
whole-grain, bran, germ or enriched	½ slice	½ slice	1 slice

[a] ¼ cup or ⅓ ounce, whichever is less.

[b] ⅓ cup or ½ ounce, whichever is less.

[c] ¾ cup or 1 ounce, whichever is less.

[d] Yogurt may be used as a meat/meat alternate in the snack only; 4 ounces or ½ cup of plain or sweetened and flavored yogurt to fulfill the equivalent of 1 ounce of the meat/meat alternate component. For younger children, 2 ounces or ¼ cup may fulfill the equivalent of ½ ounce of the meat/meat alternate requirement.

[e] This portion can meet only one-half of the total serving of the meat/meat alternate requirement for lunch or supper. Nuts or seeds must be combined with another meat/meat alternate to fulfill the requirement. For determining combinations, 1 ounce of nuts or seeds is equal to 1 ounce of cooked lean meat, poultry or fish.

Taken from U.S. Department of Agriculture, 1996.

were discussed in Chapter 18. Median daily intakes of men and of women for vitamin A, vitamin E, folate, calcium, and zinc were lower than recommended, but sodium intakes were higher than recommended. The median daily intakes of women were also lower than recommended for magnesium, iron, and copper. The vast majority of adults are physically sedentary. Depending upon the standards used, a quarter to a half of adults in various population groupings are overweight or obese.

Older Adulthood

The older adult grouping generally starts at 60 or 65 years of age, but some organizations refer to older adults as those 50+ years of age. Older adults are frequently referred to as the *elderly.* Life expectancy, as given by the National Center for Health Statistics for 1996, is 73 years for men and 79 for women. Little was known about the nutrition and exercise needs of the elderly until the last couple of decades. The nutrition and exercise habits that have been practiced over one's whole lifetime greatly influences one's health when one is in the elderly grouping. One's psychological well-being also influences one's overall health.

Energy needs generally decrease with advancing age. Older people have lower BMRs. Also, most older people have decreased their physical activity levels. Physical activity helps maintain not only energy needs, but other body functions as well. Exercise helps decrease the loss of muscular strength, endurance, and bone density generally observed in aging and may even increase it. Exercise also improves the mood of most people.

Loss of teeth, gum problems, and ill-fitting dentures influence one's food consumption and generally one's intakes of essential nutrients.

Many of the elderly lose their sense of thirst and they become dehydrated. Sometimes the dehydration leads to confusion and problems with blood pressure, body temperature regulation, and constipation.

Many of the elderly take various kinds of medications. These medications can adversely affect many of the nutrients. These medications can also interact with each other.

The elderly on the average have more problems with the functioning of the various organs than younger individuals. The organs affected include those of the gastrointestinal tract, liver, kidneys, lungs, and heart. Vision and hearing usually decline as one ages as does immune function.

Nutrient recommendations are available for older adults. Iron needs of older women are less than those of premenopausal women. Recommendations for calcium and vitamin B_6 are higher for adults over the age of 51 years than those younger than 51. Evidence exists that older adults may require more vitamin E than younger adults.

A variety of nutrient supplements are marketed for older adults. Evidence does exist, though not considered conclusive, that multivitamins/multiminerals taken at Daily Value levels may improve resistance to disease in older adults.

21

Health Benefits of Exercise

Exercise is beneficial to one's health. Exercise enables one to be physically fit. Exercise has a positive influence on the cardiovascular and musculoskeletal systems as well as the endocrine, metabolic, and immune systems. Adults with higher physical activity levels have lower *mortality rates*. Mortality rates are also lower for adults who exercise moderately than in those who are sedentary.

Beneficial Effects of Exercise on Health and Disease

Exercise has been associated with decreases in the incidence and severity of several diseases and disorders. Some of these diseases and disorders are listed below:

- Cardiovascular disease — regular exercise decreases the risk of mortality due to cardiovascular disease and coronary heart disease.
- Cancer — regular exercise is associated with decreased colon cancer risk. Insufficient and sometimes conflicting data are available to relate physical activity with other cancers.
- Noninsulin-dependent diabetes mellitus — regular exercise decreases the risk of developing this disease.
- Osteoporosis — weight-bearing exercise during childhood and adolescence has been associated with the achieving and maintaining of peak bone mass in early adulthood. Some evidence exists that strength training may slow the decrease or even increase bone density in adults.
- Osteoarthritis — regular exercise is sometimes beneficial for individuals with arthritis.
- Pulmonary function — regular aerobic exercise improves pulmonary function.
- Falling — regular exercise, particularly strength training, may reduce the risk of falling in older adults.
- Obesity — sedentary adults have a higher prevalence of obesity than those who exercise. Exercise also influences body composition and usually increases the fat-free mass of the body.
- Muscle flexibility — appropriate exercises moving the joints through their complete range of motion seems to increase muscle flexibility.
- Muscular strength — appropriate exercises increase both muscle mass and strength. Leg muscle strength influences one's independence.
- Neuromuscular function — individuals who exercise regularly move faster than those who are less active. This is particularly evident in the elderly.

Disease	Exercise decreases risk of	Exercise treats disease	Obesity increases risk of	Age during which exercise decreases disease risk (years) 0-20 20-40 40-60 60-100
Breast and female reproductive cancers	X		X	------------------▶
Claudication	X	X	X	--▶
Coronary artery disease	X	X	X	--▶
Depression	X		X	--------------------------------------▶
Diseases arising from chronic bedrest	X	X	X	--------------------------------------▶
Hypertension	X	X	X	--------------------------------------▶
Type I diabetes mellitus		X		--------------------▶
Type II diabetes mellitus	X	X	X	--------------------▶
Obesity	X	X		--------------------------------------▶
Osteoporosis (post-menopausal)	X	X		--------------------------------------▶
Severe acute pancreatitis		X	X	--------------------------------------▶
Sleep apnea associated with obesity	X	X	X	--------------------------------------▶
Stroke	X		X	--------------------------------------▶
Back pain	X	X	X	----------------------▶
Colon cancer	X		X	----------------▶
Congestive heart failure	X		X	----------------▶
Loss of independence with aging	X	X		--------------------▶
Severe gastrointestinal hemorrhage	X			----------▶
Rheumatoid arthritis		X		----------▶

FIGURE 21.1

Age ranges for which exercise is recommended to decrease risk of disease in patients. Reprinted with permission from Lippincott, Williams & Wilkins, Baltimore, MD. Booth, F. W. and Tseng, B. S., *Medicine & Science in Sports & Exercise*, 27, 463 © 1995.

- Appetite stimulation — exercise stimulates appetite. This may enable some individuals to consume adequate quantities of essential nutrients.

- Mental health — regular exercise may reduce the risk of depression and improve one's mood. Exercise has been shown to have beneficial effects on measures of anxiety, reactions to stress, and self-esteem.

- Quality of life — regular exercise seems to enhance one's overall well-being.

Good exercise habits should be practiced over one's lifetime. Research indicates that individuals should exercise in order to decrease the risk of disease. Booth and Tseng summarized research findings indicating the age ranges for which exercise is recommended to decrease risk of disease and to treat disease in patients (see Figure 21.1). Exercise habits established during the childhood years is most beneficial in decreasing disease risk. These researchers professed that "physical inactivity is a disease: exercise is a pediatric, primary care, general internal, rehabilitative, and geriatric medicine."

Exercise is not the only factor influencing health and disease. However, exercise is one of the major factors that one can control that positively influences one's health. Lack of exercise may interact with other risk factors and increase the statistical possibility of one's developing many diseases and disorders.

Adverse Effects of Exercise on Health

Musculoskeletal injuries may result from excessive or (adverse cardiovascular events can occur during exercise individual is performing strenuous exercise. High levels of exe vidual's resistance to infection. The problem observed most often in inu. cise is fluid imbalance, where the individuals simply do not consume sufficient a. fluids (primarily water).

Improved Fitness

Even modest amounts of exercise positively influences overall health and longevity. Blair et al. investigated the relationship between death rate and fitness in a group of 13,000 men and women. Other factors that influenced longevity were controlled such that fitness was isolated as the contributing factor. The subjects were subdivided into five fitness levels from low to high. The subjects in the low fitness category had more deaths per 10,000 than those in the upper four fitness categories. Thus, even the lower moderate level of fitness was beneficial with regard to increased longevity.

22

Exercise as Therapy for Degenerative Diseases

The previous chapter discussed the benefits of exercise to healthy individuals. Exercise is also being employed as therapy to individuals having degenerative diseases and even a combination of several degenerative diseases. These degenerative diseases include coronary artery diseases, hypertension, diabetes mellitus, osteoporosis, and perhaps neuromuscular disease.

Coronary Artery Disease

Many clinics, hospitals, and universities have exercise programs for individuals with coronary artery disease. The patient should have a thorough medical examination and a graded exercise test before the exercise program is initiated as well as having the permission of his or her physician to participate in the program. The availability of an onsite physician is highly recommended. The patients' behavior and vital signs should be monitored during the exercise. The exercise program for these patients is that for developing a training effect in healthy persons as modified with relation to the patients' cardiovascular and general medical status according to the American College of Sports Medicine. The exercise program is individually designed for each patient.

For many years, researchers and physicians have known that exercise increases serum HDL cholesterol concentrations in most people. Reductions in serum total and LDL cholesterol and triglyceride concentrations are frequently also observed as a result of exercise training. Exercise training increases $\dot{v}O_2$ max and functional capacity in most coronary artery disease patients by increasing the oxygen difference between arteries and veins and sometimes maximal stroke volume.

The patient with coronary artery disease usually has several risk factors including altered blood lipid concentrations, tobacco usage (particularly smoking), obesity, hypertension, diabetes mellitus, and sedentary physical activity. Improvements are generally observed when these patients quit smoking and lose weight as well as have controlled hypertension and diabetes mellitus. Patients are counselled to alter these behaviors and factors as well as participate in exercise (and dietary) programs. So, a combination of these influences usually results in health improvement. However, patients assigned to exercise-based rehabilitation programs had a 20 to 25 percent reduction in fatal cardiovascular events and total mortality as compared to control groups according to studies by O'Connor et al. and Oldridge et al. The patients participating in an exercise program usually also experience psychological benefits.

Some evidence exists that resistance exercise therapy may be beneficial in preventing glucocorticoid-induced muscle wasting and weakness. Braith et al. recommends that this exercise be initiated early after heart transplantation.

Hypertension

Endurance exercise training is recommended by the American College of Sports Medicine as a means to reduce the incidence of hypertension in susceptible individuals and those with mild to moderate essential hypertension. The exercise program is generally the same as that for developing and maintaining cardiovascular fitness in healthy adults. Evidence indicates that exercise training at slightly lower intensities (40 to 70 percent $\dot{v}O_2$ max) seems to lower blood pressure more than exercise at higher intensities.

As with coronary artery disease, the hypertension risk factors include those other than sedentary physical activity. Lifestyle behavioral counselling is generally included as part of the therapy. Aerobically fit and physically active hypertensive patients have much lower mortality rates than those who are sedentary. The exercise training usually improves the hypertension as well as several other cardiovascular disease risk factors. The exercise program generally improves the quality of life of hypertensive patients.

Diabetes Mellitus

The epidemic of Type II (also referred to as Type 2 or noninsulin-dependent) diabetes is associated with decreased physical activity and an increased prevalence of obesity. Exercise is of use in the prevention and the management of Type II diabetes, with the greatest benefit being observed early in the progression of diabetes. Patients with Type I (also known as Type 1 or insulin-dependent) diabetes can safely participate in all forms of physical activity if their therapeutic regimen is adjusted with this in mind. Exercise is important in the therapy of patients with or at risk of diabetes.

The diabetic patient should have a thorough medical examination frequently including a graded exercise test before the exercise program is initiated. Patients should also have good metabolic control of their diabetes, particularly if the exercise is vigorous. Diabetic patients should have their physicians' permission to participate in exercise programs, particularly if they are also at risk for cardiovascular disease.

Long-term exercise programs generally improve glycemic control (see Chapter 4), help prevent cardiovascular disease and hyperlipidemia, may improve hypertension, and enhance weight loss and weight maintenance in diabetic patients. Blood glucose levels of the diabetic patient should be monitored before and after exercise. According to the American College of Sports Medicine exercise should be avoided if fasting blood glucose levels are above 250 mg/dL and ketosis is present, or if blood glucose levels are above 300 mg/dL. The patient should consume carbohydrates if blood glucose levels are below 100 mg/dL. Foods rich in carbohydrates should be readily available to the diabetic at all times.

Osteoporosis

According to the American College of Sports Medicine, weight-bearing exercise is vital for the normal development and maintenance of a healthy skeleton. The types of exercise programs that best benefit the skeleton are controversial. Bone strength depends on the quantities of several minerals in bone and the architecture of the bone. The mineral content of bone can be assessed by dual energy x-ray absorptiometry (DEXA) and computed tomography (CT).

One's risk of osteoporotic fractures is mainly determined by one's peak bone mass developed during childhood and early adulthood. Proper diet and exercise are important during this time. Slow, continuous loss of trabecular bone mineral density begins when one is in their twenties. The decrease in cortical bone seems minimal until menopause. Osteoporosis is more common in women than in men. Decreased endogenous levels of estrogen and progesterone are associated with decreases in bone mineral mass. Reports exist that weight-bearing exercise combined with hormone replacement therapy seems to have an osteogenic effect or at least slow the decrease in loss of bone mineral density; exercise alone is not effective in this regard. Bone fractures are generally associated with low bone mineral density and most often occur as fractures of the vertebrae, forearm, and hip. Hip fractures usually follow a fall. Decreased balance, poor muscle strength and power in the lower extremities, and reduced soft tissue in this area as well as low bone mineral density are causative factors. An exercise program which emphasizes strength, flexibility, coordination, and cardiovascular fitness may decrease the risk of falling with resulting bone fractures.

Neuromuscular Disease

Evidence suggests that maximal aerobic power, muscle strength, and the oxygen cost of locomotion are trainable in children with neuromuscular disease. Unfortunately, training effects may be masked by the natural deterioration of function. Bar-or reported that exercise training reduced spasticity in children with cerebral palsy and polio. It also improved nonwalking motor skills in children with cerebral palsy and other neuromuscular disease.

Physical Effects

As indicated earlier exercise enhances well-being. Exercise can also help patients get their minds off their diseases/conditions, and thus, positively influence their health.

Summary

23

Interrelationships Between Nutrition and Exercise

Good nutrition and moderate exercise throughout one's life span improves the likelihood of one's having and maintaining good health. Good nutritional practices can enhance physical performance. Good exercise habits can improve the nutritional status of individuals. Exercise and nutrition are integral components of health and a healthy lifestyle.

Body Weight

Nutrition and exercise are both important in weight control. In adults the number of calories consumed should approximately equal the number of calories expended. Physical activity increases total energy expenditure.

The consumption of more calories than one expends leads to weight gain. Theoretically, a pound of body weight is gained when energy intake exceeds energy expenditure by 3,500 cal. Likewise, a pound of body weight is lost when energy expenditure exceeds energy intake by around 3,500 cal. The major components of weight loss and weight gain plans are caloric intake, physical activity, and behavioral modification.

More American children, adolescents, and adults are overweight today than ever before. Over 90 percent of the time, the reason individuals are overweight or obese is because their energy intakes exceed their energy expenditures. The majority of American adults and many children and adolescents are sedentary and perform very little physical activity. Health risks are increased in overweight individuals with even further increased risks observed in those who are obese. Some of the health complications frequently observed in obese individuals are hypertension, stroke, heart disease, respiratory diseases, cancers, and kidney diseases.

Some people are underweight. Others have eating disorders such as anorexia nervosa and bulimia. Some of the health complications frequently observed in underweight individuals are respiratory disease, digestive diseases, some cancers, and impaired immune function.

Disease

Poor nutrition and inadequate exercise are *risk factors* (also known as risk behaviors) for chronic diseases that are leading causes of adult deaths. According to the Center for Disease Control in 1998, chronic diseases are responsible for 7 out of every 10 deaths in the United States. This Center further stated that much of this chronic disease burden could be prevented by decreasing the prevalence of tobacco use, lack of physical activity, and poor nutrition. The 10 leading causes of death (see Figure 1.1) which are definitely nutrition-related are heart disease, cancers, strokes, and diabetes mellitus. Those which are definitely exercise-related include heart disease, diabetes mellitus, and perhaps cancers. The remaining top 10 causes of death — chronic obstructive lung disease, accidents, pneumonia and influenza, suicide, HIV infection, and chronic liver disease and cirrhosis — may also have some association with nutrition and with exercise. Poor nutrition and inadequate exercise likely are frequently synergistic in relation to their roles in the development of chronic disease.

Good nutrition and moderate exercise can also help prevent infectious diseases by supporting immune functioning. Thus, the body is better able to fend off some infections and keep others under control.

Healthy People 2000

Healthy People 2000 is a set of health objectives for the United States released in 1990 by the Department of Health and Human Services. The overall objective is to promote more healthy lifestyles and reduce preventable death and disability in individuals living in the United States. The nutrition-related health objectives are given in Table 23.1, and physical activity-related objectives in Table 23.2. Nutrition and exercise influences frequently are synergistic and may also relate to other health determinants such as sleep, stress, tobacco usage, alcohol usage, and environmental quality issues.

TABLE 23.1

Nutrition-Related Health Objectives for the Nation for the Year 2000

- Reduce dietary fat intake to an average of 30% of cal or less and saturated fat to 10% of cal or less
- Increase intakes of complex carbohydrates and fiber-containing foods
- Increase the proportion of overweight people taking effective steps to control their weight
- Increase calcium intakes among teenagers, pregnant women, women who are breastfeeding their infants, and adults in general
- Reduce salt intakes and purchases of foods high in salt
- Remedy iron deficiencies in children and women
- Encourage breastfeeding of infants immediately after birth and the continuation of breastfeeding for at least six months after birth
- Teach parents infant-feeding practices that will minimize the chances of tooth decay
- Promote people's learning of how best to use food labels to correctly select nutritious foods
- Make food labels more informative and complete
- Make more low-fat, low-saturated-fat foods available
- Encourage more restaurants and institutions to serve low-fat, low-calorie foods
- Improve the nutrition quality of school lunches and breakfasts and child-care foodservice meals
- Make sure as many elderly people as possible receive home food services
- Offer nutrition education in more schools from preschool through twelfth grade
- Encourage workplaces to provide nutrition education and/or weight management programs for their employees
- Support health care providers in offering nutrition assessment, nutrition counseling, and referrals to qualified nutrition experts as part of their services

Taken from U.S. Department of Health and Human Services, 1990.

TABLE 23.2

Physical Activity-Related Health Objectives for the Nation for the Year 2000

- Increase to at least 30%, the proportion of people aged 6 and older who engage regularly, preferably daily, in light to moderate physical activity for at least 30 minutes per day
- Reduce to no more than 15%, the proportion of people aged 6 and older who engage in no leisure time activity
- Increase to at least 20%, the proportion of people aged 18 and older to at least 75% the proportion of children and adolescents aged 6 through 17 who engage in vigorous physical activity that promotes the development and maintenance of cardiorespiratory fitness three or more days per week for 20 or more minutes per occasion
- Increase to at least 40%, the proportion of people aged 6 and older who regularly perform physical activities that enhance and maintain muscular strength, muscular endurance, and flexibility
- Increase to at least 50%, the proportion of overweight people aged 12 and over who have adopted sound dietary practices combined with regular physical activity to attain an appropriate body weight

Taken from U.S. Department of Health and Human Services, 1990.

Nutrition and Exercise Guidelines

Nutrition and exercise guidelines were discussed in Chapter 19. For good health, individuals are encouraged to practice good lifelong nutrition and exercise habits. Good nutrition and exercise habits are also beneficial in the maintenance of mental health and overall quality of life.

References

Books

American College of Sports Medicine, *ACSM Fitness Book*, 2nd ed., Human Kinetics, Champaign, IL, 1998.

Arnheim, D.D., and Prentice, W.E., *Principles of Athletic Training*, 8th ed., Mosby-Year Book, St. Louis, MO, 1993.

Berdanier, C.D., *Advanced Nutrition: Macronutrients*, CRC Press, Boca Raton, FL, 1995.

Berdanier, C.D., *Advanced Nutrition: Micronutrients*, CRC Press, Boca Raton, FL, 1998.

Bezkorovainy, A., and Rafelson, M.E., Jr., *Concise Biochemistry*, Marcel Dekker, New York, 1996.

Driskell, J.A., Wolinsky, I., Eds., *Macroelements, Water, and Electrolytes in Sports Nutrition*, CRC Press, Boca Raton, FL, 1999.

Federation of American Societies for Experimental Biology, *Third Report on Nutrition Monitoring in the United States*, vols. 1 and 2, U.S. Government Printing Office, Washington, DC, 1995.

Gibson, R.S., *Principles of Nutritional Assessment*, Oxford University Press, New York, 1990.

Gottfried, S.S., *Biology Today*, Mosby-Year Book, Inc., St. Louis, MO, 1993.

Harper, L.J., Deaton, B.J., and Driskell, J.A., *Food, Nutrition, and Agriculture: Textbook*, World Health Organization, Rome, 1984.

Harrison, G.G., Buskirk, E.R., Carter, J.E.L., Johnston, F.E., Lohman, T.G., Pollock, M.L., Roche, A.F., and Wilmore J., Skinfold thicknesses and measurement technique, *Anthropometric Standardization Reference Manual*, Lohman, T.G., Roche, A.F., and Martorell, R., Eds., Human Kinetics Books, Champaign, IL, 1988, pp. 55-70.

Institute of Medicine, *Dietary Reference Intakes: Thiamin, Riboflavin, Niacin, Vitamin B_6, Folate, Vitamin B_{12}, Pantothenic Acid, Biotin, and Choline*, National Academy Press, Washington, DC, 1998.

Institute of Medicine, *Dietary Reference Intakes: Calcium, Phosphorus, Magnesium, Vitamin D, and Fluoride*, National Academy Press, Washington, DC, 1997.

International Life Sciences Institute, *Healthy Lifestyles: Nutrition and Physical Activity*, ILSI Press, Washington, DC, 1998.

Jackson, C., Ed., *Nutrition for the Recreational Athlete*, CRC Press, Boca Raton, FL, 1994.

Kopple, J.D., and Swendseid, M.E., Effect of histidine intake on plasma and urine histidine levels, nitrogen balance, and N^T-methylhistidine excretion in normal and chronically uremic men, *J Nutr*, 111, 931, 1981.

Lee, R.D., and Nieman, D.C., *Nutritional Assessment*, William C. Brown Communications, Dubuque, IA, 1993.

Machlin, L.J., Ed., *Handbook of Vitamins*, 2nd ed., Marcel Dekker, New York, 1991.

Mertz, W., Ed., *Trace Elements in Human and Animal Nutrition*, 5th ed., vols. 1 and 2, Academic Press, Orlando, FL, 1986.

Minson, C.T., and Halliwill, J.R., Fluid and electrolyte replacement. In: Driskell, J.A., and Wolinsky, I., Eds., *Macroelements, Water, and Electrolytes in Sports Nutrition*, CRC Press, Boca Raton, FL, 1999.

Murray, R.K., Granner, D.K., Mayes, P.A., and Rodwell, V.W., *Harper's Biochemistry*, 23rd ed., Appleton & Lange, Norwalk, CT, 1993.

National Center for Health Statistics, *Health, United States, 1997 and Healthy People 2000 Review*, Public Health Service, Hyattsville, MD, 1993.

National Research Council, *Diet and Health: Implications for Reducing Chronic Disease Risk*, National Academy Press, Washington, DC, 1989.

National Research Council, *Recommended Dietary Allowances*, 10th ed., National Academy Press, Washington, DC, 1989.

Nieman, D.C., *Fitness and Sports Medicine: An Introduction*, Palo Alto, CA, Bull Publishing, 1990.

Rose, W.C., The amino acid requirements of adult man, *Nutr Abstr Rev*, 27, 631, 1957.

Shils, M.E., Olson, J.A., Shike, M., and Ross, C., *Modern Nutrition in Health and Disease*, 9th ed., Lippincott Williams & Wilkins, Baltimore, MD, 1998.

Simko, M.D., Cowell, C., and Gilbride, J.A., *Nutrition Assessment: A Comprehensive Guide for Planning Intervention*, Aspen Publishers, Gaithersburg, MD, 1984.

Sizer, F., and Whitney, E., *Nutrition Concepts and Controversies*, 7th ed., West/Wadsworth, Belmont, CA, 1997.

Spallholz, J.E., Boylan L.M., and Driskell, J.A., *Nutrition: Chemistry and Biology*, 2nd ed., CRC Press, Boca Raton, FL, 1999.

Strauss, R.H., *Sports Medicine*, 2nd ed., W. B. Saunders, Philadelphia, PA, 1991.

United States Department of Agriculture, *What's in a Meal? A Resource Manual for Providing Nutritious Meals in the Child and Adult Care Food Program*, 2nd ed., U.S. Government Printing Office, Food and Nutrition Service, Washington, DC, 1996.

United States Department of Health and Human Services, *Healthy People 2000: National Health Promotion and Disease Prevention Objectives*, U.S. Government Printing Office, Washington, DC, 1990.

United States Department of Health and Human Services, *Anthropometric Reference Data and Prevalence of Overweight: United States, 1976-80*, Vital and Health Statistics, Series 11, No. 238, U.S. Government Printing Office, Washington, DC, 1987.

Wardlaw, G.M., *Contemporary Nutrition: Issues and Insights*, Brown & Benchmark, Dubuque, IA, 1997.

Wolinsky, I., Ed., *Nutrition in Exercise and Sport*, 3rd ed., CRC Press, Boca Raton, FL, 1998.

Wolinsky, I., and Driskell, J.A., Eds., *Sports Nutrition: Vitamins and Trace Elements*, CRC Press, Boca Raton, FL, 1997.

Ziegler, E.E., and Filer, L.J., Jr., Eds., *Present Knowledge in Nutrition*, 7th ed., International Life Sciences Institute Press, Washington, DC, 1996.

Pamphlets

National Center for Health Statistics, U.S. Department of Health and Human Services, *Deaths: Final Data for 1996*, National Vital Statistics Reports, vol. 47, no. 9, NCHS, Hyattsville, MD, 1998. [DHHS Publ. No. (PHS) 99-1120]

National Center for Health Statistics, U.S. Department of Health and Human Services, *United States Abridged Life Tables, 1996*, National Vital Statistics Reports, vol. 47, no. 13, NCHS, Hyattsville, MD, 1998. [DHHS Publ. No. (PHS) 99-1120]

National Cholesterol Education Program, *Facts about Blood Cholesterol*, National Heart, Lung, and Blood Institute, National Institutes of Health, Bethesda, MD, 1994. [NIH Publ. No. 94-2696]

United States Department of Agriculture and of Health and Human Services, *Nutrition and Your Health: Dietary Guidelines for Americans*, 4th ed., U.S. Government Printing Office, Washington, DC, 1995. [Home and Garden Bulletin No. 232]

United States Department of Agriculture, *The Food Guide Pyramid*, U.S. Department of Agriculture, Human Nutrition Information Service, Hyattsville, MD, 1992. [Home and Garden Bulletin No. 252]

United States Department of Agriculture, *Meal Pattern Requirements and Offer Versus Serve Manual*, U.S. Government Department of Agriculture, Food and Nutrition Service, Washington, DC, 1990. [FNS-265}

Federal Register

Food and Drug Administration, Food Labeling: Serving Sizes, *Federal Register*, 58, 2229, 1992.

Food and Drug Administration, Food Labeling: Reference Daily Intakes and Daily Reference Values, *Federal Register*, 58, 2206, 1992.

Food and Drug Administration, Food Labeling: Nutrient Content Claims, General Principles, Petitions, Definition of Terms; Definitions of Nutrient Content Claims for the Fat, Fatty Acid, and Cholesterol Content of Food, *Federal Register*, 58, 2302, 1992.

Food and Drug Administration, Food Labeling, *Federal Register*, 38, 2161, 1973.

Food and Drug Administration, Food Labeling: Mandatory Status of Nutrition Labeling and Nutrient Content Revision, Format for Nutrition Label, *Federal Register*, 58, 2079, 1992.

Food and Drug Administration, Food Labeling: Statement of Identity, Nutrition Labeling and Ingredient Labeling of Dietary Supplements; Compliance Policy Guide, Revocation, *Federal Register*, 62, 49826, 1997.

Articles

American College of Sports Medicine. Position stand: Exercise and fluid replacement. *Med Sci Sports Exer*, 28, i, 1996.

American College of Sports Medicine. Position stand: Exercise for patients with coronary artery disease. *Med Sci Sports Exer*, 26(3), i, 1994.

American College of Sports Medicine. Position stand: Osteoporosis and exercise. *Med Sci Sports Exer*, 27(4), i, 1995.

American College of Sports Medicine. Position stand: Physical activity, physical fitness, and hypertension. *Med Sci Sports Exer*, 25(10), i, 1993.

American College of Sports Medicine. Position stand: The recommended quality and quantity of exercise for developing and maintaining fitness in healthy adults. *Med Sci Sports Exer*, 22, 265, 1990.

American College of Sports Medicine. The recommended quantity and quality of exercise for developing and maintaining cardiorespiratory and muscular fitness, and flexibility in healthy adults. *Med Sci Sports Exer*, 30, 975, 1998.

American College of Sports Medicine and American Diabetes Association. Joint position statement: Diabetes mellitus and exercise. *Med Sci Sports Exer*, 29(2), i, 1998.

American Heart Association, Dietary guidelines for healthy American adults: a statement for physicians and health professionals by the Nutrition Committee. *Circ*, 7, 721A, 1988.

Bar-or, O., Role of exercise in the assessment and management of neuromuscular disease in children, *Med Sci Sports Exer*, 28, 421, 1996.

Beals, K.A., and Manore, M.M., Nutritional status of female athletes with subclinical eating disorders, *J Am Diet Assoc*, 98, 419, 1998.

Blair, S.N., Kohl, H.W. III, Paffenbarger, R.S., Jr., Clark, D.G., Cooper, K.H., and Gibbons, L.W., Physical fitness and all-cause mortality: A prospective study of healthy men and women, *JAMA*, 262, 2395, 1989.

Booth, F.W., and Tseng, B.S., American needs to exercise for health, *Med Sci Sports Exer*, 27, 463, 1995.

Bouchard, C., Current understanding of the etiology of obesity: Genetic and nongenetic factors, *Am J Clin Nutr*, 53, 1562S, 1991.

Braith, R.W., Welsch, M.A., Mills, R.M., Jr., Keller, J.W., and Pollock, M.L., Resistance exercise prevents glucocorticoid-induced myopathy in heart transplant recipients, *Med Sci Sports Exer*, 30, 483, 1998.

Bray, G.A., and Gray, D.S., Obesity: Part I — pathogenesis, *West J Med*, 149, 429, 1988.

Costill, D.L., Carbohydrates for exercise: Dietary demands for optimal performance, *Int J Sports Med.*, 9, 1, 1988.

Driskell, J.A., Krumbach, C.J., Ellis, D.R., Vitamin and mineral supplement use among college athletes, *J Am Diet Assoc, 98, A, 1998.*

Drozen, M., and Harrison, T., Structure/function claims for functional foods and nutraceuticals, *Nutraceuticals World*, Nov/Dec, 18, 1998.

Glinsmann, W.H., Bartholmey, S.J., and Coletta, F., Dietary guidelines for infants: A timely reminder, *Nutr Rev*, 54, 50, 1996,

Grandjean F., Hursh, L.M., Majure, W.C., and Hauley, D.F., Nutritional knowledge and practices of college athletes, *Med Sci Sports Exer*, 13, 82, 1981.

Kurtzwell, P., An FDA guide to dietary supplements, *FDA Consumer*, 32(5), 28, 1998.

Mermelstein, N.H., A new era in food labeling, *Food Tech*, 47(2), 81, 1993.

O'Connor, G.T., Buring, J.E., Yusaf, S., Goldhaber, S.Z., and Olmstead, E.M. An overview of randomized trials of rehabilitation with exercise after myocardial infarction. *Circulation*, 80, 234, 1989.

Oldridge, N.B., Guyait, G.H., Fischer, M.E., and Rimm, A.A., Cardiac rehabilitation after myocardial infarction: Combined experience of randomized clinical trials. *JAMA*, 260, 945, 1988.

Pate, R.R., Pratt, M., Blair, S.N., et al., Physical activity and public health: A recommendation from the Centers for Disease Control and Prevention and the American College of Sports Medicine, *JAMA* 273, 402, 1995.

Position of the American Dietetic Association and the Canadian Dietetic Association: Nutrition for physical fitness and athletic performance for adults, *J Am Diet Assoc*, 93, 691, 1993.

Schulz, L.O., Factors influencing the use of nutritional supplements by college students with varying levels of physical activity, *Nutr Rev*, 8, 459, 1988.

Sherman, W.M., Costill, D.L., Fink, W.J., and Miller, J.M., Effect of exercise-diet manipulation on muscle glycogen and its subsequent utilization during performance, *Int J Sports Med*, 2(2), 114, 1981.

Sobal, J., and Marquart, L.F., Vitamin/mineral supplement use among athletes: A review of the literature, *Int J Sports Nutr*, 4, 320, 1994.

Summary of the Surgeon General's report addressing physical activity and health. *Nutr Rev*, 54, 280, 1996.

Internet

American Academy of Pediatrics, *AAP Releases New Breastfeeding Recommendations*, http://www.aap.org/advicacy/archives, December 1, 1997.

National Heart, Lung, and Blood Institute, National Institutes of Health, *Clinical Guidelines on the Identification, Evaluation, and Treatment of Overweight and Obesity in Adults: The Evidence Report*, http://www.nhlbi.nih.gov/nhlbi/news, June 26, 1998.

United States Department of Agriculture, Agricultural Research Service, USDA Nutrient Database for Standard Reference, Release 12, http://www.nal.usda.gov/fnic/foodcomp, 1998.

Index

A

Abdominal circumference, 194
Abdominal skinfold measurement, 188
Absorption of nutrients, see Digestion, absorption, and circulation of nutrients
Acetoacetate, 150
Acetone, 150
Acetylcholine, 80, 82
Acetyl coenzyme A, 148
Acid-base balance, 125
Active transport
    amino acids absorbed by, 13
    calcium absorbed by, 87
    copper absorbed by, 104
    magnesium absorbed by, 93
    Na^+K^+-pump utilized in, 95
    phosphorus absorbed by, 91
    water-soluble vitamins absorbed by, 14
Activity category, 139, 140
Actomyosin, 210
Adenosine diphosphate (ADP), 80, 145
Adenosine triphosphate (ATP), 12
Adequate Intake (AI), 55, 89
Adipose tissue, 30, 42, 56, 131
Adolescence, 245
ADP, see Adenosine diphosphate
Adrenalin, 16
Aerobic conditions, 158
Aerobic energy production, 146
Aerobic exercise, 175
Aerobic training program, 241
Aging processes, 58
AI, see Adequate Intake
Albumin, 42
Alcohol, 6, 64, 102
    calories in, 134
    intake, chronic, 42
Alcoholics, 67, 81
Aldehyde oxidase, 116
Aldosterone, 95
Alkaline phosphatase, 122
Allergic reactions, 62, 77
Amenorrhea, 89, 103
Amino acid(s), 39, 123
    branched-chain, 65, 125
    conversion of proteins to, 165
    essential, 7, 40
    glucogenic, 148
    ketogenic, 148
    limiting, 41

    nonessential, 40
    oxidases, 66
    semiessential, 7, 40
Aminopeptide, 12
Ammonia, 165
Amylase, 30
Anaerobic energy production, 146
Anaerobic glycolysis, 212
Animal proteins, 38
Anorexia nervosa, 206, 245, 259
Antacids, aluminum-containing, 92
Antibiotics, 60
Anticoagulants, 58, 60
Antidiuretic hormone, 21, 22
Antioxidants, 56, 61, 109, 127
Antirachitic vitamin, 53
Anti-scorbutic factor, 61
Appetite, 133
Arachidonic acid, 7, 37, 70
Arsenic toxicity, 121
Artificial sweeteners, 29
Ascorbic acid, 61, 101
Asparagine, 124
Aspartame, 44
Aspartate, 124
Aspartic acid, 168
Athletes, nutritional status of, 219–221
    median daily nutrient intakes of adults, 219
    nutritional status of athletes, 221
    use of vitamin/mineral supplements by athletes, 219–221
Athletic performance in humans, coenzymes, growth factors, amino acids, and buffers possibly related to, 123–125
    arginine, ornithine, and citrulline, 124
    aspartate and asparagine, 124
    bicarbonate, phosphate, and citrate salts, 125
    branched-chain amino acids, 125
    coenzyme Q_{10}, 123
    creatine, 124
    inosine, 125
Athletic performance in humans, nutrients essential for animals possibly related to, 119–123
    arsenic, 121
    boron, 122–123
    carnitine, 120
    myo-inositol, 120–121
    nickel, 121–122
    silicon, 122
    taurine, 119
    trace elements, 123

Athletic performance in humans, substances not
        determined essential possibly related to,
        125–128
    bee pollen, 128
    bioflavonoid derivatives, 127
    caffeine, 128
    carotenoids, 127
    dimethylglycine, 126
    ethanol, 128
    gamma hydroxybutyrate and
        hydroxymethylbutyrate, 126
    ginsengs, 127
    glandulars, 126
    glutathione, 127
    lecithin, 126
    octacosanol, 126
    oryzanoles and ferulic acid, 126
    smilax compounds, 126–127
    yohimbine, 127
ATP, see Adenosine triphosphate

B

Bacterial synthesis, 60
Basal metabolic index, 197
Basal metabolic rate (BMR), 138, 247
B-complex vitamins, 7, 49
Beam balance scale, 174
Bee pollen, 128
Behavior modification, 178
Beriberi, 63, 65
Betaine, 82
Bicarbonate, 11
Bicarbonate salts, 125
Biceps skinfold measurement, 188
Bile, 11, 35, 56
Biliary obstruction, chronic, 60
Biocytin, 78
Bioflavonoid derivatives, 127
Biologic membrane, 37
Biotin, 12, 78, 164, 228
Bitot's spots, 52
Blindness, 52
Blood
    clotting, 104
    coagulation, 59
    doping, 103
    glucose homeostasis, 106, 114
    pressure, 96, 213, 247, 254
BMI, see Body mass index
BMR, see Basal metabolic rate
Body
    image, 205, 245
    mass index (BMI), 171
    protein, 42, 149
    shape, 206
    size, 138
    temperature, 19, 102
    weight, desirable, 174, 175

Body composition, assessment of, 183–196
    direct assessment, 183
    indirect assessment, 183–196
        breadth measurements, 194
        girth measurements, 193–194
        hydrostatic weighing, 183–184
        methods for evaluating body density, 184–185
        skinfold measurements, 185–192
Bomb calorimeter, 134
Bond energies, 168
Bone
    density, 89, 206, 247
    fractures, 255
    mineralization, 123
    strength, 88
    turnover, 91
Boron, 122
    deficiency, 122
    toxicity, 122
Branched-chain amino acids, 65
Breast milk, 244
Brush border, 12
Buffers, 39
Bulimia, 206, 245
Burning foot syndrome, 81
Buttock circumference, 194

C

β-Carotene, 50, 53
Cadmium, 123
Caffeine, 88, 128
Calciferol, 53
Calcification, excessive, 89
Calcitonin, 87
Calcitriol, 54
Calcium, 7, 54, 122, 227
    deficiency, 221
    food sources of, 89
    -fortified orange juices, 89
    homeostasis, 88
    phosphate, 101
    toxicity, 89
Caloric density, 136
Caloric expenditures, 131
Caloric intake, 197
Calorie, 6, 31, 131
Cancer, 51, 63, 206, 249
Carbohydrate(s), 3, 6, 29–33, 147
    available, 30
    blood glucose homeostasis, 31
    carbohydrate and fiber consumption habits, 32–33
        endurance capacity, 32–33
        glycogen loading, 32
    classification, 29
    complex, 29, 30
    digestion, 30
    energy production from, 147
    functions, 30–31
    indigestible, 13, 29

intake, recommended, 31
 meal, post-event high complex, 32
 recommended intakes, 31–32
Carboloading, 32
Carbon dioxide, 27, 137
Carboxybiocytin, 168
Carboxylation, 78
Carboxypolypeptidase, 11
Cardiac sphincter, 11
Cardiovascular disease, 30, 74, 123, 249
Cardiovascular endurance, 209, 212, 213
Cardiovascular system, 22
Carnitine, 62, 120, 161
Carotenoids, 50, 127
Carrier-mediated transport
 molybdenum absorbed by, 116
 zinc absorbed by, 106
Cataracts, 57, 58, 62
Cell signaling, 88
Cellulose, 29
Central nervous system, 30, 77
Cereals, iron-fortified, 244
Cerebral palsy, 255
Ceruloplasmin, 105
CHD, see Coronary heart disease
Cheilosis, 67
Chest circumference, 193
Childhood, food preferences formed in, 5
Cholecystokinin, 11
Cholesterol, 11, 35, 231
 esterase, 11
 HDL, 114, 128, 213
 intake, 37
Choline, 81, 82, 228
Christmas factor, 59
Chromium, 7, 114
 deficiency, 115
 food sources of, 115
 picolinate, 115
 toxicity, 115
Chronic disease, 3, 223
Chylomicrons, 13, 36
Chyme, 11, 12
Chymotrypsinogen, 11
Circulation of nutrients, see Digestion, absorption, and circulation of nutrients
Circulatory system, 9, 12, 15
Citrulline, 168
Closed-circuit indirect calorimetry, 137
Cobalamins, 75
Coenzyme A, 80
Coenzyme Q_{10}, 123
Coenzymes, 49, 123
Cold intolerance, 205
Collagen, 62, 88
Colon cancer, 30, 89
Common cold, 63
Complementary proteins, 41
Complete proteins, 41
Complex carbohydrates, 29, 30
Compound lipids, 35

Conditioning, 209–214
 cardiovascular endurance training, 212–213
 fitness and health, 209
 muscle contraction, 210
 muscle endurance, 211–212
 muscular strength, 211
 principles of, 210
 resistance training programs, 211
 training programs, 213–214
Conjugated proteins, 40
Constipation, 30
Convulsions, 71
Copper, 7, 104, 68, 156
 food sources of, 105
 metabolism, 117
 toxicity, 105
Core body temperature, 23
Coronary heart disease (CHD), 38, 58, 62, 249
Corticosteroid synthesis, 62
Coumarins, 59
Creatine, 47
 catabolism, 42
 phosphate, 131, 145, 212
 supplementation, 124
 synthesis, 124
Creatinine, 42
Creeping obesity, 203
Cysteine, 7, 40, 119
Cystine, 7, 40, 95
Cytochrome reductase, 66
Cytochrome series, 61, 104

D

7-Dehydrocholesterol, 54
Daily energy allowances, 142
Daily Value (DV), 43, 234, 235
Deamination, 70
Death, causes of, 8, 260
Defecation, 12
Degenerative diseases, see Exercise, as therapy for degenerative diseases
Dehydration, 24, 44, 128
Dehydroascorbic acid, 61
Dental caries, 31
Dental fluorosis, 112
Dental topical treatments, 111
Depression, 250
Derived lipids, 35
Desulfhydration, 70
Dextrinase, 12
Dextrins, 12, 29
Dextrose, 29
Diabetes mellitus, 31, 202, 253, 254
Dicumarol, 59
Diet(s)
 histories, 135
 recommendations, 217
 sample, 232
Dietary fiber, 29

Dietary Guidelines for Americans, 3, 31
Dietary intake, 135
Dietary supplements, 223, 237
Dieting, yo-yo, 178
Diffusion, facilitated, 12
Digestion, absorption, and circulation of nutrients,
    9–16
    absorption, 12–14
        absorption of nutrients, 13–14
        absorptive mechanisms, 12–13
    circulatory system, 14–16
    GI tract function, 9–12
    intestinal microflora, 14
    lymphatic system, 14
Digestive efficiencies, 134
Digestive tract, 3
Diglycerides, 35
Diketoglutamic acid, 61
Dimethylglycine, 126
Dipeptides, 13
Direct assessment, of body composition, 183
Direct calorimetry, 134
Disaccharides, 9, 29
Disease(s)
    chronic, 3, 8, 226, 260
    degenerative, 253
    neuromuscular, 255
    respiratory, 259
Diuretic(s), 96, 128
DNA, 11, 91
    precursor, 125
    synthesis, 72, 75
Dopamine, 70, 104
Douglas bag, 137
Drinking water, 85, 105
Duodenum, 11
DV, see Daily Value

E

Eating disorders, 181, 221, 259, see also Underweight,
    eating disorders and
Ectomorphs, 200
Elbow breadth, 171, 174, 194
Elderly, 22
Electroencephalograms, 71
Electrolytes, 7, 14, 85
Electron carrier, 100, 104
Electron transport chain (ETC), 57, 147, 156, 157
Embden-Meyerhof pathway, 147, 150
Empty calories, 31
Endomorphs, 200
Endurance exercise training, 254
Energy
    allowances, recommended, 225
    anaerobic, 241
    balance, 131, 175
    content, of food, 6
    -dense lipids, 6
    formation, 63

    generation, 93
    metabolism, 76, 79, 101
    requirements, 131
    reserves, 145
    utilization, 69
    -yielding nutrients, 27
Energy expenditure, assessment of, 137–143
    body calorimetry, 137
    components of energy expenditure, 137–139
        basal and resting metabolism, 138
        thermic effect of exercise, 138–139
        thermic effect of food, 138
    estimating energy expenditure, 139–143
Energy intake, assessment of, 133–136
    caloric density of foods, 136
    calories, 133–134
    dietary intakes, 135
    hunger, appetite, and satiety, 133
Energy production, body, 145–169
    aerobic and anaerobic energy release, 146
    anaerobic and aerobic energy from foods, 146
    elimination of ammonia, 165–168
    energy, ATP, and catabolic pathways, 168–169
    energy currency, 145
    energy pathways, 147–149, 150–165
        catabolic pathways of carbohydrates, 150–160
        catabolic pathways of lipids, 161–164
        catabolic pathways of proteins, 164–165
    energy reservoir, 145
    fasting, 149–150
    feasting, 149
Enterogastrones, 9
Enterohepatic circulation, 72
Enterokinase, 11
Epiglottis, 9
Epinephrine, 16, 70
Epithelial tissues, 51
Ergogenic acids, 47, 119, 124
Ergosterol, 54
Esophagus, 11
Essential amino acids, 7, 40
Essential fatty acids, 7, 36
Essential minerals, 7, 85, 87
Essential nutrients, 3, 6
Estimated Average Requirements, 226
Estimated Minimum Requirement of Healthy Persons
    for chloride, 99
    for potassium, 96
    for sodium, 98
Estimated Safe and Adequate Daily Dietary Intake,
    225
    for chromium, 115
    for copper, 105
    for fluoride, 112
    for manganese, 113
    for molybdenum, 116
Estrogen, 38, 88, 103
ETC, see Electron transport chain
Ethanol, 128
Ethanolamine, 81
Evaporation, 21

Exercise(s)
  adaptations to, 240
  aerobic, 175
  circuit, 211
  dependency, 206
  habits, 245, 259
  -induced oxidation, 63
  moderate, 240, 259
  programs, 244
  recommendations, see Nutrition and exercise
      recommendations
  regimen, 178
  resistance, 91
  thermal effect of, 138
  vigorous, 243
  warm-up, 211
  weight-bearing, 91, 254
Exercise, health benefits of, 249–251
  adverse effects of exercise on health, 251
  beneficial effects of exercise on health and disease,
      249–250
  improved fitness, 251
Exercise, interrelationships between nutrition and,
      259–261
  body weight, 259
  disease, 259–260
  Healthy People 2000, 260–261
  nutrition and exercise guidelines, 261
Exercise, as therapy for degenerative diseases,
      253–255
  coronary artery disease, 253
  diabetes mellitus, 254
  hypertension, 254
  neuromuscular disease, 255
  osteoporosis, 254–255
  physical effects, 255
Exocytosis, 13
Expiration, 21
Extracellular fluid, 14

F

Facilitated diffusion, 14
FAD, see Flavin adenine dinucleotide
Fasting, 149
Fat
  cell number, 133
  cell size, 133
  counting grams of, 232, 233
  distribution, 201
  -free mass, 183
  mass, 183
  saturated, 231
  -soluble antioxidant, 51
  -soluble vitamins, 7, 35, 37, 49
  substitutes, 38
Fatfolds, 189
Fatigue, 146
Fats, 3, 35, 169

Fatty acid(s)
  essential, 36
  even-carbon-numbered unsaturated, 164
  long-chain, 120, 162
  odd-chain, 76
  polyunsaturated, 164
  saturated, 35
  short-chain, 30, 149
  synthesis, 64, 66, 93
Feasting, 149
Fecal weight, 30
Ferritin, 102
Ferulic acid, 126
FFAs, see Free fatty acids
Fiber intake, recommended, 31
Fibrinogen, 59
Fitness, 241
  improved, 251
  level, 213
Flavin adenine dinucleotide (FAD), 66
Flavin mononucleotide (FMN), 65, 66
Flavoprotein, 165
Flexibility, 241, 255
Fluid
  balance, potassium and, 95
  replacement, 23
  volumes, 20
Fluorapatite, 111
Fluoride, 7, 88, 111, 227
Fluorosis, 112
FMN, see Flavin mononucleotide
Folacin, 72
Folate, 7, 76, 246
  fortification, 74
  trap, 75
Folic acid, 62, 72
  food sources of, 73
  synthetic, 229
Follicular hyperkeratosis, 52
Food(s), 3, 7
  caloric density of, 136
  caloric energy of, 168
  choices, 5, 245
  composition tables, 134
  energy, 6, 27
  frequency questionnaires, 135
  habits, of children, 245
  labels, 133, 234
  models, 135
  recalls, 135
  refining of, 115
  selection, 5
  solid, 244
  thermic effect of, 139
Forearm circumference, 194
Fortification, 51
Fractures, 88
Frame size, 171, 174
Free fatty acids (FFAs), 13, 161

G

Gallbladder, 11
Galvanized containers, 107
Gamma hydroxybutyrate, 126
Gastric enzymes, 11
Gastric inhibitory polypeptide, 11
Gastric lipase, 11
Gastrin, 41
Gastrointestinal tract, 9, 10, 23
Genetic carnitine deficiency, 120
Gestational hypertension, 89
Ginsengs, 127
Girth measurements, 193
Glucagon, 11, 16
Glucocorticoids, 91
Glucogenic amino acids, 148
Gluconeogenesis, 78
Glucose, 7, 33, 64, 146
Glutamic acid, 73, 124
Glutathione, 95, 127
Glutathione peroxidase, 110, 111
Glycemic control, 254
Glycemic Index, 31
Glycerol, 35
Glycine, 40
Glycogen, 29, 32, 164
Glycolysis, 68, 150, 151, 152
Goitrogens, 108
Gout-like syndrome, 117
Green tea, 127
Gross energy expenditure, 137
Growth hormone, 124
Guanosine triphosphate, 154

H

β-Hydroxybutyrate, 150
5-Hydroxytryptophan, 62
Hallucinogenic, 127
HDL, see High density lipoprotein
Head circumference, 194
Health
    care costs, 199, 217
    claims, approved, 236, 237
    objectives, 261
    risks, 200
Healthy People 2000, 260
Healthy weight ranges, 171
Heart
    disease, 57, 90
    transplantation, 253
Heat of combustion, 134
Heat stroke, 21
Height measurement, 181
Hematuria, 103
Heme iron, 100
Hemoglobin, 101
Hemorrhaging, 60
Hereditary hemochromatosis, 103

Hexose monophosphate shunt, 64
High density lipoprotein (HDL), 36
Histamine, 7, 40, 70, 104
Homocysteine, 75
Hormones, 16
Hunger, 133
Hydrocarbon, 136
Hydrochloric acid, 11, 41, 99, 106
Hydrolysis, free energy of, 160
Hydrostatic weighing, 181
Hydroxymethylbutyrate, 126
Hypercarotenosis, 53
Hyperglycemia, 16, 31
Hyperhydration, 22
Hyperkalemia, 96
Hypernatremia, 98
Hypersensitivity, 65
Hypertension, 202
    gestational, 89
    treatment of, 95
Hypertrophy, 210
Hypervitaminosis A, 53
Hypervitaminosis D, 55
Hypoglycemia, 31
Hypohydration, 22
Hyponatremia, 98, 99
Hyposmolarity, 22
Hypothalamus, 133

I

Ileum, 11
Immune factors, of mothers' milk, 243
Immune function, 52, 62, 101
Immune response, 205
Immune system, 102, 110, 249
Immunoglobulins, 13
Incomplete proteins, 41
Index nutrient, 64
Indigestible carbohydrate, 29
Indirect calorimetry, 134
Infant formulas, 119, 121, 244
Infections, 63
Inorganic nutrients, 6
Inosine, 125
Insensible perspiration, 21
Insulin secretion, 53, 54
Insulin, 11, 95, 161
Insulin-dependent diabetes, 31
Interviewers, trained, 135
Intestinal amylase, 30
Intestinal lipases, 35
Intestinal microflora, 14, 59
    biotin synthesized by, 79
    conversion of choline to betaine, 82
Intestinal mucosa, 12
Intestinal parasites, 43
Intestinal transit time, 30
Intracellular fluid, 16
Intracellular water, 19

Intrinsic factor, 75
Iodine, 7, 108
Iodized salt, 108
Iodothyronine deiodinase, 110
Iron, 7, 100
    deficiency, 102, 221
    food sources of, 101
    -fortified cereals, 244
    poisoning, 103
    toxicity, 102
Isokinetic resistance training, 211
Isoleucine, 7, 40, 125

J

JDL cholesterol, 253
Jejunum, 11
Joint flexibility, 209, 212

K

Keshan disease, 110
Ketogenic amino acids, 148
Ketoisocaproate, 127
Ketone bodies, 30
Ketosis, 254
Kidney(s), 16
    disease, 202
    disorders, 99, 97
    stone formation, 89
Kilocalorie, 133
Kilojoules, 6
Krebs cycle, 146, 147

L

Lactase, 30
Lactate
    dehydrogenase, 107
    stacking, 212
Lactation, 243
Lactic acid, 125, 126
Lactose intolerance, 30, 87
Laxative abuse, 96
LDL, see Low density lipoprotein
Lead, 123
Lean body mass, 42, 138, 175, 184
Lecithin, 83, 126
Leucine, 7, 40, 125
Life
    expectancy, 247
    stage, 228, 229, 243
Life cycles, recommendations for individuals in
            various stages of, 243–247
    adolescence, 245
    childhood, 245
    infancy, 244
    lactation, 243–244
    older adulthood, 247

    pregnancy, 243
    young and middle adulthood, 245–246
Limiting amino acid, 41
Linoleic acid, 7, 36, 70
Linolenic acid, 7, 36–37
Lipid(s), 3, 6, 27, 35–44
    calorie-dense, 6
    classification, 35
    compound, 35
    derived, 35
    dietary, 54
    digestion, 35–36
    fat substitutes, 38
    functions, 36–37
    health effects of fats, 38
    lipid transport, 36
    malabsorption, 58, 60
    peroxidative damage, 101
    recommended intakes, 37
    simple, 35
    unsaturated, 56
Lipoic acid, 153
Lipoproteins, 36, 42
Liquid supplements, 207
Lithium, 123
Liver damage, 60, 82
Long-chain fatty acids, 35, 120, 162
Low density lipoprotein (LDL), 36, 38
Lymphatic system, 9, 12, 14, 36
Lysine, 7, 40
Lysyl oxidase, 104

M

Macerates, 9
Macrominerals, 7, 95
Macronutrients, 6
Macular degeneration, 62
Magnesium, 7, 64, 159, 227
    food sources of, 93, 94
    metabolism, 124
    toxicity, 94
Magnetic resonance imaging, 114
Malignancies, 74
Malnutrition, 43
Maltase, 30
Maltodextrins, 23, 33
Manganese, 7, 64, 113, 168
    deficiency, 114
    food sources of, 113
    toxicity, 114
Marasmus, 43
Margarines, fortified with vitamin D, 55
Meal pattern, for children, 246
Medications, 247
Medium-chain fatty acids, 35
Megaloblastic macrocytic anemia, 74, 76
Menadione, 59, 60
Menaquinone, 59
Menstruation, iron lost via, 101

Mental development, 43
Mental health, 250, 261
Mesomorphs, 200
Metabolic alkalosis, 100
Metabolic water, 20, 23
Metal toxicity, 57
Methionine, 40, 75, 95
Metropolitan height and weight tables, 173
Metropolitan Life Insurance Table, 171
Micronutrients, 6, 47
Microorganisms, 9
Microvilli, 12
Midaxillary skinfold measurement, 188
Mid-upper arm circumference, 193, 195, 196
Minerals, 3, 47, 85–117
    calcium, 87–91
        absorption and metabolism, 87–88
        deficiency, 89–90
        dietary recommendations, 89
        food sources, 89
        functions, 88–89
        needs in exercise, 90–91
        pharmacologic doses, 90
        toxicity, 90
    chloride, 99–100
        absorption and metabolism, 99
        deficiency, 100
        dietary recommendations, 99
        food sources, 99
        functions, 99
        needs in exercise, 100
        pharmacologic doses, 100
        toxicity, 100
    chromium, 114–115
        absorption and metabolism, 114
        deficiency, 115
        dietary recommendations, 115
        food sources, 115
        functions, 114
        needs in exercise, 115
        pharmacologic doses, 115
        toxicity, 115
    copper, 104–106
        absorption and metabolism, 104
        deficiency, 105
        dietary recommendations, 105
        food sources, 105
        functions, 104
        needs in exercise, 106
        pharmacologic doses, 105
        toxicity, 105
    essential, 7, 85, 87
    fluoride, 111–112
        absorption and metabolism, 111
        deficiency, 112
        dietary recommendations, 112
        food sources, 111
        functions, 112
        needs in exercise, 112
        pharmacologic doses, 112
        toxicity, 112

iodine, 108–109
    absorption and metabolism, 108
    deficiency, 109
    dietary recommendations, 109
    food sources, 108–109
    functions, 108
    needs in exercise, 109
    pharmacologic doses, 109
    toxicity, 109
iron, 100–104
    absorption and metabolism, 100–101
    deficiency, 102
    dietary recommendations, 102
    food sources, 101–102
    functions, 101
    needs in exercise, 103–104
    pharmacologic doses, 102
    toxicity, 102–103
magnesium, 93–95
    absorption and metabolism, 93
    deficiency, 94
    dietary recommendations, 94
    food sources, 93–94
    function, 93
    needs in exercise, 95
    pharmacologic doses, 94
    toxicity, 94
manganese, 113–114
    absorption and metabolism, 113
    deficiency, 114
    dietary recommendations, 113
    food sources, 113
    functions, 113
    needs in exercise, 114
    pharmacologic doses, 114
    toxicity, 114
molybdenum, 116–117
    absorption and metabolism, 116
    deficiency, 116
    dietary recommendations, 116
    food sources, 116
    functions, 116
    needs in exercise, 117
    pharmacologic doses, 117
    toxicity, 117
phosphorus, 91–93
    absorption and metabolism, 91
    deficiency, 92
    dietary recommendations, 92
    food sources, 91–92
    functions, 91
    needs in exercise, 92–93
    pharmacologic doses, 92
    toxicity, 92
potassium, 95–97
    absorption and metabolism, 95
    deficiency, 96
    dietary recommendations, 96
    food sources, 96
    functions, 95
    needs in exercise, 97

pharmacologic doses, 96
toxicity, 96
selenium, 109–111
absorption and metabolism, 109–110
deficiency, 110
dietary recommendations, 110
food sources, 110
functions, 110
needs in exercise, 111
pharmacologic doses, 111
toxicity, 111
sodium, 97–99
absorption and metabolism, 97
deficiency, 98
dietary recommendations, 98
food sources, 97
needs in exercise, 98–99
pharmacologic doses, 98
toxicity, 98
sulfur, 95
trace, 7
zinc, 106–108
absorption and metabolism, 106
deficiency, 107
dietary recommendations, 107
food sources, 106
function, 106
needs in exercise, 107–108
pharmacologic doses, 107
toxicity, 107
Miso, 44
Mitochondria, 146, 156
Molybdenum, 7, 116
Monoglycerides, 13, 35
Monosaccharides, 29
Monosodium glutamate (MSG), 44
Mortality rates, 249
Motilin, 11
MSG, see Monosodium glutamate
Mucopolysaccharide synthesis, 51
Mucus, 9, 52
Multiple 24-hour recalls, 135
Multivitamin/multimineral, 177
Muscle
contraction, 89, 97, 210
hypertrophy, 124
mass, 249
performance, anaerobic, 107
strength, 209, 249, 255
Myelin sheath, 70
Myocardial infarction, 103
Myofilaments, 210
Myoglobin, 101
Myo-inositol deficiency, 121

N

NE, see Niacin equivalent
Nervous system, 9, 56, 65, 119
Neural tissues, 37

Neural transmission, 93
Neural tube syndrome, 74
Neuromuscular disease, 255
Neuromuscular function, 249
Neuropathies, 71, 77
Neuropeptides, 62
Neurotransmitters, 9
Niacin, 7, 54, 67, 228
equivalent (NE), 68
food sources of, 68
toxicity, 69
Niacinamide, 68
Nickel
deficiency, 121
toxicity, 122
Nicotinamide adenine dinucleotide, 68
Nicotinic acid, 49, 67
Night blindness, 52
Nitrogen balance, 41, 164
Nitrosamines, 62
Nonessential amino acids, 40
Non-insulin-dependent diabetes, 31, 249
Nonnutrients, 7
Nonweight bearing activities, 138
Noradrenalin, 16
Norepinephrine, 16
Nucleic acids, 64, 70
Nutrient(s), 5–8
absorption, 9
assessment, 221
classes of, 6–7
content descriptors, 236
deficiencies, 8
definition of, 5
disease relationships, 7–8
energy-yielding, 6, 131, 149
essential, 3, 6
Facts, 133
good sources of, 50
habits, 5, 247, 261
inorganic, 6
labile, 64
nutritional habits, 5
organic, 6
practices, 3
rich sources of, 50
supplements, 6
toxicities, 8
Nutrition and exercise recommendations, 223–242
dietary recommendations, 223–239
dietary guidelines for Americans, 230
Dietary Reference Intakes, 225–229
dietary supplements, 237–239
Food Guide Pyramid, 231–233
nutritional labeling, 234–237
Recommended Dietary Allowances, 223–225
exercise recommendations, 240–242
evolution of physical activity guidelines, 240
physical activity guidelines, 241–242

O

β-Oxidation, 161, 162, 163
Obesity, 27, 131, 249, see also Overweight, obesity and
    creeping, 203
    determinants of, 201
    health complications of, 202
Octacosanol, 126
Odd-chain fatty acids, 76
Oils, 35
Oligosaccharides, 9
Open-circuit indirect calorimetry, 137
Opsin, 51
Orange juices, calcium-fortified, 89
Organic nutrients, 6
Ornithine, 168
Oryzanoles, 126
Osmosis, water absorbed by, 14
Osteocalcin, 60
Osteomalacia, 53, 55, 89
Osteoporosis, 89, 94, 249, 254
Other Substances in Foods, 47, 119
Overweight, obesity and, 197–203
    body fat distribution, 200
    determinants of obesity, 201–203
    health concerns of overweight individuals, 200
    obesity as familial trait, 200
    obesity as lifestyle, 203
    treatment of obesity, 203
Oxalic acid, 88, 101
Oxidant:antioxidant balance, 58
Oxidation
    exercise-induced, 63
    -reduction reactions, 101
Oxidative phosphorylation, 20, 123, 158
Oxygen
    carrier, 100
    consumption, 137
    transport, 22

P

Palatability, 23, 37
Pancreas, 11
Pancreatic amylase, 11, 30, 88
Pancreatic lipase, 11, 35
Pantothenic acid, 7, 81, 153, 228
Parasites, intestinal, 43
Parathyroid hormone (PTH), 54, 87, 91
Parietal cells, 11
Passive absorption, 12
Passive diffusion
    calcium absorbed by, 87
    copper absorbed by, 104
    magnesium absorbed by, 93
    molybdenum absorbed by, 116
    phosphorus absorbed by, 91
    water-soluble vitamins absorbed by, 14
    zinc absorbed by, 106
Pellagra, 67, 69

PEM, see Protein-energy malnutrition
Penicillamine, 71
Pepsinogen, 41
Peptide bond, 39
Percent body fat, 184, 197
Perifollicular hyperkeratosis, 63
Peripheral neuropathy, 111
Peripheral obesity, 200
Peristalsis, 11, 12, 20
Peroxidation, 58
Perspiration, 19, 21
Pesticide, 105
Phagocytosis, 13
Pharmacologic agents, 47
Pharmacologic functions, 50
Phenolic antioxidants, 127
Phenylalanine, 7, 40
Phosphatases, 91
Phosphate loading, 125
Phosphatidylcholine, 82
Phospholipids, 91
Phosphorus, 7, 54, 227
    food sources of, 91, 92
    inorganic, 91
Photophobia, 67
Photoreceptor cells, 51
Photosynthesis, 168
Phylloquinone, 59, 60
Physical activity, 199, 240
Physical Activity and Health, 3
Physical fitness, 217
Phytates, 91, 92, 113
Phytic acid, 88
Phytochemicals, 7
Pinocytosis, 13
Polio, 255
Polypeptidase, 12
Polysaccharides, 29
Polyunsaturated fatty acids, 57, 164
Portable spirometry, 137
Portal vein, 36
Post-event high complex carbohydrate meal, 32
Potassium, 7, 95, 96
Prealbumin, 42
Precompetition meal, 32
Pregnancy, 243
Presenile cataracts, 67
Proconvertin, 59
Progesterone, 103
Prohormones, 54
Proline, 40
Prostaglandin metabolism, 57
Protein(s), 3, 6, 27, 39–44
    amino acids, 39
    animal, 38
    body, 42, 149
    carrier, 12
    catabolism, 42–43
    classification of amino acids by function, 40
    complementary, 41
    complete, 41

conjugated, 40
conversion of to amino acids, 165
deficiency, 52
digestion, 41
-energy malnutrition (PEM), 43
functions of proteins in body, 42
incomplete, 41
processed proteins, 44
quality, 41
recommended intakes, 43–44
   excessive protein intakes, 44
   protein consumption habits, 44
status, 41–42
structure, 39–40
translation, 62
vegetable, 38
zinc-DNA binding, 106
Prothrombin, 59, 88
Psychiatric treatment, 205
Psychoanalysis, 181
Psychologic problems, 43
Pteroylmonoglutamic acid, 72
PTH, see Parathyroid hormone
Ptyalin, 9
Public health issue
  current
    iron classified as, 102
    sodium as, 98
  potential
    copper classified as, 105
    fluoride classified as, 112
    selenium classified as, 110
    zinc classified as, 107
Pulmonary circulation, 14
Pulmonary function, 249
Purine, 42, 72
Pyloric sphincter, 11
Pyridoxal, 70
Pyridoxamine, 70
Pyrimidine, 72, 78
Pyruvate, 153, 154
Pyruvic acid, 147

Q

Quality of life, 181, 217, 261

R

Racemization, 70
RBP, see Retinol-binding protein
RDA, see Recommended Daily Allowance
RE, see Retinol equivalent
Recommended carbohydrate intake, 31
Recommended Daily Allowance (RDA), 43
Recommended Dietary Allowances, 223, 224, 225, 227
Recommended energy allowances, 225
Recommended fiber intake, 31
Rectal cancer, 89

Reduction-oxidation carrier, 123
Rehydration, 23
Relative humidity, 23
Religion, 5
Rennin, 11
Residual air, 183
Resistance exercise, 253
Resistance training, 178, 214, 241
Respiratory diseases, 259
Respiratory oxygen debt, 153
Resting energy expenditure, 140
Resting metabolism, 137
Resting pulse, 213
Retinoids, 50, 51
Retinol-binding protein (RBP), 51
Retinol equivalent (RE), 52
Rhodopsin, 51
Riboflavin, 7, 66, 228
Rickets, 53, 55, 89
Risk behaviors, 259
RNA, 11, 91
  precursor, 125
  synthesis, 72, 75

S

Saliva, 9
Salivary amylase, 9, 30
Salt
  iodized, 108
  table, 97, 99
Satiety value, 37
Saturated fat intake, 37
Saturated fatty acids, 35
Scurvy, 61, 62
Seaweeds, 109
Secretin, 11
Selenium, 7, 58, 109
  foods sources of, 110
  toxicity, 111
Selenocysteine, 109
Selenomethionine, 109
Selenoproteins, 110
Semiessential amino acids, 7, 40
Semiessential fatty acid, 7
Sensory attributes, 5
Serine, 73
Serotonin, 70, 104
Serum cholesterol, 69
Serving, what counts as, 232
Short-chain fatty acids, 30, 35, 149
Silicon toxicity, 122
Similax compounds, 126
Simple lipids, 35
Skeletal muscle degeneration, 110
Skeletal tissues, 51
Skin disorders, 52, 53
Skinfold(s)
  calipers, 185, 186
  measurements, 185, 189

sum of, 189
    thickness, 185, 186
Sleep apnea, 202
Slow twitch, 210
SLPs, see Substrate-level phosphorylations
Smoking, 38
Social behavior, eating as, 5
Social customs, 133
Sodium, 7, 231
    citrate, 125
    -dependent active transport, 13
    food sources of, 97
    homeostasis, 97
    intakes, high, 88
Solvent, inorganic, 19
Somatostatin, 11
Sports beverage, 32, 98, 100
Stainless steel containers, 115
Starch, 6, 12, 169
Strength training, 249
Stroke, 96, 260
Structure-function claims, 237
Stuart-Prower factor, 59
Subcapular skinfold, 187, 191, 192
Substrate-level phosphorylations (SLPs), 153
Succinic dehydrogenase, 66
Sugar, 6, 29, 231
Sulfite oxidase, 116
Sulfur, 95
Sun, 145
Sunlight, overexposure to, 55
Suprailiac skinfold, 187, 188
Surimi, 44
Sweat, 21
    hypotonic, 98
    potassium lost in, 95
Systematic conditioning, 63
Systemic circulation, 14

T

Table salt, 97, 99
Taste
    perception, 106
    receptors, 9
Taurine, 70, 119
TCA, see Tricarboxylic acid
Teenagers, food choices of, 245
Temperature shock, 36
Testosterone, 88, 89
Tetany, 89
Tetrahydrofolate, 75
Thermodynamic efficiency, 158
Thiamin, 7, 63, 95, 228
Thiamin pyrophosphate (TPP), 64
Thigh
    circumference, 194
    skinfold measurement, 188
Thoracic duct, 12, 14
Threonine, 7, 40

Thrombin, 88
Thyroid-stimulating hormone (TSH), 108
Thyroxine synthesis, 205
TIBC, see Total iron-binding capacity
Tin, 123
Tobacco usage, 63
Tocopherol, 56
Tocotrienols, 56
Tofu, 44
Tolerable Upper Intake Levels
    for calcium, 229
    for choline, 229
    for fluoride, 229
    for magnesium, 229
    for niacin, 229
    for phosphorus, 229
    for synthetic folic acid, 229
    for vitamin B_6, 229
    for vitamin D, 229
Tooth decay, 29
Toothpastes, 111
Total cholesterol, 253
Total fat intake, 37
Total iron-binding capacity (TIBC), 102
Total parenteral nutrition (TPN), 82–83, 92, 122
Toxic intake levels, 50
TPN, see Total parenteral nutrition
TPP, see Thiamin pyrophosphate
Trace elements, 7, 85
Trace mineral, 7, 100
Training effects, 194
Transamination, 40, 70
Transcellular fluid, 19
Transcobalamins, 75
Trans-fatty acids, 38
Transferrin, 101, 113
Transpiration, 19
Transthyretin, 51
Tributyrin, 11
Tricarboxylic acid (TCA), 64, 153
Triceps skinfolds, 189, 190
Triglycerides, 35, 148, 164, 200
Triiodothyronine, 108
Trypsin, 11, 88
Trypsinogen, 11, 88
Tryptophan, 7, 40, 68
TSH, see Thyroid-stimulating hormone
Type I diabetes, 31
Type II diabetes, 31
Tyramine, 104
Tyrosine, 7, 40

U

Ultraviolet light exposure, 54
Underwater weighing, 183
Underweight, eating disorders and, 205–207
    anorexia nervosa, 205
    bulimia, 206
    exercise dependency, 206

health concerns, 205
nutritional and exercise therapy, 206–207
Urea cycle, 165, 166, 167
Uric acid, 116
Urine, 16

V

Valine, 7, 40, 125
Vanadium, 123
Vegetable(s)
cruciferous, 108
proteins, 38
Very low density lipoprotein (VLDL), 36
Vitamins, 3, 7, 47, 49–83
B-complex, 7, 49
biotin, 77–79
deficiency, 79
dietary recommendations, 79
food sources, 78
forms, 78
functions, 78
needs in exercise, 79
pharmacologic doses, 79
toxicity, 79
choline, 81–83
deficiency, 82–83
dietary recommendations, 82
food sources, 82
form, 82
function, 82
needs in exercise, 83
pharmacologic doses, 83
toxicity, 83
fat-soluble, 7, 35, 37, 49
folic acid, 72–74
deficiency, 74
dietary recommendations, 73
food sources, 73
forms, 72
functions, 72–73
needs in exercise, 74
pharmacologic doses, 74
toxicity, 74
niacin, 67–69
deficiency, 69
dietary recommendations, 68
food sources, 68
forms, 68
functions, 68
needs in exercise, 69
pharmacologic doses, 69
toxicity, 69
pantothenic acid, 79–81
deficiency, 81
dietary recommendations, 81
food sources, 80
forms, 80
functions, 80
needs in exercise, 81

pharmacologic doses, 81
toxicity, 81
riboflavin, 65–67
deficiency, 67
dietary recommendations, 66–67
food sources, 66
forms, 66
functions, 66
needs in exercise, 67
pharmacologic doses, 67
toxicity, 67
thiamin, 63–65
deficiency, 65
dietary recommendations, 64–65
food sources, 64
forms, 64
functions, 64
needs in exercise, 65
pharmacologic doses, 65
toxicity, 65
vitamin A, 50–53
deficiency, 52
dietary recommendations, 52
food sources, 51–52
forms, 51
functions, 51
needs in exercise, 53
pharmacologic doses, 52–53
toxicity, 53
vitamin B_6, 69–72
deficiency, 71
dietary recommendations, 70–71
food sources, 70
forms, 70
function, 70
needs in exercise, 72
pharmacologic doses, 71
toxicity, 71
vitamin B_{12}, 75–77
deficiency, 76–77
dietary recommendations, 76
food sources, 76
forms, 75
functions, 75–76
needs in exercise, 77
pharmacologic doses, 77
toxicity, 77
vitamin C, 61–63
deficiency, 62–63
dietary recommendations, 62
food sources, 62
forms, 61
functions, 61–62
needs in exercise, 63
pharmacologic doses, 63
toxicity, 63
vitamin D, 53–56
deficiency, 55
dietary recommendations, 55
food sources, 55
forms, 54

functions, 54
needs in exercise, 56
pharmacologic doses, 55
toxicity, 55
vitamin E, 56–59
deficiency, 58, 60
dietary recommendations, 57, 60
food sources, 57, 60
forms, 56
functions, 56–57, 59–60
needs in exercise, 58–59, 60
pharmacologic doses, 58, 60
toxicity, 58, 60
vitamin K, forms, 59
water-soluble, 7, 49
VLDL, see Very low density lipoprotein

W

Waist circumference, 174, 176
Waist-to-hip ratios, 200, 201
Warm-up exercises, 211
Waste products, 14, 21
Water, 3, 12, 19–24
absorption of by osmosis, 14
body distribution, 19
content, of selected food, 21
dietary recommendations, 22–24
exogenous, 19
functions, 19–21
intoxication, 22
intracellular, 19
metabolic, 20, 23
-soluble vitamins, 7, 49
supply, fluoridated, 111
water balance, 21–22
Weight
-bearing activities, 138, 254
gain, 178, 207

loss, 177, 203
measurement, 181
-reduction diets, 37
values, ideal, 171
Weight control, 171–178
behavior modification, 178
caloric intake and body weight changes, 176–178
weight gain, 178
weight loss, 177–178
energy balance, 175–176
healthy body weight, 171–175
Weight training, 241
Wheat germ oil, 126
Whole body density, 183
Wound healing, 62, 104, 105

X

Xanthine oxidase, 66
Xerophthalmia, 52

Y

Yohimbine, 127
Yo-yo dieting, 178

Z

Zinc, 7, 103
deficiency, 107
-DNA binding proteins, 106
food sources of, 106
toxicity, 107